W9-DGI-109

PSYCHOLOGICAL PERSPECTIVES OF HELPLESSNESS
AND CONTROL IN THE ELDERLY

ADVANCES
IN
PSYCHOLOGY

57

Editors:

G. E. STELMACH

P. A. VROON

NORTH-HOLLAND
AMSTERDAM · NEW YORK · OXFORD · TOKYO

PSYCHOLOGICAL PERSPECTIVES OF HELPLESSNESS AND CONTROL IN THE ELDERLY

Edited by

Prem S. FRY
The University of Calgary
Calgary, Alberta, Canada

1989

NORTH-HOLLAND
AMSTERDAM · NEW YORK · OXFORD · TOKYO

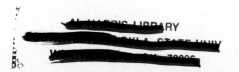

ISBN: 0 444 70546 5

Publishers:
ELSEVIER SCIENCE PUBLISHERS B.V.
P.O. Box 1991
1000 BZ Amsterdam
The Netherlands

Sole distributors for the U.S.A. and Canada:
ELSEVIER SCIENCE PUBLISHING COMPANY, INC.
52 Vanderbilt Avenue
New York, N.Y. 10017
U.S.A.

PRINTED IN THE NETHERLANDS

Warmly dedicated to

Bhag and Yudhishter Malik

in appreciation of many years

of their support and encouragement

TABLE OF CONTENTS

PART 1
PRECONCEPTIONS AND EMERGING ISSUES
OF CONTROL AND AGING

PART II
LIFE-SPAN DEVELOPMENT AND CONTROLLABILITY

PART III
PERSON-ENVIRONMENT FIT AND INTERACTION
MODEL OF CONTROL AND COPING

Chapter 5.   **PERSON-ENVIRONMENT TRANSACTIONS RELEVANT TO CONTROL AND HELPLESSNESS IN INSTITUTIONAL SETTINGS**   **121**

Eva Kahana, Boaz Kahana and Kathy Riley

Chapter 6.   **SITUATIONAL PERCEPTIONS OF CONTROL IN THE AGED**   **155**

Virgina L. Fitch and Lee R. Slivinske

Contents

Chapter 10.   THE IMPLICATIONS OF GENDER AND SPEECH FOR THE
               EXPERIENCE OF CONTROL IN AGING   291

               Adrienne Harris and Naomi Miller

PART V
PSYCHOSOCIAL ANTECEDENTS AND SOCIOLOGICAL
PERSPECTIVES OF CONTROL AND AGING

Chapter 11:   POWER, CONTROL AND WELL-BEING OF THE ELDERLY:
               A CRITICAL RECONSTRUCTION   319

               Prem S. Fry, Lee R. Slivinske and Virginia L. Fitch

CONTRIBUTORS

Fredda Blanchard-Fields, Department of Psychology, Louisiana State University, Baton Rouge, Louisiana, U.S.A. 70803-5501.

Elaine S. Elliott, Center for Cognitive Therapy, Newton, Massachusetts, U.S.A. 02159.

Virginia L. Fitch, Department of Social Work, College of Fine and Applied Arts, The University of Akron, Ohio, U.S.A. 44325.

Prem S. Fry, Department of Educational Psychology, The University of Calgary, Calgary, Alberta, Canada. T2N 1N4.

Mary Gergen, Department of Psychology, The Pennsylvania State University, Delaware County Campus, Media, Pennsylvania, U.S.A. 19063.

Steven H. Goldfinger, VA Outpatient Clinic, Boston, Massachusetts, U.S.A. 02108.

Adrienne Harris, Department of Psychology, Newark College of Arts and Sciences, Rutgers-The State University of New Jersey, Newark, New Jersey, U.S.A. 07102.

Friedrich E. Heil, Department of Psychology, University of Trier, Postfach 3825, D-5500 Trier, FRG.

Jon Hendricks, Department of Sociology, Oregon State University, Corvallis, Oregon, U.S.A. 97331.

Boaz Kahana, Department of Psychology, College of Arts and Sciences, Cleveland State University, Cleveland, Ohio, U.S.A. 44115.

Eva Kahana, Department of Sociology, Case Western Reserve University, Cleveland, Ohio, U.S.A. 44106.

Günter Krampen, Department of Psychology, University of Trier, Postfach 3825, D-5500 Trier, FRG.

Margie E. Lachman, Department of Psychology, Brandeis University, Waltham, Massachusetts, U.S.A. 02254.

Cynthia A. Leedham, College of Arts & Sciences, University of Kentucky, Lexington, Kentucky, U.S.A. 40506-0027.

John **A. Meacham,** Department of Psychology, State University of New York at Buffalo, Buffalo, New York, U.S.A. 14260.

Naomi Miller, Department of Psychology, Rutgers-The State University, Newark College of Arts & Sciences, Newark, New Jersey, U.S.A. 07102.

Richard **A. Monty,** U. S. Army Engineering Laboratory, Aberdeen Proving Ground, Maryland, U.S.A. 21005

Paul **A. Munson,** Health and Welfare Canada, Ottawa, Ontario, Canada.

Lawrence C. Perlmuter, VA Outpatient Clinic, Boston, Massachusetts, and Tufts University School of Dental Medicine, Boston, Massachusetts, U.S.A. 02108.

David **W. Reid,** Department of Psychology, York University, North York, Ontario, Canada. M3J 1P3.

Kathy Riley, Department of Psychology, College of Arts and Sciences, Cleveland State University, Cleveland, Ohio, U.S.A. 44115.

Nancy R. Sizer, VA Outpatient Clinic, Boston, Massachusetts, U.S.A. 02108.

Lee R. Slivinske, Department of Sociology, Anthropology, and Social Work, Youngstown State University, Youngstown, Ohio, U.S.A. 44555.

Gloria Stirling, Department of Psychology, York University, North York, Ontario, Canada. M3J 1P3.

ACKNOWLEDGEMENTS

Many friends and colleagues have reviewed various chapters or parts of chapters of this volume. First, I would like to thank these reviewers for their constructive criticism of individual chapters. Most of them wished to stay anonymous and hence I have tried to thank them along the way. I would like to give special thanks to my colleagues Roy I. Brown, Barry P. Frost, Clifford M. Christensen, Dorothy L. Harris and Daniel Perlman who perhaps unknown to them have contributed to this volume by sharing intellectual insights in the past. Second, I would like to acknowledge with gratitude and appreciation the contribution of each author to this volume. All of them are extremely busy and committed individuals and I thank them for struggling to meet the deadline for submission of chapters and for making the changes and revisions suggested to them. Without their timely cooperation I doubt that the 1988 volume of *Advances in Psychology* would have been possible. My heartfelt thanks to each of the contributing authors listed on pages xv-xvi of this volume.

Special compliments and thanks are due to Margaret J. Samuelson who assisted me ably and reliably in typing, format-editing, and proof-reading the chapters with dedication and care. The present volume owes much to Margaret J. Samuelson and Dagmar Walker for their determined struggle at the site of word production. Val Nicholson kindly helped in proof-reading and library searches. Ms. Titia Kraaij, technical editor with North-Holland publishers, assisted me ably with advice on technical aspects of formatting; I thank her for her help.

My husband David Fry and son Shaun Fry have taught me that self-control and self-discipline are at the core of any significant achievement. I am grateful to them for their encouragement and support.

Finally, I acknowledge with gratitude the assistance of the Killam Resident Fellowship Committee at The University of Calgary. The completion of this volume was facilitated, in part, by an assisted leave period funded by this Fellowship Committee.

P. S. Fry

PREFACE AND SUMMARY

The central topic of this special volume of *Advances in Psychology* is a study of core concepts and perspectives related to older persons' experiences of the positive and negative impact of control or loss of control.

In the 10 to 15 years since studies of personal control or helplessness have begun to appear in the gerontological literature, the field of gerontology also has undergone many changes. The past few years have witnessed widespread acceptance of the notion that few elderly individuals are willing to stand silently in the process of growing, and to relinquish whatever actual controls, autonomy or control beliefs they had in the past. Increasingly, old age is viewed as the dynamics of growth in mastery, control and self-efficacy, on the one hand, and a relative decline in psychological and physical resources on the other hand. It is the intent of this volume to communicate both aspects of these changes, and to offer a comprehensive review of the cross-fertilization of the field of gerontology and the psychology of reactance, freedom and control. Although the meanings and usage of control-related constructs have increased correspondingly with the number of gerontological researchers attending to them, there still are a number of unifying themes concerning the influence of control ideology and control constructs which can be discerned in the growing body of gerontological literature and research addressing these concepts.

It is these psychological consequences of control beliefs, the desire for control, the threats to control and the implications of these for the well-being of older adults with which the present volume is concerned.

Rationale For The Present Volume

As seen in the growing body of gerontological literature, questions and concerns about the bases, consequences and manipulation of control are being examined, discussed and applied in a number of major laboratories in the Western world. Leading psychologists and social science researchers from the United States, Canada and Europe were asked to give their views on the meaning and application of control-related constructs having specific implications for the field of human aging. The contributors were invited to develop chapters representing their most recent theoretical work, with an explicit request that they be bold, innovative, and free in theorizing varying concepts of "personal control," "power," or "mastery" having relevance to the psychological functioning of older persons. Many contributors have chosen to include research data to substantiate their views and to share specific conclusions and interpretations. Some contributors have presented critical reconstructions of the ethical, practical and conceptual limitations and strengths of studies and interventions specifically developed to enhance control in older persons. The space allotted to the authors has been very limited and all of them would have liked to say more. For every contributor whose work is included and recognized in this issue, there are others equally deserving who were omitted. Some were missed in the asking, while others were missed in the responding. Space and time limitations, however, have required a somewhat selective consideration of the work of certain contributors. Those ultimately invited address themselves to one or more of the major themes, issues or concerns which currently figure in discussions of control beliefs and control constructs as they apply to aging and old age. Throughout, the authors highlight some of the issues, controversies and challenges occupying the minds of social psychologists, developmental theorists and researchers involved in the study of aging.

Specific Objectives

Although most of the contributors have subscribed to the fundamental notion that a high degree of personal control and desire for autonomy are vital attributes for well-adjusted and mentally healthy elderly individuals, there are some authors who have also challenged the traditional notion of the autonomous individual and argued for intergenerational dependencies and person-environment negotiations and transactions for control. Individual and gender-linked differences in helplessness and control processes are also considered as well as age-related and developmental components involved in the relationship between controllability, coping and adjustment. In the main, individual development has been viewed by most of the contributing authors as being the central target of personal action and control. The emphasis invariably has been on the individual or groups of individuals contributing to their own control development. Overall, the goal has been to provide a holistic view of control constructs and beliefs having implications for present and future research, practice and interventions for older adults.

It is not the aim of this volume to furnish a full introduction or review of the multidimensional aspects of control and helplessness as associated with old age. The scope of such an analysis can hardly be envisioned. Instead the volume has assembled chapters that call attention to critical problems of control in gerontology and do so in a way that gives them special identity and function. What is illustrated in this volume are some aspects of the theoretical, developmental and clinical utility of control concepts for aging and well-being. It is the intention of the contributing authors to both challenge and affirm that the constructs of control as they have been previously studied in cradle to grave populations are robust enough to withstand the many demands made upon them by gerontologically-oriented researchers. Some chapters represent innovations that extend the utility of the control constructs to areas of the practitioner's concerns. In both cases it is assumed that the reader is already familiar with the basic literature in the psychology of control and the psychology of aging.

Although written primarily for scholars, researchers and developmental theorists interested in the complexities and generativity of control constructs and their applications for the psychological well-being of older adults, the data and issues are presented in a very straightforward style and will be equally informative to gero-psychologists and mental health professionals concerned with healthy adaptive functioning of the elderly. As editor of the volume, I am convinced that you, the reader, are embarking on the study of a controversial and complex topic. The contributing authors would agree with me that our efforts cannot yield definitive conclusions regarding the positive or negative effects of control with aging. Nonetheless, we hope they will encourage further inquiry.

Organization of This Book

Each chapter in this volume stands on its own, and readers may wish to sample them selectively or proceed on the basis of their own interests. However, a reading of the chapters in the published sequence does provide one organization of the work that is perhaps more useful to those readers who are interested in focusing on (1) preconceptions and emerging issues of vulnerability and control in aging, (2) life-span conceptualizations of control and controllability factors and their place in human development, (3) the person-environment fit model of aging and controllability, (4) reconceptualizations and reconstructions of well-known control-related constructs with a primary and renewed emphasis on the cultural dialectic of sex and gender differences within a feminist critique; and lastly (5) the psychosocial antecedents and sociological perspectives on control and aging. Not all possible topics of theoretical interest or research projects in the psychology of control and aging are included, but the selected chapters are intended to be exemplars of the nature of theoretical

analysis, reconstructions and research considerations that characterize the aforegoing domains.

   The contributors have presented both diverse and complementary
approaches to the conceptualizing of control orientations and
perspectives of the aged and they bring varied theoretical and
methodological resources to bear. Although each author was invited to
write a personal statement on important concepts of control and aging,
there are several themes that are somewhat similar and familiar, and
echo reassuringly throughout the text.

Part 1:

Preconceptions and Emerging Issues of Control and Aging

In *Chapter 1*, Fry prepares the groundwork for this book. First she
draws attention to the several myths, stereotypes and preconceptions
surrounding the development or the need for control in aging.
Subsequently she highlights meanings, definitions and preconceptions
inherent in concepts of vulnerability and control as related to aging
and the functioning of older adults. An adapted model of vulnerability having specific implications and applications for older adults is
proposed. Predisposing factors, risks and precipitants of vulnerability in late adulthood are discussed. The value of various
vulnerability and control constructs is reviewed with special
reference to their implications for intervention programs for older
adults. This chapter touches on a number of psychosocial perspectives
leading to and emanating from later chapters of this volume.

Part II:

Life-Span Development and Control

In *Chapter 2* Blanchard-Fields discusses the relationship between
controllability and coping in the elderly from a developmental
perspective. After summarizing the empirical evidence to support the
notion that there is an adult developmental component to aging and a
developmental component to appraised controllability and coping, she
attempts to analyze (1) how these two processes change with respect to
each other, (2) the theoretical issues pertaining to the developmental
components of controllability and coping in adulthood and aging, and
(3) the implications of both the theoretical issues and the research
evidence for healthy adaptive functioning in the elderly. Blanchard-
Fields presents data from a number of ongoing research projects to
support the notion that the dimensionalization of internality and its
relationship to self-blame differ across age groups and that older
adults compared to younger adults more effectively balance both
instrumental and emotional/palliative coping strategies depending on
the appraised controllability of the specific situation. This chapter

speaks to the greater maturity of older adults who respond more differentially to various forms of external control, as compared to younger adults.

In *Chapter 3* Meacham proffers a second way of conceptualizing the life-span developmental components of helplessness and loss of control by turning to a reexamination of the life-course perspective of Erik Erikson. Meacham articulates the quest for a life-long evolution of control-related beliefs in terms of Erikson's sequence of stages and resolution of crises at each stage of development. In its concern for understanding helplessness and lack of control in aging in the broadest sense the Meacham chapter turns to Erikson's eighth stage of ego integrity *versus* despair in late adulthood, and inquires into the antecedents of despair. Meacham introduces a notation system for representing the formal aspects of Erikson's theory in late adulthood and aging and uses this notation system as a tool to show how the stage of generativity versus stagnation in middle adulthood is a crucial foundation for the maintenance or loss of feelings of autonomy, perceived personal control and self-containment in late adulthood.

In *Chapter 4* by Heil and Krampen the theme is the increasing evidence on the relationship between self-efficacy and action control. The authors are proponents of the action-theoretical approach in the study of life-span development. Although similar in part to the action-focused theory advocated by a number of authors on the American scene (e.g., Frese & Sabini, 1985; Miller, Gallanter & Pribram, 1960), Heil and Krampen represent a more European tradition in which action control is seen as a dominant force in development. Within this perspective which emphasizes the individual's own contribution to development, person and personality variables are specified in terms of self-related cognitions, emotions and actions. Control-related actions are embedded in a life-span perspective which has as its basis the subjective beliefs about the individual's contribution to control of the life-span development. The more European action-theoretical approach adopted by Heil and Krampen permits them to review firstly the action-theoretical approaches of E. A. Skinner (1985) which focuses on the relationship between action frequency and control judgments and the structure of control experiences, and secondly the dialectic theory of L. Seve (1972) in which human development is reconstructed in terms of temporal structures and action structures. Heil and Krampen present evidence to show causal links among (1) development-related actions and control efforts, (2) affective emotional evaluations of personal development and aging, and (3) cognitive motivational antecedents of these development-related actions and emotions. The results converge on the conclusion that there are significant relationships between adults' action frequency and action control orientations, on the one hand, and life satisfaction and psychological well-being on the other hand. This view of control beliefs about the individual's own contribution to present and future development squares well with other chapters in this book, especially the chapters by Blanchard-Fields and Meacham who both argue for a "controllability of life-span development" perspective.

Part III:

Person-Environment Interactional Model of Aging and Control

The substantive concern in the person-environment interactional model is how individuals differing in their control expectancies exert control over environmental factors or are controlled by them. The thesis advocated follows that of the person-environment congruence approach first proposed by Watson and Baumal (1967). The congruence thesis is two-fold and argues that individuals who believe they can control their environment adapt better to environments that respond to their control efforts than to environments that are unresponsive; and individuals who believe they have little control over their environments adapt better to environments that are not responsive to individual control attempts than to environments that are controllable (Sandler, Reese, Spencer & Harpin, 1981).

Four chapters presented in this volume are conceptualized within a person-environment interaction framework.

In *Chapter 5* Kahana, Kahana and Riley move the discussion of personal control and expectancies of the elderly to the formal institutional sector of long-term care in nursing homes. The chapter critically reviews empirical evidence concerning the Person *X* Environment congruence hypothesis on the issue of control for elderly living in controlled environments. It examines the effects of long-term institutional care on personal control of elders, and concludes that the social world of long-term institutional care provides little support for independent or autonomous behaviors. Alternative formulations which focus on learned helplessness and environmentally-induced deficits are proposed as accounting for adverse mental health effects on elderly residents. Physical environmental features, institutional policies and staff attitudes are proposed as exerting influence on the control beliefs of residents. These are mediated through staff behaviors. A congruence model of personal and environmental control is advocated whereby it is proposed that congruence between patient needs and staff behaviors with respect to control and compliance are major determinants of well-being and self-efficacy in frail elderly. Lack of congruence may be diminished through coping (primary control) efforts of residents in environments where staff response is made more contingent on the behaviors of the residents. It is postulated that secondary dependency may represent a useful coping response in such environments. Based on the assumption that there is a relational quality to control, Kahana, Kahana and Riley advocate direct observation of the nature and temporal sequence of resident-staff interactions and argue that the staff and elderly residents influence one another in the course of long-term care.

In *Chapter 6* Fitch and Slivinske also support the congruence model discussed by Kahana, Kahana and Riley but move the discussion to explore the person-environment fit paradigm for understanding situation-specific control beliefs of the elderly. They argue that more attention needs to be paid to both intrinsic factors (abilities, illness, efforts and perseverance) and extrinsic factors (uncontrollability of the environment, hostile individuals in the setting) which may singly or collectively lead to a decrease in situational controls for vulnerable elderly persons. Although control-enhancing interventions for elderly persons may focus primarily on one or more of these factors, both actual control and control beliefs should be evaluated in order to create a reasonable degree of the person-environment fit. The authors caution that the degree of fit or misfit that can or should be tolerated must be determined on an individual basis. Although a match or fit between abilities and demands of the individual and the resources in the environment is associated generally with desirable consequences, too perfect a fit may tend to promote stagnation, lack of growth and passivity in certain situations for certain individuals. Fitch and Slivinske advocate that research efforts should be directed toward examining what degree of misfit would maintain an acceptable level of tension-reduction, comfort and well-being and at the same time keep the individual working towards personal growth and development. Consistent with the views of Kahana, Kahana and Riley in Chapter 5, Fitch and Slivinske emphasize that the coping skills available to the individual may do much to determine the nature of the interaction between the person and the environment. Thus the authors of Chapters 5 and 6 agree that an understanding of the agents and interactional processes involved in the person-environment fit is crucial to the development of control-enhancing interventions for elderly persons.

In *Chapter 7*, Munson concentrates on the role of long-term care facilities in generating, maintaining, and shaping control-related beliefs and behaviors in older adults. The chapter summarizes the existing research on planned control-enhancing interventions and provides a critical examination of the control constructs used and the validity of the findings, and their implications for the management of residential care-settings. Munson argues that the presently available corpus of data on the psychology of control in individuals in residential care settings is associated with poorer psychological adjustment and physical health. However, he concludes that although various control-enhancing interventions have been designed, their beneficial effects on psychological or physical health and well-being have not been demonstrated. The social world of residential settings is found to be one of reinforcement for dependent behavior with little direct support for autonomy. Munson studies the regulation of social interaction, privacy and health-care activities in elderly individuals and discusses the prospects for potential entry points for intervention activities. Particular emphasis is given to the caregiver/recipient interaction as a potential therapeutic modality. Munson argues that by providing the care staff with alternatives for promoting choice the social world of residential care settings can be made more growth-oriented for residents and management.

Not unlike the Munson chapter, *Chapter 8* by Reid and Stirling is also concerned with studying the relationship of control and aging in elderly individuals in long-term care settings. The authors argue that past conceptualizations of psychological control have not explained why control is relevant to the process of aging and how existing psychological constructs such as choice, behavioral controls and predictability apply to the process of becoming old. Reid and Stirling discuss the ethical, practical and conceptual limitations of previous studies designed to enhance controls in elderly residents and subsequently propose a reconceptualization of the psychological control construct that is more dynamic and accommodating to the multitude of psychosocial variables affecting the aging process. The authors advance a reinterpretation of the control construct and psychological adjustment within a cognitive social learning framework which has also guided their previous research in locus of control and aging. Using a person-environment fit framework, Reid & Stirling define psychological adjustment as any alteration of functioning an individual makes so as to become both better fitted and more content within his/her environment. However, psychological adjustment is predicated on the notion of participatory control which emphasizes that all persons, regardless of age, manage to retain an acceptable sense of control that encourages them to take initiative to part-icipate in the system. Expanding on the notion of participatory control, the authors explain how interpersonal transactions between older persons and their health-care professionals can maintain the experience of being in control in situations where changes in health and situational pressure would otherwise erode the older patients' control. Reid and Sterling conclude their chapter by reporting on two recent studies which illustrate the application of the participatory control concept to facilitate the adjustment of hospitalized geriatric patients. The authors emphasize that advances in psychological control and aging research require reconceptualizations of control that are more readily applicable to natural field settings in which elderly persons reside.

In short, the two chapters by Munson and Reid and Stirling examine and challenge the implications of learned helplessness for intervention efforts with geriatric clients. Munson argues that helplessness in elderly persons living in long-term residential care is dependent in part on the willingness of the care staff to tolerate the core index of helplessness. By contrast, Reid and Stirling argue that helplessness can be reduced by allowing clients more participat-ory control to contribute to their own well-being. Although it is assumed that the style of participatory control maintained varies from individual to individual, the major contention of these authors is that the provision of participatory control in long-term care settings makes it possible for chronically ill elderly persons both to perceive more controls and also to adjust more readily to the reality of being dependent on the care of others.

Part IV:

Reconstructions of Control Within A Cultural Dialectic of Feminism, Language and Gender

In *Chapter 9* Gergen articulates a view of control that is primarily informed by social psychology and is proffered within a social constructionist paradigm. Her critique of the existing literature on personal control and the aging person is presented from a philosophy of science perspective. The chapter commences with a review of the major research literature and theory which associates increasing psychological distress and impairment with increasing loss of control in aging individuals. Research which avoids this positivistic approach is then presented. Using a discourse analysis approach, the author stresses the limitations of the rhetoric of personal control and well-being. Sociological critiques that discount the value of the self-controlled and autonomous individual are presented. In particular, Gergen emphasizes recent writings of feminist scholars who resist the cult of the self-reliant (i.e., internally controlled) individual. Using a feminist critique, Gergen argues that the autonomous individual with a high degree of personal control and well-being is a masculine idea in which interdependencies of people and ages can be easily denied. In sum, the author challenges the traditional notion of the autonomous individual as being well-adjusted and healthy. The chapter is controversial because it does not assume that the positivist traditions upon which the notions of personal control and well-being of elderly individuals are based, are well-fixed. Gergen views aging persons as being socially embedded and dependent upon their interpersonal relations for their psychological well-being. The chapter closes with the vision of a social world in which men and women can freely acknowledge the mutuality of their needs and support capabilities. The author presents a viewpoint that is uniquely different from the viewpoints expressed in earlier chapters wherein it is suggested that a high degree of personal control is a vital attribute for a well-adjusted and healthy person. Gergen reinforces the idea that instead of urging aging persons to become optimally self-regulated and self-controlled, it might be more profitable to aim toward enhancing the interdependence between persons and the socio-cultural ecologies.

In *Chapter 10* Harris and Miller use a discourse analysis approach similar to Gergen's approach in Chapter 9. Harris and Miller consider the impact and force of gender socialization on the process of aging in respect to feelings or attributions of helplessness, coping and self-regulation. The authors concentrate on gender differences in adaptive capacities, in life continuities, and reactance to loss of control, separation and dependency. Their approach to these issues is dialectical in the sense that they consider aging and gender in a contradictory and reciprocal setting, both as internally lived experiences and as socially inscribed and culturally constituted phenomena. Focusing on the work of Luria and Vygotsky, Harris and Miller discuss the self-regulatory function of the speech of men and women. Using a feminist critique, they argue that these speech functions are potentially adaptive for women in mediating experiences of helplessness and loss of control, and in carrying out relations with others. Clinical anecdotal evidence is offered in support of this perspective. Harris and Miller take the position that the particular function of women's communicative competence makes their language use a potentially adaptive factor in aging and promotes a better adjustment to loss of control and autonomy. Drawing on interview data designed to provide a more phenomenological account of aging, gender development and helplessness, they propose a model of psychological functioning in which autonomy and separateness are not stressed at the expense of interpersonal dispositions and relational styles.

Part V:

Psychosocial Antecedents and Sociological Perspectives of Control and Aging

What are the psychosocial antecedents of control in aging? How can the normative course of control during adulthood be altered with respect to power resources, power relationship and influences? Can the normative course of cognitive functioning in older adults be modified by control-enhancing interventions? Assuming that the need for control and influence relationships does not diminish with age, is there an interface between individuals' needs and societal forces? The chapters which follow address some of these issues and offer a few insights.

In *Chapter 11* Fry, Slivinske and Fitch address the question of an interface between the need for power relationships and environmental influences of older adults and the societal forces which work to reduce power resources and influences. The authors show how the power construct in old age is often synonymous with the constructs of locus of control, self-efficacy, identity and knowledge. Power resources are used in social exchange with agents of change and agents of external control. Societal forces which are the source of power-lessness and power deflation in the later years are identified. Ways and means for maintaining and promoting the power resources and control of older people are discussed both at the personal-instrumental level and at the level of public policy and governmental control.

In *Chapter 12* Elliott and Lachman elucidate the relationship of helplessness and control beliefs to facets of memory functioning in elderly subjects. The authors show that very little work has been done to examine the role of attributions and control beliefs regarding memory. They propose that dysfunctional self-conceptions of memory ability and control may, in part, affect cognitive performance regardless of actual impairment or loss. A self-conception of memory as a shrinking entity opens the door to a constellation of other attributions, control beliefs and perceived performance that impact negatively on memory performance. As people age they may believe that their memory abilities decrease, and that memory losses are irreversible and uncontrollable. Elliott and Lachman advance intervention programs for enhancing memory by modifying control beliefs, attributions, and performance goals of participants. Within their reconceptual framework of control beliefs and performance goals, memory capacity is viewed to be controllable and subject to increases through targeting self-conceptions of change using cognitive restructuring techniques. The intervention approach they advocate is unique in that it is rooted in a framework that elucidates a constellation of cognitive, affective and behavioral factors contributing to the so-called performance loss in memory with increasing age. The authors show a subsequent increase in memory is possible through the use of cognitive restructuring techniques that attempt to modify the aging individual's cognitions, affects and perceptions. In doing so, Elliott and Lachman report evidence on the relationship between self-efficacy, mastery beliefs, attributions and performance of elderly persons in memory tasks. They infer that there may be a causal linkage from change in perceived control to change in cognitive performance which can be brought about by modeling techniques of cognitive restructuring of control beliefs and attributions.

Chapter 13 by Hendricks and Leedham illustrates nicely how our personal conception of what is desirable or ideal in individual development is, in the final analysis, controlled and modulated by the values, social policies and resultant social structures which shape the control beliefs of aging individuals. Rather than focus on the internal dynamics of control or psychological dependency Hendricks and Leedham advance an adaptation model to examine ways in which shared cultural values and social policies reinforce dependency or empowerment in old age. Hendricks and Leedham advocate a position of intergenerational dependency for successful aging to occur. Opportunities for active participation of older persons in problem solutions and policy decisions are proposed as a means of empowering persons in late life. Rather than framing the debate over control versus dependency in terms of inequity among the young and old, these authors propose that social policies directed specifically to the elderly should seek to maximize potentials for autonomous functioning by providing adequate services and resources sufficient to forestall dependency while avoiding overprotectiveness. The position advocated in this chapter is similar in a number of respects to the position taken by Fry, Slivinske and Fitch in Chapter 11. Both chapters recognize the interface between the individual's need for power relations and power resources and the societal pressures which work against the maintenance of these resources in old age. Both chapters propose that social policies directed to the elderly should seek to replenish the personal and social power and control resources of older individuals.

In *Chapter 14* Perlmuter, Goldfinger, Sizer and Monty summarize research and theory which demonstrates the effectiveness of choice in enhancing motivation and cognitive function in both young and old subjects. The authors define choice as the act of distinguishing in action between available options. They argue that availability of control and related choice in the selection of even small components of a task enhances motivation and performance. Based on their key findings they conclude that diminished levels of control and choice reduce motivation, and in turn, degrade cognitive performance. Even among frail elderly subjects with chronic disease, the opportunity to make some choices significantly improves cognitive performance (e.g., recall, retention, reaction time). However, decreased concentration on relevant information and increased interference from less relevant (background) information are characteristic of age-related decline in the cognitive performance of older subjects. The authors conclude that with advancing age, problems such as chronic disease and related depression and dependency may attenuate motivation levels and adversely affect differentiation in laboratory tasks requiring a high degree of precision. Like the chapter by Heil and Krampen (Chapter 4), the approach of Perlmuter et al. stresses cognitive performance in the context of action. Consistent with the approach of Elliott and Lachman (Chapter 12), however, they articulate a theoretical view of control that is primarily informed by cognitive psychology.

In *Chapter 15* (the concluding chapter) Fry presents an overview and appraisal of the areas of helplessness and control as related to aging, and attempts to elucidate the degree of integration that has been achieved hitherto between the areas. Fry reviews a number of areas of deficits in the psychology of control in aging that must be encountered in future theorizing, research, applications and health care interventions for older persons. Additionally, Fry notes areas of control and aging within which significant conceptual advances have been made. Implications of these conceptual advances in control processes are discussed in terms of their relevance to the clinical psychology of aging, social and developmental psychology of aging, and the sociology of aging.

References

Frese, M., & Sabini, J. (Eds.) (1985). *Goal-directed behavior: The concept of action in psychology*. Hillsdale, NJ: Lawrence Erlbaum Associates.

Miller, G. A., Galanter, E., & Pribram, K. H. (1960). *Plans and the structure of behavior*. New York: Holt, Rinehart & Winston.

Sandler, I., Reese, F., Spencer, L., & Harpin, P. (1983). Person X environment interaction and locus of control: Laboratory, therapy, and classroom studies. In H. M. Lefcourt (Ed.), *Research with the locus of control construct, Volume 2: Development and social problems* (pp. 187-251). New York: Academic Press.

Seve, L. (1972). *Marxismus und Theorie der Persönlichkeit.* Frankfurt, FRG: Verlag Marxistische Blätter.

Skinner, E. A. (1985). Action, control judgments, and the structure of control experience. *Psychological Review, 92,* 39-58.

Watson, D., & Baumal, E. (1967). Effects of locus of control and expectation of future control upon present performance. *Journal of Personality and Social Psychology, 6,* 212-215.

PART I

PRECONCEPTIONS AND EMERGING ISSUES
OF CONTROL AND AGING

Psychological Perspectives of Helplessness
and Control in the Elderly, P.S. Fry (ed.)
© *Elsevier Science Publishers B.V. (North-Holland), 1989*

Chapter One

PRECONCEPTIONS OF VULNERABILITY AND CONTROLS IN OLD AGE: A CRITICAL RECONSTRUCTION

Prem S. FRY

The University of Calgary

Abstract

Preconceptions, myths and stereotypic beliefs concerning control capabilities, control motivations and performance expectancies of older adults are addressed. It is postulated that these myths and stereotypic preconceptions of the effects of aging on performance and outcome expectancies contribute significantly to a sense of vulnerability in late life. The unifying meanings, definitions and preconceptions inherent in concepts of vulnerability and control are discussed with reference to aging and the functioning of older adults. An adapted model of vulnerability having specific implications for older adults is proposed, and predisposing factors, risks and precipitants of vulnerability and decline in control are considered. Strengths and limitations of varying control constructs and vulnerability constructs are discussed with special reference to their implications for intervention programs for older adults.

Introduction

First chapters are usually written last and this chapter is no exception. In these first and "last words" I attempt to place the chapters that follow in context, and to describe and integrate preconceptions of vulnerability and controls in aging and old age. I will attempt to lay the ground and will describe what I take to be the unifying meanings, definitions and preconceptions inherent in vulnerability and control and the implications of these for interventions designed to reduce elements of vulnerability. Inextricably linked to the notion of successful aging and adaptation are myths about controls in old age. Some of these myths will be addressed in the earlier section of this chapter.

The Psychological Bases of Control Through the Life-Span

A number of researchers including some who are gerontologically-oriented, have been concerned to present acceptable definitions of control having relevance for understanding the development of strengths and vulnerabilities throughout the life-course. Lazarus and Folkman (1984) introduce the notion of reversibility and coping. A person has power or control if he can reverse the state of affairs, if he so desires. Baron and Rodin (1978) and Rodin (1979) operationally define control as the ability to regulate or influence intended outcomes through selective responding. The crucial component of this view is the assumption, held in varying degrees of conviction by different people and in different situations, that they are responsible for the outcomes that accrue to them through their own efforts. Mandler (1975) draws attention to similarities between competence (White, 1959) and Bandura's (1982) concept of self-regulation and self-efficacy. Competence and self-efficacy is an individual's "felt-control" in executing responses that are organized. Other writers (e.g., Rotter, 1966) have emphasized that the tendency to perceive whether control is or is not possible is a personality disposition that varies between individuals. Seen in this light, attitudes about the presence or absence of control may reflect not only ideological beliefs but also the nature of life-events and life-history experiences of aging individuals (Fisher, 1984). The perception of control will be likely to depend on assessments made in advance of or during an experience, and in these circumstances they should add to the mental workload. The decision-making load for aging individuals throughout the life-span may vary as a function of the uncertainty about whether control is possible.

Although the meaning of psychological control is not universally shared by theorists or researchers working in life-span development and aging, the field of study has emerged with much force to command the attention of social psychologists and developmental theorists in western society (Perlmuter & Monty, 1979; Schaie, 1983; Schulz, 1976; Sorensen, Weinert, & Sherrod, 1987; Weisz, 1983). Subject populations from cradle to grave have been examined in order to identify control-related constraints having specific implications for the field of human aging.

The psychology of control in human aging, however, has been long on data and short on ideas. Based on empirical and experimental evidence various models of perceived and actual control (learned helplessness: Seligman, 1975; self-efficacy: Bandura, 1982) have been proposed to explain the potential role that various psychological factors associated with reduced control might have in the acceleration of the aging process. The theory of learned helplessness has particular relevance to aging and developments in late adulthood. The learned helplessness view suggests that passivity in old age is an

iatrogenic disease brought about by the severe deprivations of the
constrained environments in which the elderly live and especially the
presumed noncontingent behavior-environment relationship thrust on the
elderly.   The causal chain that seems to be implicated in current
conceptualizations of vulnerability with regard to late life developments is as follows: (1) deprivation of control, (2) perceived loss
of control, (3) motivational deficit, (4) performance deficit, (5) and
accelerated aging (see Langer & Rodin, 1976; Schulz & Hanusa, 1980;
Seligman, 1975).

Other applications of vulnerability models, especially the
learned helplessness model have been proposed, largely in medically
relevant areas of psychology of aging (e.g., Peterson, 1982; Taylor,
1979) where it has been argued that long-term hospitalization may lead
to loss of both actual and perceived control, in part because
hospitals require patients to forfeit control over most of the tasks
they can normally perform.   This surrender of control may result in
increasing feelings of depression, apathetic reactance and long-term
sense of vulnerability.   While the majority of earlier studies
concerning helplessness or control or loss of control have used
youthful research subjects and argued for the psychological importance
of maintaining a strong sense of personal control and self-efficacy,
recently the exact same concepts of control are being applied to the
well-being and adjustment of older persons.   The hypothesis guiding
most of the research and writing is that it is important to preserve a
strong sense of efficacy in later life because low levels of perceived
personal efficacy can have negative implications for performance and
for the status of elders in society (Bandura, 1977; Siegler & Gatz,
1985; Kuypers & Bengtson, 1973; Lachman, 1985).   Taken together there
is an overwhelming body of literature that characterizes personal
control and mastery as being the critical ingredients determining
successful aging.   It is argued that personal control and mastery
expectation will determine both the initiation and the persistence of
coping behavior in later life.

In most discussions of the psychological importance of personal
controls, the theme generally holds that to have freedom, autonomy and
control is good and psychologically beneficial to the health and
outlook of the aging individual while not to have control or autonomy
is potentially harmful to the mental well-being of the older adults.
This assertion is practically a truism for the more youthful subjects
studied in the psychology of control literature and may also be a
fairly accurate representation of the experimental evidence emanating
from earlier studies with older subjects.

Studies (cf. Lachman, 1986; Lachman & McArthur, 1986) describe
unflattering attributional patterns of controls reflecting a stereotypic view of elderly adults as being less competent than the young.
Such expectancies for control and efficacy in later adulthood,
however, do not necessarily square well with the perceptions of the
elderly themselves, and have given rise to many anxieties and fears

about adjustment in old age. Younger adults' preconceptions about the aging process and the expectancies for control have also contributed to the development of a number of myths and stereotypic views of risks, crises and vulnerability factors associated with aging and old age. Some of these myths and preconceptions about control and aging are the subject of major concern and need to be addressed.

Aging: A Downward Trajectory of Controls?

The aging process is viewed as a gradual downward trajectory with ever increasing decline in psychological and cognitive functioning and lack of control over bodily resources (Farberow & Moriwaki, 1975; Verwoerdt, 1976; Weinberg, 1975). The process of growing older into late adulthood is characterized as a cumulative experience of increased social and emotional vulnerability, and helplessness and loss of control over the psychological environment (Goodstein, 1981; Palmore, 1980). Typically, aging is viewed as a period of diminutions in functioning and ability (Cerella, Poon, & Williams, 1980). This has led to a myth surrounding the elderly individuals' inevitable decline in cognitive control in a number of domains such as memory (Craik, 1977; Walsh, 1975), information-processing and action control (Oyer & Oyer, 1978). It is postulated that older persons having limited personal-cognitive resources and capacities will characteristically surrender to anxieties and fears about their inability to maintain control over their activities. It is assumed that even after the experience of many decades of autonomy and independence, the potential for illness or bodily decline will induce a serious reduction in the level of perceived control in many elderly persons. This raises the hypothesis that fear or anxiety associated with loss of control is a factor that may influence performance and level of actual control (Roth & Kubal, 1975).

Aging: A Depressive Attitude Towards One's Own Development?

The elderly are an *at risk* population especially endangered by the commonly accepted view that loss of perceived control or mastery in old age is inevitably accompanied by a corresponding increase of a depressive attitude toward one's own development.

Kuhl's (1986) theoretical analysis of various models suggests that perceived loss of control may accelerate the mental and physical concomitants of aging by reducing the individual's motivation to exercise control functions whenever possible. A person who decides that he/she is never likely to have control may, irrespective of reason, be less mentally loaded in terms of decision making about control, but more likely to incur the punishment attached to being helpless and to the consequences of failure. The demands made upon older individuals to retain control may thus be more tension-producing in light of the declining physical energies and declining motivations for self-efficacy, and increasing needs for dependency on *powerful others*.

Moreover, there are other prevalent stereotypes and widespread expectations for change, largely negative, in intellectual functioning, physical health and psychological well-being associated with age. Some of Lachman's (1986) data support the stereotypic view that the elderly compared to younger age groups are more likely to expect a decline in controls over intellectual aging. More specifically, Lachman's (1986) data show that the elderly, compared to younger adults, are less likely to believe that they are responsible for maintaining their level of intellectual functioning or for effecting improvement in performance. Consistent with prevalent stereotypes about old age, the elderly in Lachman's research were more likely to expect decline and to believe that decline is inevitable in later life (Chance). Finally, the elderly believe more strongly than younger groups that they cannot succeed in cognitive tasks without assistance. Krampen's (1982) overview of developments through the life-cycle for a consistent pattern of external control beliefs during adulthood shows that evidence is sketchy and inconclusive up to now. However, the cross-sectional findings produced by Brandtstädter, Krampen and Heil (1986) contribute to aspects of the prevalent stereotypic view. Their data show a rather consistent developmental pattern indicating a perceived and experienced loss of personal control over relevant outcomes. According to these authors there is an age-related perceived loss of control especially marked in areas such as occupational efficiency, intellectual efficiency, physical fitness, self-esteem and self-development. From the perspective of an emotional evaluation of self-development, the cross-sectional findings observe potentials for a more depressive outlook with a successive increase with age, in feelings of depression, resignation and exhaustion.

Aging: A Time of Increasing Social and Environmental Constraints?

A number of gerontologists (Baltes & Willis, 1979; Kuypers & Bengtson, 1973) have expressed concern about the potential for a serious decline in the perceived control of older adults, due to the numerous constraints associated with aging. They suggest a direct linkage between the tenets of the social constraints policy in old age and the potential for decline in controls. In the American culture, for example, the elderly are faced with involuntary retirement, a lack of respect, an absence of participatory control, and lack of defined roles. Such experiences could contribute to a loss in personal control in later life (Kuypers & Bengtson, 1973) and increase the likelihood of a greater sense of vulnerability and helplessness associated with aging. Such emotional states and evaluations may negatively affect the individual's motivation to actively intervene in the course of developmental events or to remedy the conditions that have led to diminished control. Although the occurrence of these depressive and apathetic reactions is not universal nor do they exhibit universal patterns of onset, duration, constellation or sequencing, nevertheless a study of the social policy of increasing social and environmental constraints in old age is likely to explain much of the large interindividual variability in the downward trajectory associated with late life.

Aging: Is There Too Heavy an Expectancy for Control and Performance?

The prototheoretical notions of differential development and intellectual and control plasticity inherent in current life-span thinking provide some support for the rationale that expectancies for control functioning in late adulthood are inconsistent with the actual goals for performance in old age. The basic position that is deserving of attention is that a discussion of controls and expectancies for controls in developmental aging must include an examination of the ecological context as well as the intraorganismic factors of control in developmental aging.

Even in the face of weaknesses and losses associated with aging high control is viewed to be a necessary prerequisite for the optimization of human potential in later life. This has contributed to the notion that high personal control is an expectancy and a desirable state for all individuals regardless of age or circumstances. The vantage point for such an approach is a conception of late life development which emphasizes the individual's active contribution to personal development. Self-efficacy expectations are necessary to the individual's persistence in the face of obstacles. Self-efficacy expectations require self-discipline and "mastery of knowledge and skills that can be attained only through long hours of arduous work" (Bandura, 1982, p. 142). The notion of self-efficacy expectations as essential to "successful aging" further contributes to the myth that the elderly as a group are especially *at risk* because of lowered perceptions of self-efficacy which will stand in the way of their trying to bring about environmental changes even if these are easily attainable.

Since the value of personal control throughout the life-cycle is associated with energy, vitality, robustness and action, it follows that *disengagement* is not a desirable state of being at any juncture of the life-cycle. Theoretical developments in gerontology have argued that older individuals choose to retreat or disengage because of a realistic awareness of their diminishing capacities and the short time left to them before death. Geropsychologists concerned with aspects of control, however, might argue that *disengagement* is a form of *quitting*. This is a response to perceived loss of control and competence and is best likened to a state of helplessness. The important message for late life development from the perspective of the control model is that a person must maintain vigilance in the face of all emotional declines and as far as possible resist the centripetal movement inherent in *disengagement*. This contributes to a social preconception that the characteristic of a reflective attitude in adulthood is not necessarily a sufficient attribute for life satisfaction and "successful aging." Kuhl (1986) proposes that most older adults faced with a choice between acceptance and reflective attitude (wisdom), on the one hand, and action and innovation on the other hand would accede to the social pressure to give up "reflective acceptance" and stay active and invested.

Most action-control models would also argue that for the vast bulk of older persons, the continuance of a robust and active lifestyle is an important factor which by itself will have a marked preservative effect on their sense of well-being. The role of personal control and vigilance throughout the life-cycle has spurred this line of interest in gerontology. Various social psychologists, for example, Rodin (1986) and Schulz (1976) have studied the influence of perceived personal control on measures of well-being and mortality among aged subjects. The basic theme of their work has been to propose innovative intervention studies designed to assess if older persons can be helped to become more vigorous and active by increasing their actual or their perceived personal control. Perlmuter, Monty, & Chan (1986) have also concluded that with the strengthening of the perception of control comes a variety of beneficial effects for individuals including an increase in motivation, a decrease in stress and facilitation of problem solving. The conclusions of these studies, however, ignore the historical or cultural context in which control-related constructs have developed. In other words, there has been rather limited focus on the societal contexts of aging due to a strong personal psychological cast to the field of aging and control.

In studying the impact of high or low control in the aged, investigators have measured outcomes of control in terms of health factors, social participation, and emotional evaluation of their own development and efficacy. Against this theoretical background, there is a push to support a conception of adult development that emphasizes the individual's active contribution and self-regulation in the course of personal development (cf. Brandtstädter, Krampen & Heil, 1986). Various notions of control-related issues as they apply to social problems of the aged and to social controls governing late-life development have not been examined from the perspective of social gerontology. Simultaneously, the emphasis on individual control has ignored context in various ways and older individuals have all too often been seen in isolation. If the context is ignored it may be argued that social psychologists may be placing increasingly heavy demands for self-regulatory functions as an end in itself. Reduced physical strength of the aged may render the enactment of self-directed and self-generated activities increasingly difficult and subsequently lead to a reduction in both actual and perceived control (Kuhl, 1985).

Thus the theme of personal control over development and self-efficacy expectancy outcomes (although very promising for the developmental psychology of adulthood and old age) is likely to create much tension for many elderly who lack motivation or desire for control or who have already experienced reduced control expectations concerning their physical and emotional health. This may further perpetuate anxiety resulting from the expectation that staying active and vigilant under all circumstances is the only respectable way to be. The notion that competence and sense of personal mastery are a required ingredient of successful aging may unduly accelerate feelings of depression and despaired resignation. Such prescribed expectancies for old age are especially pernicious because of their potential for generating guilt and shame in many older persons who have tangible declines in sensory-motor functioning and are incapable of solving their own problems or living independently. Moral pressures on older persons to stay active and in control under most situations are more demoralizing and behaviorally self-debilitating than are external impediments in the physical environment.

These considerations, admittedly speculative, raise issues about vulnerability factors in old age and risk and crises factors accompanying the aging process. These issues are developed further in later sections of this chapter.

Aging: Is there a Danger or Advantage in Relaxing Expectancies for Control?

What about the opposite side of the coin? Is there potential danger in suggesting to older persons that if they reduce their controls or freedom that they are inevitably yielding to helplessness, debilitation and depressive development? In some quarters it is argued that the psychological consequences of struggling to maintain mastery and control in the face of emerging vulnerabilities and loss of physical and psychological resources in approaching old age may be not only *harmful* but *destructive*.

The review of relevant existing literature on the basis of personal control in aging has generally suggested that exercise of personal control, personal choice and decision making has a definite and positive role in sustaining life (Glass, 1977; Perlmuter, Monty & Chan, 1986; Rodin; 1983). However, other gerontologically-oriented writers have argued some of the negative effects of high level control expectancies. Misapplied moral and compensatory models that set unrealistic expectations for control and efficacy can have catastrophic results for elderly individuals when the demands of their problem or the pressures of their environment are beyond their capacity (Lawton & Nahemow, 1973). Fostering the myth of self-reliance capabilities or putting pressure on the elderly individuals to perform beyond their declining capacities and capabilities can result in essential resources being withheld as unnecessary (Karuza, Rabinowitz & Zevon, 1986). Based on the attribution literature of control and aging (cf. Janoff-Bulman & Brickman, 1982)) it is postulated that perpetuating a myth of control and responsibility can lead to feelings of anger, loss of self-esteem, and eventually to depression and vulnerability. Many elderly persons may become convinced of their moral responsibility to be totally self-reliant and self-regulated in their functioning. In the end, elderly persons may feel guilt and shame for their lack of self-sufficiency and may become so overwhelmed by negative emotions that their effective coping is threatened. Under these conditions older persons may become so victimized by unrealistic expectations they set for themselves and persist fruitlessly on problems for which there is little or no control facility or skills needed to do the task (cf. Janoff-Bulman & Brickman, 1982).

These myths and preconceptions about patterns of controls in aging and their implications for risks, crises and vulnerability factors in late life raise the question of understanding the antecedents of vulnerability. What are the predisposing environments and precipitants which lead to apathetic reactions, helplessness depressions and stressful experiences in old age? One of the terms commonly used to describe these pathological conditions ranging from depression to somatic impairment in older persons is "vulnerability states." Certainly "vulnerability states" in old age are both genetically and environmentally induced and deserving of detailed study and empirical investigation. The sections which follow will examine various concepts of vulnerability in aging and discuss the predisposing and precipitating factors in the development of vulnerability.

Meaning and Definition of Vulnerability in Late Life

A dictionary definition of vulnerability normally involves the term "susceptibility" and implies that the individual who is vulnerable perceives a reduction in controls and will succumb to affects of depression in certain situations where control may be socially expected or is personally desirable. It remains possible that vulnerability in older adults is both very *general*, so that a person is at risk for a number of different precipitants such as adverse life circumstances, loss of cognitive functions, and loss of social networks and also *specific*, so that only certain configurations such as bereavement or specific stressors will be relevant.

This concept of vulnerability squares well with explanations offered by Rabkin (1982) who delineated evolving models of stress that contribute to the individuals' state of mental and emotional fragility and helplessness. According to the earliest and simplest "innocent victim" model, adverse circumstances may induce mental disorder in otherwise perfectly healthy individuals. This conception of stress as leading to long-term vulnerability is now acceptable only in sufficiently intense situations such as post-traumatic disorders occurring in later life, but not in most other circumstances.

A second more current model having wider applicability to old age developments is based on the "vulnerability hypothesis" (Brown & Birley (1970), according to which helplessness, depressive reactance and erosion of self-esteem and self-concept are triggered only when *already* vulnerable persons are exposed to crises and stressful situations. Vulnerability factors mediate the impact of later stressors and influence the probability of the individual becoming more depressed, helpless and lacking in motivations or ability to control or cope. Brown and Harris (1978) differentiated between vulnerability factors and provoking factors which interactively increase the risk of emotional disorders resulting in chronic depressive states, motivational deficits and deficits in controllability. In their specific research they utilized major vulnerability factors such as deprivation, environmental impoverishment, losses in support networks that both increase the risk of depression and decrease the probability of help-seeking behaviors.

The third "interactive model" considers all of the interacting factors: individuals' proneness, life-event characteristics and environmental influences in terms of constraints, powerful others and absence of sanctions.

This interactive model, along with the "vulnerability hypothesis" model (Brown & Harris, 1978), seems to be the most appropriate model in terms of its wider applicability to developments in old age. Various factors from these vulnerability models will be considered with reference to their potentials for explaining vulnerability in late life.

Environments of Older Persons as Predisposing Factors in Vulnerability

The strong emphasis in the psychology of aging on the adjustment of the individual to society has served to decontextualize the aging experience by treating social institutions of the aged and social arrangements as comparatively noninfluential and nonproblematic. According to social control theory (see Janowitz, 1978) social institutions and social arrangements are by no means nonproblematic. They have a system of built-in coercion, and although the coercion is circumscribed by legitimate norms, it nevertheless elicits in the elderly residents a primary helplessness. The helplessness arising from the superordinate decision that nothing can be done preserves the person's mental and biological resources but leaves him/her exposed to accelerated feelings of vulnerability. It is supposed that the greater vulnerability in the aged is the result of various failures experienced in situations where control over the environment was expected. The question of greater interest is environmental factors which make most adults in their later years at greater risk for depressive feelings, resignation and motivational deficits in psychological functioning. A number of critical questions are involved.

The first concerns the deterministic and absolute nature of most of the physical environments in which the aged persons live in relation to social institutions and the maintenance of social systems (Rosow, 1974). McClure (1985) notes that in deterministic environments, the contingencies are more uncontrollable and inescapable and there is greater potential for both personal and universal helplessness to occur. Universal helplessness occurs when outcomes are not contingent on one's own responses or the responses of other persons whereas personal helplessness occurs when there are responses that can produce the desired outcome in other persons' repertoires but not in one's own (Abramson, Seligman & Teasdale, 1978). For example, universal helplessness among an older adult is illustrated by the case of a terminal illness or threatened loss of cognitive functioning. No one, including surgeons or physicians or family members can help the older person. In most cases, however, the ailing person must forfeit control to the medical institution for maintenance of physical life and the preservation of basic mental functions (Parkes, 1978). Personal helplessness is illustrated by the case of an older woman who struggles to a point of desperation to tackle a problem because of the clear social expectancy that the control facility is available and the capability to exercise control is possible. If she perceives herself as failing she is then open to added punishment because she must consider the notion that her intellectual or cognitive functioning is declining. Alternatively, she may console herself with the thought of having tried. These different attitudes might variously flavor the state of helplessness and vulnerability the elderly person experiences.

Having little money, poor opportunity for independent living and low mobility are additional environmental factors for elderly individuals that contribute to lowered levels of actual or perceived control. Brown and Harris (1978) showed that the prevalence of "clinical-like" states of depression often characterizing the lives of poor and older persons may predispose against resisting the transmission of helplessness (Davis, 1970). What emerges among many older adults is a slowly evolving pattern of control by avoidance and a mental condition which predisposes against seeking help or acquiring actual control over life-events (Schless, Schwartz, Goetz, & Mendels, 1974). These findings fit in well with the model of negative cognitions emphasized by Beck (1970) as being central to helplessness and vulnerability.

Control Ideologies of Older Persons as Precipitants of Vulnerability

The hypothesis that older persons, not unlike other age groups from cradle to grave, are motivated to achieve a sense of mastery and control over the environment has been put forth by numerous social psychologists (Bandura, 1977, 1982; Gurin & Brim, 1984; Rodin & Langer, 1977). Although concepts and terms related to motivations and behaviors of self-efficacy have varied (e.g., personal control, competence, mastery, internal locus of control) the general thrust of the arguments has been that individuals across ages desire a sense of effectiveness (Janis & Rodin, 1979) and an ability to influence intended outcomes. The need to foster and preserve development-related control beliefs through adulthood and old age thus contrast a loss of sense of individual control, or reduction in potentials for cognitive control (e.g., through information seeking or decision making) or proxy control (i.e., receiving external support). These needs have been seen to result in pathologies ranging from depression to generalized trauma, and these summate in determining vulnerability.

Brandtstädter (1984a, 1984b) has postulated that greater vulnerability and helplessness in old age may be interrelated with control ideology and emotional and actional tendencies or predispositions. If, for example, the individual believes that his/her anticipated developmental situations or circumstances are unsatisfying, and at the same believes that no chances exist to effect positively the course of development, then the individual will make no active attempts to control relevant developmental outcome. Feelings of resignation, depression or despair in an elder may be connected with a constellation of cognitive, motivational and behavioral deficits in controls or potentials for controls.

(a) *Beliefs About Personal Control.* In applying these concepts to older individuals and in understanding the potentials for increasing vulnerability and helplessness in old age, it is important to understand the role played by the person's control ideology in the decision to engage or not to engage in situations eliciting stress or anxiety. Today's cohorts of elderly persons have typically subscribed to control ideologies which *are not strongly polarized*, thus increasing the probability of helplessness as an immediate response. Gore and Rotter (1963) have hypothesized that in individuals or groups where the control ideology is not strongly polarized the potential for emotional vulnerability is greater because individuals' decision to engage in problem events might depend on a deeper analysis of the situation confronting them, for example, consideration of a religious commitment. The older person's belief in the control of a higher authority may logically lead to passivity, or if praying is used as a response to a problem still the individual may consider his/her own control potentials insufficient. For some older individuals, the religious dictate "God helps those who help themselves" may require that they become engaged in a problem concerning raising money for charities. However, the same religious dictate may not determine their other decisions about control facility or personal capability concerning their health or income or cognitive functioning. In the latter cases, the pattern of behavior in a stress scenario could be much the same as a person who believes in chance and fate. The elderly person may become engaged but still see no chance of augmenting his/her *personal control potential* (e.g., through information seeking or skill training) nor of acquiring *proxy control* (Bandura, 1977) through the instrumentality of external supports.

(b) *Beliefs About Proxy Control.* An elderly person's decision to engage in difficult events may also depend on a consideration of the anticipated effects or developments that a given course of action may have on other family members or persons in authority. If stressful experiences with poor outcomes are anticipated for lack of support from external sources, the probability of helplessness as an immediate response increases, thus precipitating greater risk of stress, deprivation and environmental impoverishment. Some of these vul-nerabilities may be self-confirming results precipitated by the elderly persons' avoidance to become engaged in a problem or to encounter the information that would tell them whether they could have succeeded.

Understanding the control ideologies of adults and elders is helpful in predicting their anxiety reactions. Understanding the differences in control ideology should also help caregivers of older persons to determine whether decisions to engage or not to engage in a stressful circumstance are likely to occur. It is then possible for professionals, family members or caregivers to examine the possibility of preparing influences in the environment that reduce the risk of precipitants to have negative outcomes for the older person.

Incidence and Frequency of Precipitants of Control or Vulnerability

Studies of stress, coping and vulnerability in aging have been based on the hypothesis that higher levels of perceived vulnerability may be induced by the higher incidence of precipitants; precipitants may lead to a worsening of conditions under way or trigger immediate admission to the hospital. Precipitants may take the form of severe depriva-tions of social and emotional supports, loss of intimate relationships shortly before a stressful episode and might trigger severe reactions in an older person.

A probabilistic model of vulnerability developed by Schulberg and Sheldon (1968) has clear implications for older adults' expectancies for helplessness and levels of perceived control in stressful circumstances. This model assumes that the probability that a hazardous event will occur, that the individual will be exposed to the event, and of counterharm resources combine multiplicatively to determine outcome and perceived levels of control. The implicit assumption is of a reciprocal relationship between (a) vulnerability determined by previous history on the one hand, and (b) current factors of medical illness, loss of mobility, unavailability of social and external support, and the number of powerful others residing in the immediate environment of older persons on the other hand (cf. Levenson's (1974) three-dimensional measure of control: Internal, Chance and Powerful Others). For most purposes, the precipitant of Powerful Others (i.e., influential and powerful persons such as adult children, family physician or hospital staff) is very influential in determining the older person's decision to engage or not to engage in external events. Thus the vulnerable and nonvulnerable elderly person's control profile could, in theory, appear similar in the phenomenology of perceived controls, but it is the current state of precipitants present at the time of the occurrence of severe events which will be expected to affect a high proportion of elderly individuals' decision for engagement or nonengagement in life-events. Even less intense experiences would often affect those elderly persons who are already vulnerable with respect to beliefs about their personal inefficacy and control by powerful others.

As seen in Figure 1 a useful distinction is between two sets of risk factors prevalent in the natural environment of all older adults: (1) the individual's perceptions of proxy control facility as represented by amplifying factors of the individual's social support systems and (2) primary aetiological factors such as genetically determined medical conditioning, and major genetic problems in intellectual capacities, physical energies and sensory-motor functioning.

Current medical and gerontological studies of aetiological factors and amplifying factors governing vulnerability perceptions of control in aging are based on the hypothesis that the elderly may be doubly vulnerable to both processes just considered.

Genetic factors and life-history experiences of older adults as shown in Figure 1 may moderate the risk of depression and negative outcomes, and enhance perceptions of control for similar situations in the future. In the model of vulnerability proposed the older person's experiential history of trauma, loss of relationships, social and cultural belief systems, and control ideology are all identified as key factors in the development of vulnerability. Helplessness, passivity, dependency, excess disability are often seen to be outcomes or deficits brought about by severe threats to individuals' sense of control summating in their vulnerability. Reactive depression and apathetic behaviors may therefore be viewed both as *outcomes of vulnerability* or *predisposing factors to vulnerability* in old age.

These situations of vulnerability in late life can be explained by means of both an "obstacle theory" or "big bang" theory. Whereas "obstacle theory" assumes that low expectancies for control develop as a function of unpleasant circumstances and lead to apathetic behavior and a learned helplessness depression, the "big bang" theory assumes that a number of deprivations or motivational deficits that develop in later life result from earlier losses and deprivations. Inability to deal with trauma (illness) and crises in later life is often a result of loss of perceived control in the earlier stages of development. Such situations would create increased perceptions of zero control, especially for older individuals living in health care or highly

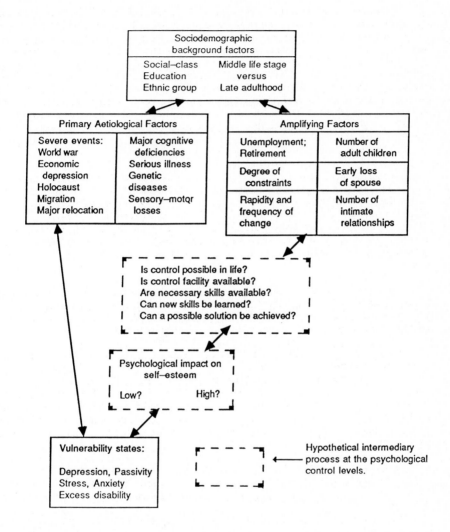

Figure 1. Illustration of possible ways in which sociodemographic factors and environmental factors interacting with control orientations predispose the individual to vulnerability states.

constraining institutions, such as nursing homes. In highly constraining environments, high or moderate levels of vulnerability might
result from predisposing factors in the constrained environments which
demand passive and dependent behaviors in elderly residents (Taylor,
(1979).

Circumstantial Factors in Vulnerability

A number of important studies (e.g., Dohrenwend & Dohrenwend, 1974;
Jarvis, 1971) have implicated the role social factors might play in
the development of vulnerability in the later years. Several studies
(Brandtstädter, 1984a; Bourestom & Pastalan, 1981; Brand & Smith,
1974) have emphasized the importance of impoverished environments in
which deprivations of activity, reinforcements and social stimulation
cause vulnerability. The consequence is a poor psychological state
(helplessness and morbidity), a likely outcome of an impoverished
environment in which a complex mixture of deprivation, social stress,
and lack of intimacy in relationships weaken the beliefs of the older
person that he can exercise control.

A particular combination of circumstantial factors where there
are stresses and problems but lowered capacities for solving them
should result in increased vulnerability (Brown & Harris, 1978) and a
sense of lowered self-esteem and self-denigration arising from such
circumstances. Lower self-esteem in many older adults may predate
rather than arise from the consequences of helplessness in aging. In
this case the older person is vulnerable not only because of deprivation and lack of intimacy but also because he may be causing these
types of experiences to occur through responses of avoidance and
withdrawal. This point needs investigating.

Dohrenwend (1973) attempted to separate (a) *undesirability of
events*, and (b) *rapidity of change* as factors of stress and vulnerability in later life and reported that generally the two were
confounded, with both stress and control reactions being attributed to
undesirability and change as main features; individuals with low life
changes reported more positive categories of control than did those
who scored high. Analysis suggested that high degree of life change
is most highly correlated with stress among older individuals (Kiyak,
Liang, & Kahana, 1976; Sarason, Johnson, & Siegel, 1978) and may be a
more important variable than undesirability in determining perceptions
of helplessness or control.

Goodstein (1981) notes that by the nature of sheer longevity
elderly persons face multiple stresses acting in tandem across social,
psychological and biological parameters. In view of the overlap of
stresses in various life spheres and also in view of the rapidity of
life changes, the elderly may be at greater risk for reactions of
resigned helplessness (i.e., taking on the sick role or letting
powerful others control stressful events). Verwoerdt (1976) proposed

that psychological decompensation may occur as a result of accumulated and cumulative stress states, hastening in elderly individuals a process of withdrawal and lowered perceptions of control. Similarly, Suls (1982) found that uncontrollable events were associated with psychological distress or ill-health, but only if they were also undesirable. Uncontrollable positive events had no negative effects on perceived control levels, suggesting an important modification of Seligman's (1975) view that exposure to all uncontrollable events, either positive or negative in nature, leads to helplessness or loss of control.

Fisher (1984) has argued that variations in degree of undesir- ability and variations in degrees of change may significantly influence whether difficult events are even appraised as stressful. Wack (1981) reported that even chronically ill older persons assoc- iated controllable events with fewer perceptions of psychological undesirability than with uncontrollable events, thus arguing that high levels of perceived control were associated with low levels of undesirability of events. The main focus of this research was to show that the degree of control individuals perceive themselves as having over their life circumstances is based on their cognitive appraisals and that these are important antecedents of adaptive or unadaptive coping. In summary, the rapidity of change, the number of stressful precipitants present, and the individuals' perceptions of the aversiveness of events will collectively influence the degree of vulnerability in later life (see Figure 1).

Biological Links in Vulnerability of the Elderly

Any cognitively based model of vulnerability would be incomplete if it failed to take into account the biological vulnerability factor. The presumption is that older persons are biologically and physiologically more vulnerable to the effects of uncontrollability (Rodin, 1986). Krantz, Glass, Contrada, & Miller (1981) have argued that pathophysio- logical concomitants of uncontrollability are believed to result from activation of both the sympathetic adrenal medullary system and the pituitary adrenal cortical axis. Catecholamines, secreted by the sympathetic nervous system are associated with increased blood pressure, elevation of blood lipids, induction of myocardial lesions, and provocation of ventricular arrythmias. The genetic vulnerability factor suggests a form of biological memory, a "biological tuning" which determines the differential intensity of experiences or lability of biological response at each stage of development. Vulnerability in old age may be influenced by compatibility or incompatibility of the physiological system with incoming influences. The genetic factor may determine for each individual the outcomes of the stress scenarios.

In summary, old age vulnerability as portrayed in Figure 1 is a genetically tuned metamemory that comes to represent deprivations and trauma, impoverished social circumstances, undesirable life-history

experiences, and both gradual and abrupt changes in life. This
cognitive model must provide a basis for understanding both the
psychology of control in aging and psychology of helplessness and
depression in aging. The basic idea developed about vulnerability in
old age is that it is a form of risk (extrinsic risk) of inappropriate
response patterns to stress scenarios, and will center on decisions
concerned with perceptions of control availability in the living
environment and personal control capabilities evaluated with respect
to needed skills, cognitions and beliefs. These combine interactively
with stressful circumstances of ill-health, declining physical
energies, and motivational deficits in old age to determine outcomes
of helplessness or control.

Spheres of Control in Aging as Related to Vulnerability

Using Paulhus and Christie's (1981) conceptions of control, it has
been argued by a number of theorists (cf. Bandura, 1977; Levenson,
1973, 1974) that aging adults will vary along the dimensions of
expectancies of control in general and specific domains of functioning. Paulhus and Christie's spheres of control (SOC) framework holds
that personal efficacy, interpersonal control, and sociopolitical
control are conceptually independent dispositions. As portrayed in
Figure 2 it could well be that vulnerability for older adults, unlike
younger adults, is the summation of the pattern of low expectancies
for control in a number of behavioral-cognitive domains such as the
following:

(a) *Personal Efficacy*. Due to invariably poor communications and
misinformation, older adults may have difficulty in maintaining
harmony between their dependency and interdependency needs with family
members and caregivers (Gurin & Brim, 1984). As a result they may
settle for relinquishing control over the most trivial daily activities, when to sleep, wake, visit, perform toileting activities or
when to eat (Janis & Rodin, 1979) and be subject to infantilization in
daily activities.

(b) *Interpersonal Control*. Perceived control in the sphere of
personal efficacy may act to reduce further the individual's self-
esteem. Low self-esteem may have self-confirming results in other
areas of influence such as interpersonal interactions with friends or
caregivers. The decline of controls in the sphere of personal
efficacy and interpersonal interactions might precipitate perceptual
changes in the individual's ability to control the whole nature of the
subsequent course of events of life history.

(c) *Sociopolitical Control*. Most older adults may come to
experience conflict between personal goals and social policy factors
governing their retirement, pension plans, insurance, etc. Attempts
to obtain necessary action by means of demonstrations, writing letters

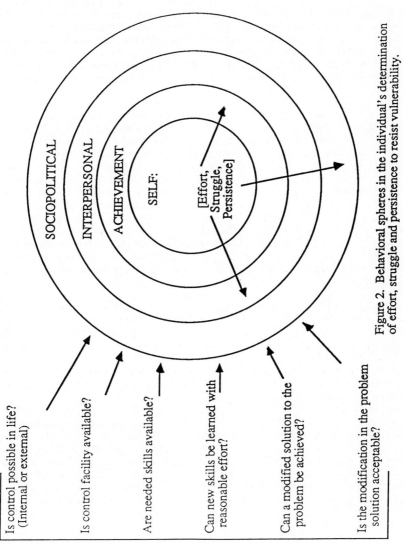

Figure 2. Behavioral spheres in the individual's determination of effort, struggle and persistence to resist vulnerability.

etc. may fail.   Perceived control in this sphere is termed sociopolitical control and perceived loss of control in the sociopolitical
sphere may contribute further to the vulnerability in several aspects
of the functioning of older adults (Marshall, 1986).

(d) *Self-Control and Self-Regulation*. A fourth possible level of
control conflict for most older adults involves the individual against
himself (as in conflicts of self-regulation and self-actualization).
As will be explained later, much evidence has been found for the
validity and integrity of this conflict in older adults characterized
by a vulnerability control profile.

Other general dimensions of control beliefs such as chance,
powerful others, difficult world, just world, etc. (see Levenson,
1973, 1974) may also cut across the SOC factors to contribute to the
older person's more pessimistic errors of judgments concerning control
facility and personal capabilities.   While the struggle to resolve
potential conflicts between dependency needs and the desire for self-
regulation is characteristic of all individuals at various stages of
the developmental cycle, it is hypothesized that the debilitating
effects of this conflict of the individual against himself and against
other spheres of control are greater among older individuals (see
Figure 2), especially those living in constrained environments
(Bourestom & Pastalan, 1981; Brand & Smith, 1974; Carstensen &
Whitbourne, 1978) who are at greater risk for primary helplessness
rather than adaptive responding.   Those most at risk for developing a
vulnerability profile across several spheres of cognitive-behavioral
control are the depressed elderly living in highly constraining
environments with low latitude of choice controls.   With declining
levels of perceived control in the various spheres and between the
self and the other spheres, the potential for vulnerability increases
with increasing constraints in the environment.

Given the relatively weaker abilities of older adults to handle
problems by means of selective efficacy controls, they may often
choose to cope with them by (a) dependency and avoidance; or (b) by
overly pessimistic or overly optimistic and unrealistic endorsement
for challenge and attack.   As such, vulnerability for some older
adults might be defined as difficulty in decision making: a tendency
to struggle *unrealistically* as a response to impending threat of
physical illness, financial and environmental impoverishment, and the
conscious decision to engage in stressful problems for which they lack
the skills.   Vulnerability for the older person is defined therefore,
in terms of the negative results accruing from conflict between self-
efficacy and interpersonal controls and the *overly pessimistic* or
overly optimistic errors which occur as a consequence of older
individuals attempting to restore control.

Interventions For Reducing Vulnerability and Enhancing Controls of Older Adults

Several reviews of the literature (cf. Averill, 1973; Miller, 1980; Thompson, 1981) have suggested potential advantages stemming from elderly recipients retaining control in the spheres of personal efficacy, interpersonal relationships and the sociopolitical arena. For example, Brickman, Rabinowitz, Karuza, Coates, Cohn and Kidder (1982) have argued that models which hold individuals responsible for action are likely to increase individuals' actual and perceived competence in the domain of self-esteem and self-concept. Schulz (1976) and Thompson (1981) have shown that effective exercise of responsibility for decision making and information seeking also results in a more predictable and informative environment and contributes to improved well-being and ability to tolerate stress and conflict.

Returning to the Spheres of Control model postulated by Paulhus and Christie, it becomes clear that vulnerability, feelings of depression and accelerated decline in the interpersonal effectiveness might be related to loss of controls and decision-making skills. Thus a possible solution to the problem of age-related vulnerability is the introduction or reintroduction of control-enhancing intervention. Interventions need then to focus on ways of reassigning primary and secondary control to older adults living in impoverished environments characterized by boredom, low latitude of choice and environmental unresponsiveness with their concomitant implications for the sense of the competent self (Taylor, 1979).

Especially with reference to institutional settings for older persons it has been argued that passivity, dependency and powerlessness is multiple. Chanowitz and Langer (1980) and White and Janson (1986), for example, note that boredom is inherent in routine and brings about a behavioral passivity that promotes depression and the "sick role." Conceptually, both iatrogenic factors (lack of environmental responsiveness) and adaptive factors (the individual's adaptation to environments stressing compliance) can explain helplessness (White & Janson, 1986). What are the implications of these findings of control to the question of facilitating purposeful decision making and increased self-esteem? A number of different viewpoints have emerged in the literature on gerontology. The implications of a few of the more well-formulated theoretical perspectives of intervention are discussed here.

Action Control Theorists

Generally speaking, regaining personal control through engagement, involvement and action has been stressed by a number of researchers (e.g., Brandtstädter, 1984a, 1984b, 1985) who believe encouraging older individuals to take active charge of their present lives will promote a sense of personal control and self-efficacy for future developments. The vantage point for such an approach to aging is a conception of adult development that emphasizes the individual's active contribution to personal competence, interpersonal effectiveness and assertiveness in the sociopolitical sphere. An action perspective on development is assumed also to influence values and beliefs related to a sense of personal competence in the other related spheres of control such as interpersonal control. The major argument presented by action theorists (e.g., Brandtstädter, Krampen & Heil, 1986) is that old age need not be characterized by experienced loss of control over developmental outcomes or by increased depressive tendencies or loss of self-esteem if adults can be encouraged to engage in ongoing personal evaluations of such developmental goals as their health, assertiveness, self-assurance, personal independence in decision making, harmonious interdependencies in relationships and commitments to ideals (e.g., humanistic, sociopolitical or religious ideals). The viewpoints of action-theoretical proponents contribute to a philosophy for aging and old age where exercise of personal control, decision making and information seeking becomes a valued goal. This set of literature offers support for modern gerontology's emphasis on activity theory. It is argued that while disengagement leads to behavioral passivity and increases potentials for depression and apathetic affects, high levels of action control and evaluation promote well-being of older adults.

Implications for Intervention

The action-theoretical proponents make a case for counseling and intervention programs that on a preventive and corrective base may help aging individuals to cope with crises and problems of self-esteem loss associated with vulnerability in later adulthood.

Action control theorists advocate that the individual's involvement in high levels of self-regulated and self-validated activity are likely to open opportunities for self-efficacy and mastery that comes with engagement and activity.

From the perspective of several other social psychologists also (cf. Karuza, Zevon, Rabinowitz, & Brickman, 1982; Rodin & Langer, 1980; Schulz, 1980) corrective interventions aimed at restoring older individuals' sense of competence, control and responsibility lay the foundations for assisting vulnerable and frail elderly in their problems of low self-esteem, helplessness and depression. These viewpoints square well with those of social learning theorists who advocate the early development of productive roles and skills.

Self-Efficacy Theorists

Self-efficacy theorists have provided empirical support for the development of interventions that promote feelings of success,

personal competence and self-regulation. Self-efficacy has had its
critics who have argued that such perceptions are simply an epiphenom-
ena and not a cause of adaptive or unadaptive behavior (Borkovec,
1978; Eysenck, 1978). On the other hand, Goldfried and Robins (1982)
have summarized evidence concerning self-perceptions of efficacy as a
reflection of high levels of coping ability across the life-span.
Bandura (1977) would argue quite explicitly that corrective or
preventive interventions should directly address older individuals'
perceptions of helplessness and deal directly with their levels of
fear, anxiety and avoidance in decision making and exercising personal
controls.

Implications for Intervention

Bandura postulates *four sources of information* for improving self-
efficacy of vulnerable individuals:

(a) *Past and present performance accomplishments*. In the case of
older individuals this sense of past and present accomplishments could
be attained through constructive reminiscence and constructive
cognitive restructuring and cognitive reappraisals of past and present
achievements (Fry, 1983). Reminiscence as a self-reflective process
may have an adaptive value for the elderly to the extent that it
allows them to identify accomplishments and identities in a way that
adds to self-esteem and dispels the belief of some cohorts that
advanced age is a social disgrace. Group participation in reminiscence may help to reinforce the sense of competence by encouraging
individuals to recount life experiences and accomplishments of
satisfaction in a creative and self-enhancing way (Fry, 1986).

(b) *Vicarious experience of observing others perform*. Based on
the idea that the older adults are well-functioning individuals with
ability to manage their own affairs, intervention programs which open
up opportunities for elderly individuals to observe other elderly
persons engaged in meaningful activities and leadership roles can be
directed toward enhancing the social consciousness of the individual
concerned.

(c) *Verbal persuasion and other kinds of social influence*. This
social-interactionist viewpoint assumes a fusion between the older
adults' level of perceived and actual control and the social group's
expression of trust, acceptance and confidence in the individual's
ability to be autonomous and independent. The social-interactionist
framework allows the older person to function from a perception of
control and mastery. Such a model when implemented from a perspective
of reciprocity and symbiotic interaction between the older person and
the social network, has a wide appeal for community elders who may
formulate their own goals in an existential desire to fulfill their
needs for self-esteem.

(d) *States of physiological arousal.* This consideration is of primary importance when implemented with respect to frail and vulnerable older adults who may manifest pathophysiological concomitants of uncontrollability and physiological agitation responses associated with uncontrollable stress. The sensations and experiences that older adults encounter may be unfamiliar and frightening, and they may be confused about how to make sense out of them or cope with their state of physiological arousal (Janis & Rodin, 1979). The older persons' sheer inability to regulate their physiological processes may be threatening thus resulting in an enhanced state of helplessness, depression and vulnerability. The caregivers' assistance and medical doctor's cooperation in helping older individuals to mobilize their energies more constructively and to regain control over their physiological responses may help to restore a sense of self-confidence and self-control ultimately contributing to the enhancement of self-efficacy.

The self-efficacy model when translated into interventions for older persons would suggest programs for subjects' active involvement (as compared to passive listening) in tasks pertinent to life satisfactions. For example, obtaining specific information and skills needed to make a decision about relocation, health interventions, etc. can give a sense of successful performance attainment.

The self-efficacy model would also suggest more presentations by and interactions with other older individuals who are recovering from states of depression, lowered self-esteem or uncontrollable pathophysiological reactions, to provide vicarious models of coping with old age transitions.

The limited gains in planfulness, independent functioning or autonomous decision making found to result from most interventions designed for frail elderly may not be as problematic as it appears on first analysis, if it can be shown generally that intervention increases their sense of efficacy even if it does not increase their planfulness or autonomy in decision making. In so far as a low sense of self-efficacy is seen to be the best predictor of depression, apathy and vulnerability in a number of studies using older persons (cf. Taylor, 1979; Ziegler & Reid, 1983), it is argued that interventions promoting even minimal levels of planfulness, information processing and acquisition of skills in decision making may contribute to the enhancement of older persons' morale, life satisfactions and self-esteem.

Since a social-interactionist perspective is adherent in self-efficacy, the caregivers' positive attitudes, social and emotional support and reinforcement beyond the simple dispersal of information, are intrinsic ingredients of intervention programs for physically and emotionally frail and vulnerable elderly persons.

Person-Environment Fit Theorists

The thesis advocated in the person-environment fit model of intervention for older persons advocates that congruence between older persons and their environment needs to be achieved at two levels. At level one the congruence thesis states that risks for vulnerability can be reduced by helping older individuals to control their environments so that the latter can be made to become more responsive to their needs. At level two the congruence thesis states that individuals who have little control over their environment adapt better to environments that are not responsive to individual control attempts. The two-process model of control in the person-environment fit concept postulates that control may involve either "attempts to change the world so that it fits the self's needs" (primary control) or "attempts to fit in with the world and to flow with the current" (secondary control) (Rothbaum, Weisz, & Snyder, 1982, p. 8).

Implications for Intervention

When this two-process model of control is applied to older persons it follows that personal satisfaction with care, better mental health and a sense of competence are all expected to result from the fit between the elderly person's dependency and autonomy needs and characteristics. It should be noted that the person-environment fit model when applied to older persons stresses that the concept of fit is not static. It is anticipated that needs and capabilities of older adults will change just as environmental resources will change.

Interventions must ensure that there are opportunities for *transactions* to occur. As older individuals' personal resources decline, dependency needs will increase and correspondingly while certain need-meeting resources of the environment may become scarce, others will increase. Ongoing transactions between personal resources of individuals and environmental resources accessible to them are central to the concept of the person-environment fit. The significant factor is the environment's potential for meeting the older resident's needs for both autonomy and dependence.

It is increasingly recognized that the kind of primary control implied in the attempts to change the environment so that it fits the self's need is less possible with frail elderly persons (cf. Karuza & Karuza, 1984). However, it is proposed that the competence or sense of self-esteem of frail older persons may be best maintained or enhanced when their dependency needs or autonomy needs are met and where no value judgments are attached to the older person's preference for dependency or autonomy.

Recent work of Baltes and Werner-Wahl (1987) draws a useful distinction between two types of dependency, one type which suggests the need to be assisted with all functional needs of daily living and assistance in all forms of decision making. This type of dependency reflects outcomes of total compliance and helplessness. The second type of dependency may comprise a proactive coping modality (getting others to provide help) especially when the older person does not have sufficient personal resources to change the environment. The proactive coping modality of dependence implies a kind of instrumental control in which an illusion of control is maintained by elderly persons who call upon "significant others" in the environment for serving their dependency needs.

General Implications of Control Constructs
for Interventions with Elderly Adults

Having derived the three models and discussed the potential value of these for application to elderly persons, our next step is to consider some of the adverse effects or the limitations of control constructs for intervention programs designed for the elderly.

From a number of studies (e.g., Gurin & Brim, 1984; Lachman, 1986) it is not clear whether persons can change their locus of control or sense of personal efficacy over time or situations. Investigations using control-relevant interventions with ill, frail and psychologically vulnerable elderly persons have suggested that interventions stressing expectations of self-efficacy, personal action control and congruence with the environment may be detrimental because individuals are made to feel in control, and failing to achieve primary control will more likely precipitate negative reactance and depressive affects following failure.

It is recommended therefore that several other distinctions in control constructs need to be considered and implemented in programs and interventions because of their significance to the well-being of older adults and because of their vicarious effect in enhancing perceived controls.

The Value of Anticipatory Control

Intervention programs that assist older persons with information about the possible positive or negative outcomes of their choices, their behaviors or stressful experiences prepare them for the psychological and physiological impact of the difficult events. This provides them a form of anticipatory control which is useful in coping with similar or later transitions. Krantz and Schulz (1980) demonstrated that interventions designed to increase the sense of predictability of the environmental influences or outcomes brought about significant improvement in the psychological status of older participants in the program.

It is postulated that interventions that increase perceptions of anticipatory control over future events, both positive and negative, have the effect of reducing depression and the risk of further debilitation in the psychological status of *at risk* elderly persons. Even though such interventions do not produce any change in control availability or control facility, they have the benefit of producing at least temporary alterations in levels of perceived control over later events.   Certainly emotionally and physically frail elderly persons residing in rather constrained environments need to develop a sense of anticipatory control over routines and also over the amount of social support or reinforcements they can expect to receive in stressful transitions.

The Value of Secondary Control

When the primary-secondary control distinction is implemented in intervention programs for older individuals *at risk* for vulnerability and learned helplessness depression, it is argued that acquiring primary control over the environmental changes, powerful others in the environment and the unresponsiveness of a deterministic environment, is a relatively more difficult goal to be achieved by frail elderly persons.   By contrast, secondary control described as a form of control in which the individual does not attempt to alter the environmental influences but to accept the environment, has greater potential for being useful to older individuals in coping with transitions (Alloy & Abramson, 1979; Felton & Kahana, 1974; Wolk, 1976).

Secondary control mechanisms would help older persons to cope better by shielding themselves against the harsher impact of the powerful others in the environment.

Generally speaking the giving up of control inferred from passive behavior has a depressing effect on most older persons.   By contrast progressions of therapy and counseling which offer support for behavioral passivity in stressful situations and dependency on "significant others" in the environment have the benefit of creating the illusion of control in the self, and avoid the negative consequences of feeling dependent, passive and frail.   Within a social cognitive-behavioral framework of intervention, the cognitive restructuring and cognitive reinterpretation by a counselor of the meaning and purpose of difficult and stressful events has the effect of keeping the older person's self-perceptions intact.   For example, the loss of a spouse or a significant other may be deemed as designed to be part of God's larger scheme and part of the universal good.

In summary, it is argued that it is rather doubtful that corrective interventions oriented toward helping older individuals attain primary control over the environmental influences will have a high ratio of long-term success.   The nature of the aging process itself and the concomitant results as evidenced in the sensory-motor losses and declines in health accompanying late life makes it relatively difficult for older persons to exercise primary control or to achieve mastery of the environmental influences. By contrast, supportive interventions that provide encouragement and reinforcements for coping with situations of stress, helplessness and dependency have the effect not only of reducing depression (Lieberman, 1982) but also of increasing passive mastery and positive perceptions of control over environmental events that are intrinsically stressful and uncontrollable.

The Value of Instrumental Control

This is a type of vicarious control which helps older individuals in their attempts to modify their situation by seeking the help of friends, family members and "significant others" in the environment to accomplish the necessary change.

Instrumental control may not be possible or adaptive in situations where there is a high degree of environmental or external control or where the older person has experienced a severe depletion of personal resources to react or respond to the demand for compliance.

In most situations of daily living, however, the concept of instrumental control is adaptive in that it helps the older person faced with diminished personal resources to regain the illusion of control by seeking solutions to personal problems in decision making, information seeking and organization through the mediation of powerful persons.

The Value of Participatory Control

As a further extension of the concept of secondary control, a number of researchers and practitioners have proposed the concept of participatory control as a means of helping depressed and vulnerable elderly persons to overcome, as optimally as possible, a sense of helplessness, hopelessness and self-denigration associated with living in highly controlled environments.

The underlying assumptions of the proposed participatory control model (cf. Reid & Ziegler, 1981) is that self-esteem can be enhanced and a general uplifting of spirits can be achieved by helping older persons to gain control over their environment through the abilities and efforts of others. The provision of participatory control makes it possible for frail and dependent elderly, at risk for depression, to express their needs and fears and also to communicate in an effective way either their pleasure or displeasure to caregivers. The idea of having participatory control reassures the person he/she has input into the decisions that affect the self. Even weak, feeble and depressed older persons although clearly surrendering control to their caregivers acquire secondary control through the knowledge that they have a right to be consulted in decisions that affect their well-being.

A number of studies (Rodin & Langer, 1977; Reid, Haas, & Hawkings, 1977; Schulz, 1980) have advocated participatory control as a way of reducing the older person's total reliance on powerful others in the environment. Furthermore it is argued that participatory control by definition, should lead to better physical and emotional health care, for it should facilitate a better information exchange and better cooperation between older persons and their caregivers (Reid, 1984). This implies, of course, that the provision of participatory control will give rise to individual differences in the way that people choose to exercise their right to participate, to acquire information about their world, to organize the information, and use it to develop behavioral responses. It can be speculated that older persons who are more internal and less external will hold high reinforcement values for participation and as a way to nourish their vulnerable self-esteem (cf. Kahana, 1975; Lawton, 1975; Magnusson & Engler, 1977).

Conclusions

It seems reasonable to conclude that vulnerability in late life is inextricably linked to older persons' perceptions of personal control and sense of mastery or efficacy. It is postulated that vulnerability in old age is the result of various experiences in the life-cycle concerned with loss of control over the environment. The over-emphasized need to foster and preserve control beliefs throughout adulthood and old age imposes sufficient strain on the functioning and performance expectancies so as to cause stress, depression and decline in sensory-motor functioning. At each step in the sequence of adult development individuals may have conflicts between surrendering controls or struggling and persisting in the face of impending dependencies and limited physical and emotional energies. Difficulty in maintaining harmony among their autonomy, dependency and inter-dependency needs may typically contribute to older persons' sense of vulnerability and helplessness. Predisposing and precipitating factors such as the frequency and intensity of undesirable events and the rapidity of environmental change in the later years may all take their toll on the emotional energies of older adults.

Levels of perceived control in decision making, information processing and self-esteem enhancement may be central to the composition of helplessness and vulnerability in late life. Feelings of resignation or despair in elders may be multiplicatively connected with a constellation of cognitive, motivational and behavioral deficits in skills or personal control capabilities. It is important to understand the role played by older persons' control ideology in the development of depression or the potentials for increasing difficulty in coping with life stresses. What emerges among many older adults is a slowly evolving pattern of control by avoidance and a mental condition of resignation which predisposes against seeking help or acquiring actual control over life events. This combination of performance decrements and motivational deficits results ultimately in an all-prevailing sense of vulnerability.

Therapy and intervention programs for older adults need to establish the precise personal attributions and environmental conditions and factors which contribute to a sense of helplessness so that potentially debilitating consequences such as depression, lack of motivation, lack of effort or poor subsequent performance can be either prevented or modified.

In summary, the main approach that needs to be developed in therapy programs is that although vulnerability, in part, is associated with lack of personal control over the environment it also comes from a lack of knowledge about control facilities available or absence of metamemory. Intervention programs that teach older persons to make logical assessments of realistic control facilities and capabilities accessible to them may help vulnerable elderly to resist the transmission of helplessness. The hypothesis that needs to be pursued in therapy with elderly persons is that all adverse life experiences with negative outcomes should be reassessed in order to prepare the individual to change his/her expectancies about control in subsequent situations. In other words, the main concern should be with each individual assessing and reassessing life history sequential dependencies. It is then possible for each participant in therapy to examine and identify influences in the immediate environment that increase or reduce the risk for precipitants to have a negative outcome.

Acknowledgments

Preparation of this chapter was facilitated, in part, by a research grant received from the Social Sciences and Humanities Research Council of Canada, Strategic Grants Program (Grant No. 492-83-0020).

References

Abramson, L. Y., Seligman, M. E. P., & Teasdale, J. D. (1978). Learned helplessness in humans: Critique and reformulation. *Journal of Abnormal Psychology, 87,* 49-74.

Alloy, L. B., & Abramson, L. Y. (1979). Judgements of contingency in depressed or non-depressed students: Sadder but wiser? *Journal of Experimental Psychology (General), 108,* 441-485.

Averill, J. R. (1973). Personal control over aversive stimuli and its relationship to stress. *Psychological Bulletin, 80,* 286-303.

Baltes, M. M., & Werner-Wahl, H. (1987). Dependence in aging. In L. L. Carstensen & B. A. Edelstein (Eds.), *Handbook of Clinical Gerontology* (pp. 204-219). New York: Pergamon Press.

Baltes, P. B., & Willis, S. L. (1979). Life-span developmental psychology, cognitive functioning and social policy. In M. W. Riley (Ed.), *Aging from birth to death* (pp. 15-46). Boulder, CO: Westview Press.

Bandura, A. (1977). Self-efficacy: Toward a unifying theory of behavioral change. *Psychological Review, 84,* 191-215.

Bandura, A. (1982). Self-efficacy mechanism in human agency. *American Psychologist, 37,* 122-147.

Baron, R., & Rodin, J. (1978). Perceived control and crowding stress. In A. Baum, J. E. Singer, & S. Valins (Eds.), *Advances in environmental psychology* (pp. 145-190).

Beck, A. T. (1970). The core problem in depression: The cognitive triad. *Science and Psychoanalysis, 17,* 47-55.

Borkovec, T. D. (1978). Self-efficacy: Cause or reflection of behavioral change? *Advances in Behavioral Research Therapy, 1,* 163-170.

Bourestom, N., & Pastalan, L. (1981). The effects of relocation on the elderly: A reply to Borup, J. H., Gallego, D. T., & Heffernan, P. G. *The Gerontologist, 21,* 4-7.

Brand, F., & Smith, R. (1974). Life-adjustment and relocation of the elderly. *Journal of Gerontology, 29,* 336-340.

Brandtstädter, J. (1984a). Personal and social control over development: Some implications of an action perspective in life-span developmental psychology. In P. B. Baltes & O. G. Brim, Jr. (Eds.), *Life-span development and behavior, Volume 6* (pp. 1-32). New York: Academic Press.

Brandtstädter, J. (1984b). Action development and development through action. *Human Development, 27,* 115-118.

Brandtstädter, J. (1985). Individual development in social action contexts: Problems of explanation. In J. R. Nesselroade & A. von Eye (Eds.), *Individual development and social change: Explanatory analysis* (pp. 243-264). New York: Academic Press.

Brandtstädter, J., Krampen, G., & Heil, F. E. (1986). Personal control and emotional evaluation of development in partnership relations during adulthood. In M. M. Baltes & P. B. Baltes (Eds.), *The psychology of control and aging* (pp. 265-296). Hillsdale, NJ: Lawrence Erlbaum Associates.

Brickman, P., Rabinowitz, V. C., Karuza, J., Jr., Coates, D., Cohn, E., & Kidder, L. (1982). Models of helping and coping. *American Psychologist, 37,* 368-384.

Brown, G. W., & Birley, J. L. T. (1970). Social precipitants of severe psychiatric disorders. In E. H. Hare & J. K. Wing (Eds.), *Psychiatric epidemiology; Proceedings of the International Symposium* (Aberdeen, June/July, 1969). New York: Oxford University Press.

Brown, G. W., & Harris, T. H. (1978). *Social origins of depression: A study of psychiatric disorders in women.* Great Britain: Tavistock.

Carstensen, L., & Whitbourne, S. (1978, November). *Variations in locus of control and morale by institutional totality in an elderly sample.* Paper presented at Annual Meeting of the Gerontological Society of America, Dallas, TX.

Cerella, J., Poon, L. W., & Williams, D. M. (1980). Age and the complexity hypothesis. In L. W. Poon (Ed.), *Aging in the 1980s* (pp. 332-340). Washington, DC: American Psychological Association.

Chanowitz, B., & Langer, E. J. (1980). Knowing more (or less) than you can show: Understanding control through the mindlessness-mindfulness distinction. In J. Garber & M. E. P. Seligman (Eds.), *Human helplessness* (pp. 97-129). New York: Academic Press.

Craik, F. I. M. (1977). Age differences in human memory. In J. E. Birren & K. W. Schaie (Eds.), *Handbook of the psychology of aging* (pp. 384-420). New York: Van Nostrand Reinhold Co.

Davis, D. R. (1970). Depression as an adaptation to crisis. *British Journal of Medical Psychology, 43,* 109-116.

Dohrenwend, B. P., & Dohrenwend, B. S. (1974). Social and cultural influences on psychopathology. *Annual Review of Psychology, 5,* 417-452.

Dohrenwend, B. S. (1973). Life events as stressors: A methodological inquiry. *Journal of Health and Social Behaviour, 14* (June), 167-175.

Eysenck, H. J. (1978). Expectations as a causal element in behavior change. *Advances in Behavioral Research Therapy, 1,* 171-175.

Farberow, N. L., & Moriwaki, S. Y. (1975). Self-destructive crises in the older person. *The Gerontologist, 15,* 333-337.

Felton, B., & Kahana, E. (1974). Adjustment and situationally-bound locus of control among institutionalized aged. *Journal of Gerontology, 29,* 295-301.

Fisher, S. (1984). *Stress and the perception of control.* Hillsdale, NJ: Lawrence Erlbaum Associates.

Fry, P. S. (1983). Structured and unstructured reminiscence training and depression among the elderly. *Clinical Gerontologist, 1,* 15-37.

Fry, P. S. (1986). *Depression, stress, and adaptations in the elderly: Psychological assessment and intervention.* Rockville, MD: Aspen.

Glass, D. C. (1977). Stress, behavior patterns, and coronary disease. *American Scientist, 65,* 177.

Goldfried, M. R., & Robins, C. (1982). On the facilitation of self-efficacy. *Cognitive Theory and Research, 6,* 361-380.

Goodstein, R. K. (1981). Inextricable interaction: Social, psychologic and biologic stresses facing the elderly. *American Journal of Orthopsychiatry, 51,* 219-229.

Gore, P. S., & Rotter, J. B. (1963). A personality correlate of social action. *Journal of Personality, 31,* 58-64.

Gurin, P., & Brim, O. G. Jr., (1984). Change in self in adulthood: The example of sense of control. In P. B. Baltes & O. G. Brim, Jr. (Eds.), *Life-span development and behavior, Volume 6,* (pp. 281-322). New York: Academic Press.

Janis, I. L., & Rodin, J. (1979). Attribution control and decision making: Social psychology and health care. In G. C. Stone, F. Cohen, & N. E. Adler (Eds.), *Health psychology* (pp. 487-521). San Francisco, CA: Jossey-Bass.

Janoff-Bulman, R., & Brickman, P. (1982). Expectations and what people learn from failure. In N. T. Feather (Ed.), *Expectancy, incentive and action* (pp. 77-92). Hillsdale, NJ: Lawrence Erlbaum Associates.

Janowitz, M. (1978). *The last half-century: Societal change and politics in America.* Chicago: University of Chicago Press.

Jarvis, E. (1971). *Insanity and idiocy in Massachusetts: Report of the Commission of Lunacy 1855.* Cambridge: Harvard University Press.

Kahana, E. (1975). A congruence model of person-environment interaction. In P. G. Windley, T. Byerts, & E. G. Ernst (Eds.), *Theoretical developments in environments for aging* (pp. 181-214). Washington, DC: Gerontological Society of America.

Karuza, J. Jr., & Karuza, C. M. (1984, November). *Models of helping: Effects of age and problem type*. Paper presented at the Gerontological Society of America meeting, San Antonia, TX.

Karuza, J. Jr., & Rabinowitz, V. C., & Zevon, M. A. (1986). Implications of control and responsibility on helping the aged. In M. M. Baltes & P. B. Baltes (Eds.), *The psychology of control and aging* (pp. 373-396). Hillsdale, NJ: Lawrence Erlbaum Associates.

Karuza, J. Jr., Zevon, M. A., Rabinowitz, V. C., & Brickman, P. (1982). Attribution of responsibility by helpers and recipients. In T. A. Wills (Eds.), *Basic processes in helping relationships* (pp. 107-129). New York: Academic Press.

Kiyak, A., Liang, J., & Kahana, E. (1976). *A methodological inquiry into the schedule of recent life events*. Paper presented at Symposium on Life Events, American Psychological Association, New York.

Krampen, G. (1982). *Differentialpsychologie der Kontrollüberzeugungen*. Göttingen, FRG: Hogrefe.

Krantz, D. S., Glass, D. C., Contrada, R., & Miller, N. E. (1981). Behavior and health. In *The National Science Foundation's Five Year Outlook on Science and Technology: 1981*. (Source material, Vol. 2). U. S. Government Printing Office.

Krantz, D. S., & Schulz, R. (1980). A model of life crisis, control, and health outcomes: Cardiac rehabilitation and relocation of the elderly. In A. Baum & J. E. Singer (Eds.), *Advances in environmental psychology: Applications of personal control, Volume 2*, (pp. 25-59). Hillsdale, NJ: Lawrence Erlbaum Associates.

Kuhl, J. (1985). Volitional mediators of cognition-behavior consistency: Self-regulatory processes and action versus state orientation. In J. Kuhl & J. Beckmann (Eds.), *Action control: From cognition to behavior* (pp. 101-128). New York: Springer.

Kuhl, J. (1986). Aging and models of control: The hidden costs of wisdom. In M. M. Baltes & P. B. Baltes (Eds.), *The psychology of control and aging* (pp. 1-33). Hillsdale, NJ: Lawrence Erlbaum Associates.

Kuypers, J. A., & Bengtson, V. L. (1973). Social breakdown and competence: A model of normal aging. *Human Development, 25*, 181-201.

Lachman, M. E. (1985). Personal efficacy in middle and old age: Differential and normative patterns of change. In G. H. Elder, Jr. (Ed.), *Life-course dynamics: From 1968 to the 80's* (pp. 188-213). Ithaca, NY: Cornell University Press.

Lachman, M. E. (1986). Locus of control in aging research: A case for multidimensional and domain-specific assessment. *Psychology and Aging, 1*, 34-40.

Lachman, M. E., & McArthur, L. Z. (1986). Adulthood age differences in causal attributions for cognitive, physical and social performance. *Psychology and Aging, 1*, 127-132.

Langer, E. J., & Rodin, J. (1976). The effects of choice and enhanced personal responsibility for the aged: A field experiment in an institutional setting. *Journal of Personality and Social Psychology, 34*, 191-198.

Lawton, M. P. (1975). The impact of the environment on aging and behavior. In J. Birren & K. W. Schaie (Eds.), *Handbook on the psychology of aging* (pp. 276-301). New York: Van Nostrand Reinhold.

Lawton, M. P., & Nahemow, L. (1973). Ecology and the aging process. In C. Eisdorder & M. P. Lawton (Eds.), *Psychology of adult development and aging* (pp. 619-674). Washington, DC: American Psychological Association.

Lazarus, R. S., & Folkman, S. (1984). Coping and adaptation. In W. D. Gentry (Ed.), *The handbook of behavioral medicine* (pp. 282-325). New York: Guilford Press.

Levenson, H. (1973). Multidimensional locus of control in psychiatric patients. *Journal of Consulting and Clinical Psychology, 41*, 397-404.

Levenson, H. (1974). Activism and powerful others: Distinctions within the concept of internal-external control. *Journal of Personality Assessment, 38*, 377-383.

Lieberman, M. A. (1982). The effects of social supports on response to stress. In L. Goldberger & S. Breznitz (Eds.), *Handbook of stress* (pp. 764-784). New York: Free Press.

Magnusson, D., & Endler, N. S. (1977). *Personality at the crossroads: Current issues in interactional psychology.* Hillsdale, NJ: Lawrence Erlbaum Associates.

Mandler, G. (1975). *Mind and emotion*. New York: Wiley & Sons.

Marshall, V. (1986). *Later life: The social psychology of aging*. Beverly Hills: Sage.

McClure, J. (1985). The social parameter of "learned" helplessness: Its recognition and implications. *Journal of Personality and Social Psychology, 48*, 1534-1539.

Miller, S. M. (1980). Why having control reduces stress: If I can stop the roller coaster, I don't want to get off. In J. Garber & M. E. P. Seligman (Eds.), *Human helplessness* (pp. 71-95). New York: Academic Press.

Oyer, H. J., & Oyer, E. J. (1978). Social consequences of hearing loss for the elderly. *Allied Health and Behavioral Sciences, 2*, 123-138.

Palmore, E. (1980). The social factors in aging. In E. W. Busse & D. G. Blazer (Eds.), *Handbook of geriatric psychiatry* (pp. 222-248). New York: Van Nostrand Reinhold.

Parkes, C. M. (1978). *Bereavement*. New York: International Universities Press.

Paulhus, D., & Christie, R. (1981). Spheres of control: An interactionist approach to assessment of perceived control. In H. M. Lefcourt (Ed.), *Research with the locus of control construct, Volume 1, Assessment methods* (pp. 161-188). New York: Academic Press.

Perlmuter, L. C., & Monty, R. A. (Eds.) (1979). *Choice and perceived control*. Hillsdale, NJ: Lawrence Erlbaum Associates.

Perlmuter, L. C., Monty, R. A., & Chan, F. (1986). Choice, control and cognitive functioning. In M. M. Baltes & P. B. Baltes (Eds.), *The psychology of control and aging* (pp. 91-118). Hillsdale, NJ: Lawrence Erlbaum Associates.

Peterson, C. (1982). Learned helplessness and health psychology. *Health Psychology, 1*, 153-168.

Rabkin, J. G. (1982). Stress and psychiatric disorders. In L. Goldberger & S. Breznitz (Eds.), *Handbook of stress: Theoretical and clinical aspects* (pp. 566-685). New York: The Free Press.

Reid, D. W. (1984). Participatory control and the chronic-illness adjustment process. In H. M. Lefcourt (Ed.), *Research with the locus of control construct, Volume 3: Extensions and limitations* (pp. 361-389). New York: Academic Press.

Reid, D. W., Haas, G., & Hawkings, D. (1977). Locus of desired control and positive self-concept of elderly. *Journal of Gerontology, 32*, 441-450.

Reid, D. W., & Ziegler, M. (1981). The desired control measure and adjustment among the elderly. In H. M. Lefcourt (Ed.), *Research with the locus of control construct: Assessment methods, Volume 1* (pp. 127-159). New York: Academic Press.

Rodin, J. (1979). Managing the stress of aging: The role of control and coping. In S. Levine & H. Ursin (Eds.), *Coping and health* (pp. 171-202). New York: Plenum Press.

Rodin, J. (1983). Behavioral medicine: Beneficial effects of self-control training in aging. *International Review of Applied Psychology, 32*, 153-181.

Rodin, J. (1986). Health, control, and aging. In M. M. Baltes & P. B. Baltes (Eds.), *The psychology of control and aging* (pp. 139-165). Hillsdale, NJ: Lawrence Erlbaum Associates.

Rodin, J., & Langer, E. J. (1977). Long-term effect of a control-relevant intervention. *Journal of Personality and Social Psychology, 35*, 897-902.

Rodin, J., & Langer, E. J. (1980). Aging labels: The decline of control and fall of self-esteem. *Journal of Social Issues, 36*, 12-29.

Rosow, I. (1974). *Socialization to old age.* Berkeley: University of California Press.

Roth, S., & Kubal, L. (1975). Effects of non-contingent reinforcement on tasks of differing importance: Facilitation of learned helplessness. *Journal of Personality and Social Psychology, 32*, 680-691.

Rothbaum, F., Weisz, J. R., & Snyder, S. S. (1982). Changing the world and changing the self: A two-process model of perceived control. *Journal of Personality and Social Psychology, 42*, 5-37.

Rotter, J. B. (1966). Generalized expectancies for internal versus external control of reinforcement. *Psychological Monographs, 80*, 609.

Sarason, I. G., Johnson, J. H., & Siegel, J. M. (1978). Measuring the impact of life changes: Development of the *Late Life Experiences Survey. Journal of Consulting and Clinical Psychology, 46*, 932-946.

Schaie, K. W. (Ed.) (1983). *Longitudinal studies of adult psychological development.* New York: The Guilford Press.

Schless, A. P., Schwartz, L., Goetz, C., & Mendels, J. (1974). How depressives view the significance of life events. *British Journal of Psychiatry, 125,* 406-410.

Schulberg, H., & Sheldon, A. (1968). The probability of crisis and strategies to preventative intervention. *Archives of General Psychiatry, 18,* 553-558.

Schulz, R. (1976). The effects of control and predictability on the psychological and physical well-being of the institutionalized aged. *Journal of Personality and Social Psychology, 33,* 563-573.

Schulz, R. (1980). Aging and control. In J. Garber & M. E. P. Seligman (Eds.), *Human helplessness* (pp. 261-277). New York: Academic Press.

Schulz, R., & Hanusa, B. (1980). Experimental social gerontology: A social psychological perspective. *Journal of Social Issues, 36,* 30-46.

Seligman, M. E. P. (1975). *Helplessness: On depression, development, and death.* San Francisco: Freeman.

Siegler, I. C., & Gatz, M. (1985). Age patterns in locus of control. In E. Palmore, E. W. Busse, G. L. Maddox, J. B. Nowlin, & I. C. Siegler (Eds.), *Normal aging III* (pp. 259-267). Durham, NC: Duke University Press.

Sorensen, A., Weinert, F., & Sherrod, L. (Eds.) (1987). *Human development and the life course: Multidisciplinary perspectives.* Hillsdale, NJ: Lawrence Erlbaum Associates.

Suls, J. (1982). Social support, interpersonal relations and health: Benefits and liabilities. In G. Sanders & J. Suls (Eds.), *The social psychology of health and illness* (pp. 57-71). Hillsdale, NJ: Lawrence Erlbaum Associates.

Taylor, S. E. (1979). Hospital patient behavior: Reactance, helplessness, or control. *Journal of Social Issues, 35,* 156-184.

Thompson, S. C. (1981). Will it hurt less if I can control it? A complex answer to a simple question. *Psychological Bulletin, 90,* 89-101.

Verwoerdt, A. (1976). *Clinical geropsychiatry.* Baltimore: Williams & Wilkins.

Wack, J. (1981). *Appraisals and patterning of affect and coping in encounters with everyday stressors.* Unpublished doctoral dissertation, Yale University.

Walsh, D. A. (1975). Age differences in learning and memory. In D. S. Woodruff & J. E. Birren (Eds.), *Aging: Scientific perspectives and social issues* (pp. 125-200). New York: Van Nostrand Reinhold.

Weinberg, J. (1975). Geriatric psychiatry. In A. M. Freedman, H. I. Kaplan & B. J. Sadock (Eds.), *Comprehensive textbook of psychiatry-/II* (pp. 2405-2420). Baltimore: Williams & Wilkins.

Weisz, J. R. (1983). Can I control it? The pursuit of veridical answers across the life span. In P. B. Baltes & O. G. Brim (Eds.), *Life-span development and behavior, Volume 5* (pp. 233-300). New York: Academic Press.

White, C. B., & Janson, P. (1986). Helplessness in institutional settings: Adaptation or iatrogenic disease? In M. M. Baltes & P.B. Baltes (Eds.), *The psychology of control and aging* (pp. 297-313). Hillsdale, NJ: Lawrence Erlbaum Associates.

White, R. W. (1959). Motivation reconsidered: The concept of competence. *Psychological Review, 66,* 297-333.

Wolk, S. (1976). Situational constraint as a moderator of the locus of control-adjustment relationship. *Journal of Consulting and Clinical Psychology, 43,* 420-427.

Ziegler, M., & Reid, D. W. (1983). Correlates of changes in desired control scores and in life-satisfaction scores among elderly persons. *International Journal of Aging and Human Development, 16,* 135-146.

PART II

LIFE-SPAN DEVELOPMENT AND CONTROL

*Psychological Perspectives of Helplessness
and Control in the Elderly, P.S. Fry (ed.)*
© *Elsevier Science Publishers B.V. (North-Holland), 1989*

Chapter Two

CONTROLLABILITY AND ADAPTIVE COPING IN THE ELDERLY: AN ADULT DEVELOPMENTAL PERSPECTIVE

Fredda BLANCHARD-FIELDS
Louisiana State University

Abstract

The relationship between controllability and coping is discussed from a developmental perspective. For example, one such developmental framework is proposed by Labouvie-Vief who argues that adult cognition represents a major reorganization in thinking which is reflected in increasing self-control and self-regulation. Given this emphasis, the author discusses empirical research findings suggesting that (a) patterns of coping vary across age groups with younger individuals endorsing more defensive strategies than older adults, (b) there are age-related differences and changes in internal locus of control, and (c) older adults more effectively balance both instrumental and emotional/palliative coping strategies depending on the appraised controllability of the situation. These findings are discussed in terms of methodological issues for studying controllability and coping in the elderly, theoretical issues pertaining to developmental components of controllability and coping in adulthood and aging, and implications for healthy adaptive functioning in the elderly.

Introduction

A considerable amount of research has suggested that there is an adaptive relationship between attributions of control and coping (Folkman & Lazarus, 1980; Parkes, 1984; Stone & Neale, 1984). More recently, this relationship has been reexamined in the context of adult developmental maturity. For example, there is a growing area of work demonstrating major developmental reorganizations in adult cognition which equates intellectual functioning and adaptation with areas of self-control and self-regulation (Commons, Richards, & Armon, 1984; Labouvie-Vief, 1985; Sinnott, 1984). This suggests that there may be a developmental component involved in the relationship between appraised controllability and coping responses.

Therefore, in this chapter I would like to discuss the relation-ship between controllability and coping from this developmental perspective. First, what is meant by adaptive cognition or cognitive-developmental maturity in adulthood and aging will be briefly discussed. Second, empirical research suggesting that there is an adult developmental component to coping as well as a developmental component to controllability will be presented. Third, several studies I have recently conducted will be reviewed supporting the notion that developmental differences in coping and controllability may be more profitably examined in relation to each other. These findings will be discussed in terms of methodological issues for studying controllability and coping in the elderly and theoretical issues pertaining to developmental components of controllability and coping as they relate to healthy adaptive functioning in the elderly. Finally, two applied contexts in which controllability and the relationship between controllability and coping will be presented. They include primary and secondary control in institutionalized elderly and attributions of control and adaptive coping in caregivers of impaired elderly.

Adaptive Cognition in Adulthood

The recent literature on adult cognition reflects an emerging theoretical framework placing the domain of cognitive development in adulthood within a context of adaptive functioning. For example, Labouvie-Vief (in press) argues that adult cognition represents a major reorganization in thinking that has profound adaptive sig-nificance. This reorganization involves the integration of more rational, analytical modes of thinking with more concrete and contextually embedded thoughts and feelings. In turn, this integra-tion leads to what she calls a prototypical state of healthy adult functioning.

This perspective suggests that intellectual development in adulthood and aging is demonstrated best in more socio-emotional domains of reasoning. This has yielded a proliferation of research demonstrating progressions from less mature to more mature adult thinking that reflect (a) the ability to integrate and regulate both cognitive and affective systems (Blanchard-Fields, 1986; Cavanaugh, Kramer, Sinnott, Camp, & Markley, 1985; Labouvie-Vief, 1984); (b) a decrease in defensiveness when confronted with emotional issues (Greenspan, 1979); (c) a more autonomous self that is less dependent on external authority and social conventions (Labouvie-Vief, 1984; Loevinger, 1980); (d) increased cognitive complexity in adulthood in the form of more relativistic and integrative reasoning styles (Kramer, 1983; Labouvie-Vief, 1984; Sinnott, 1984); and (e) the ability of adults at higher levels of social-cognitive maturity to exhibit more cooperative and engaging communications in marital conflicts than those at lower levels of social-cognitive maturity (Kramer & Levine, 1987).

For example, in a recent study I conducted, developmental differences in reasoning in the context of emotionally salient social dilemmas were examined (see Blanchard-Fields, 1986). In order to assess these differences, ambiguously structured information of high to low emotional saliency was introduced to individuals ranging in age from adolescence through middle adulthood. The tasks consisted of two divergent accounts of the same event sequence. Subjects were questioned as to how they perceived the discrepancies. Each of the accounts was written from the perspective of a biased party. For example, two conflicting perspectives of an adolescent and his parents describing a trip to the grandparents' house was described. The adolescent's unwillingness to attend and the resolution of the problem was described from the perspectives of coercion (the adolescent's perspective) and compromise (the parents' perspective). There were three such tasks in all ranging from low to high emotional saliency. A significant upward progression of mean scores was found over the three age groups. Whereas, younger individuals constructed the event situation from one perspective with an unquestioning acceptance of one side or the other, more mature individuals realized that thinking is influenced by subjective and interpersonal factors, therefore resolution of conflict was in terms of mutually negotiated solutions.

Even more interesting about this finding was an interaction between age group and emotional saliency of the task. Adolescents' performance on the social reasoning task was comparable to that of more mature adults if the problem situation was low in emotional saliency. However, for problems high in emotional saliency, adolescents were less effective at deriving appropriate resolutions than their adult counterparts. This finding, again relates back to the inability on the part of the youthful thinker to integrate and regulate both cognitive and affective systems. Less mature cognitive systems may be less stable and less differentiated in ambiguous and emotional contexts. Given limitations of youthful thinking as indicated by the age trend discussed above, emotionally salient contexts may be more disruptive for younger individuals and, thus, affecting their performance on the task. With increasing cognitive maturity, affective contexts may pose less of a disruption on performance.

Emotionally salient contexts are well-represented in the stress and coping literature. In another study I conducted, it became apparent that the nature of the stressful situation (threat or challenge) influenced how an individual constructed a situation as controllable or noncontrollable (Blanchard-Fields & Irion, in press). Whereas, challenging situations were seen as controllable, threatening situations were not. Age differences in coping (to be discussed later) were more apparent in the threat situation. Perhaps, the effect of age or a developmental progression in coping was observed because the threat situation can be characterized as highly emotionally salient.

Of particular interest to this chapter, is the notion that a component of these cognitive advances in adulthood, i.e., the ability to effectively negotiate problems in highly emotional situations, is the issue of controllability and its relationship to coping. For example, Labouvie-Vief (in press) reports that younger as compared to older adults tend to externalize judgment processes and use external criteria such as social convention or "objective" authority to determine what is right or wrong. In other words, they are extremely vulnerable to external sources that define reality and handle stressful problem situations. This would suggest that they would attribute the cause of a stressful situation to external sources or allocate blame for a stressful outcome to others or circumstances in the environment (e.g., external locus of control). They would not take personal responsibility for the role they played in a stressful conflict. On the other hand, with maturity comes the ability to consciously reflect and appraise each stressful situation and make a decision or evaluation on the basis of autonomous standards and values (Labouvie-Vief, Hakim-Larson, & Hobart, 1987). Mature adults, in turn, would take personal responsibility for their role in the stressful encounter reflecting an internal control orientation. This suggests that perceived controllability, as a part of the appraisal process that an individual may use to assess a stressful situation, varies with developmental changes in cognitive complexity.

Given the evidence reviewed above, it appears that controllability and coping are influenced by social-cognitive maturity of the individual. However, level of developmental complexity has been relatively ignored in the traditional controllability and coping literature. At this point, I would like to review some of the relevant research on developmental differences in coping and controllability, and second, discuss some research I have conducted in this area.

Adult Development, Coping, and Controllability

Coping

There is a growing interest in the coping literature as to the stability of or developmental changes in adaptive coping throughout adulthood. A relatively recent approach to this issue is derived from the concept of cognitive maturity or cognitive-developmental reorganizations in adulthood discussed above. This approach suggests that systematic differences in coping in adulthood can be ordered along dimensions of developmental maturity.

The traditional developmental dimension, age, has resulted in findings that demonstrate a unique pattern of coping behaviors differentiating adolescents and young adults from older adults (Irion & Blanchard-Fields, 1987; Felton & Revenson, 1984; McCrae, 1982). This research is based on two competing theoretical positions, the growth hypothesis of coping (Vaillant, 1977) and the regression hypothesis (Gutmann, 1970; Pfeiffer, 1977). The regression hypothesis asserts that with increasing age adults adopt more rigid and ineffective coping strategies, moving from active to passive modes of solving problems (i.e., strategies based on distortion and denial).

Proponents of the growth hypothesis argue that age-related changes in coping are incremental and that older adults become more effective copers and distort reality less often than younger adults. McCrae (1982) reported decreases with age in the use of such stategies as hostile reaction and escapist-fantasy. More recently, Aldwin and Revenson (1985) reported similar findings that support an incremental theory of adaptive coping. Older adults in their study were less likely to use immature, maladaptive mechanisms such as escapism and self-blame, which have been associated with increases in emotional distress (Aldwin & Revenson, 1985; Felton & Revenson, 1984).

In a recent study, we examined developmental differences in coping and perceptions of efficacy of coping strategies (Irion & Blanchard-Fields, 1987). Ninety-six adolescents, young adults, middle-aged adults, and older adults were administered a *Ways of Coping* questionnaire (Folkman & Lazarus, 1980) and a defensive coping scale. Patterns of coping were examined in both threatening and challenging contexts. In addition, perceived effectiveness of each coping strategy was assessed. Coping strategies included confrontive coping, distancing, self-controlling, seeking social support, self-blame, escape-avoidance, planful problem-solving, positive reappraisal, hostile reaction, and altruism. In support of the growth hypothesis, we found that adolescents and young adults endorsed more immature strategies significantly more often than middle-aged and older adults. These include more defensive and reality distorting mechanisms such as confrontive coping, hostile reaction, escape-avoidance, and self-blame.

The growth hypothesis alone may not be the only interpretation of these findings. In line with the previous discussion on adaptive cognition in adulthood, the coping with stress paradigm reflects a domain in which demands are made on an individual's cognitive and self-regulatory behaviors. The results of this study suggest that adolescents and young adults use more defensive and reality distorting mechanisms in handling stressful demands as defined by various theorists and researchers (Aldwin & Revenson, 1985; Felton & Revenson, 1984; McCrae, 1982; Vaillant, 1977). In fact, these age differences in the use of these more theoretically immature strategies were the most consistent among reported findings.

Further, the differences in perceived effectiveness ratings between age groups followed a pattern similar to differences in use scores. More interesting, however, were the correlations between use and perceived effectiveness of strategies. Across all age groups and in both threatening and challenging situations, there were significant correlations between use and perceived effectiveness of positive reappraisal, altruism, seeking social support, and distancing. Conversely, use and perceived effectiveness of hostile reaction and escape-avoidance were not correlated for any age group in either situation. This finding suggests that even when these immature, defensive strategies are used, they are not necessarily perceived as being effective, even among adolescents and young adults who use them more frequently. Thus, all age groups recognized the differential effectiveness of particular coping strategies.

However, there were age differences in the ability to apply this knowledge in the selection of adaptive coping mechanisms. Specifically, there was no correspondence between use and perceived effectiveness of planful-problem solving approaches for adolescents in a threatening situation. Again, this lends support to the notion that adolescents may have greater difficulty dealing with both the cognitive and emotional demands of a situation that is highly emotionally salient. In sum, this study suggests that developmental differences exist in patterns of adaptive coping across the adult life span.

Recent findings in the adult developmental literature suggest that another dimension, cognitive developmental maturity, may be a better index of developmental changes in coping (Blanchard-Fields & Irion, 1988; Labouvie-Vief et al, 1987). Congruent with this notion, Labouvie-Vief et al. (1987) found that individuals scoring low on a composite developmental dimension reflecting conceptual complexity and consisting of age, ego level, and source-of-stress level used less mature coping strategies. In sum, the findings on coping support the contention of a developmental component to stress and coping in adulthood and aging. Next, I will examine the literature suggesting a developmental component to controllability.

Controllability

The majority of research on controllability and aging has treated controllability as a "style" (i.e., internal or external orientation) in which individuals report the manner in which they would bring about change in the environment through differential responding (i.e., passive versus instrumental behaviors). Accordingly, there appears to be a general consensus that internality is the more desirable of the two styles and is associated with more education, health, wealth, and youth (White & Janson, 1985). Using age as the primary developmental marker of change, there is a considerable amount of research suggesting that there are age differences and changes in internal locus of

control. In Lachman's (1986) review of these findings, she found the
results to be less than consistent. Whereas some studies find older
adults to be more internally oriented than younger adults (Gatz &
Siegler, 1981; Lachman, 1985), other studies find older adults to be
less internally oriented (Lachman, 1983; Saltz & Magruder-Habib, 1982;
Siegler & Gatz, 1985). Finally, a comparable number of studies find
no age differences in internal control (Blanchard-Fields & Irion, in
press; Nehrke, Hulicka, & Morganti, 1980). The discrepancy in
findings has been attributed to methodological inconsistencies
(Lachman, 1986) as well as the multidimensionality of control
(Blanchard-Fields & Robinson, 1987; Blanchard-Fields & Irion, in
press; Lachman, 1986). Multidimensionality will be discussed later in
the context of some current research I have conducted in this area.

What is important at this point is to consider the treatment of
the concept of controllability. Instead of treating it as a "style"
which has basically been defined by the psychometric instruments used
extensively in the literature, perhaps controllability, as with
coping, is better defined in the context of increasing cognitive
complexity of the developing individual. In other words, controllability represents a process that varies with developmental changes
in cognitive complexity. In this case, youthful thinkers are depicted
as quite vulnerable to the influence of external sources which define
reality for them (i.e., they are expected to be more externally-
regulated). Thus, they display a high degree of "conceptual dependence" (Blanchard-Fields, 1986; Labouvie-Vief, in press; Labouvie-Vief
et al., 1987; Perry, 1970). In turn, mature thinkers are expected to
be more autonomous and internally-regulated in their appraisal of
reality.

Controllability and Coping

Given evidence for age differences in both coping and internal
control orientation and their apparent relationship to changes in
cognitive complexity of the maturing adult, it may be more profitable
to examine how these two dimensions change in relation to each other.
Together they may reflect a similar developmental process. This view
is supported by several research projects I have conducted examining
the relationship between controllability and coping. Each of these
studies was cross-sectional in nature and examined age differences
from adolescence through older adulthood (e.g., 14-90 years of age).
The studies are based on the assumption that less mature individuals
have difficulty in regulating both cognitive and affective systems,
particularly in contexts high in emotional saliency (Blanchard-Fields,
1986; Sinnott, 1984). With increased maturity, affective contexts,
such as stressful situations, pose less of a disruption. Finally, the
studies address various methodological and theoretical issues
pertaining to developmental components of controllability and coping
in adulthood and aging.

Study 1. Current research in the areas of controllability and coping has either studied the relationship between these variables in a nondevelopmental context (Folkman & Lazarus, 1980; Parkes, 1984) or, from a developmental perspective with respect to age differences in coping alone (Aldwin & Revenson, 1985; Billings & Moos, 1980; McCrae, 1982). Therefore, we (Blanchard-Fields & Robinson, 1987) examined how attributions of controllability relate to coping in two separate coping contexts (achievement and relationship) using both general and domain-specific measures of controllability (i.e., control in the specific coping context).

We administered Lazarus' (see Folkman & Lazarus, 1980) *Ways of Coping* (revised) questionnaire to a total of 436 individuals consisting of 95 adolescents between the ages of 14 and 16, 99 young adults between the ages of 18 and 25, 81 adults between the ages of 29 and 39, 71 middle-aged adults between the ages of 45 and 55, and 90 older adults between the ages of 60 and 91. The Coping questionnaire assesses a broad range of cognitive and behavioral mechanisms that individuals use in an effort to manage specific stressful encounters and includes the coping scales described above in the Irion and Blanchard-Fields' (1987) study with the exclusion of hostile reaction and altruism. It was completed twice for both a relationship and achievement situation. Stressful relationship situations included marital conflicts, relationship break-ups, parent-child conflicts, etc. Achievement stressful situations included academic problems, work-related conflicts, and financial pressure. Participants were asked to indicate how frequently on a 4-point scale they used the various coping strategies. In addition, they were asked to indicate on a 9-point scale the controllability of the outcome of the stressful encounter. A causal dimension scale was also administered to assess domain-specific controllability of the cause and the stability of the stressful situation. Finally, in addition to a general vocabulary scale, a general *Attributional Style Questionnaire* (Seligman, Abramson, Semmel, & von Baeyer, 1979) was given as a global, cross-situational assessment of people's attributional style. *The Attributional Style Questionnaire* indexes the content of individuals' attributional style and consistency across situations and time. Two general attributional style scores were computed for internality and stability, each to serve as parallel generalized measures to the domain-specific measures of internality and stability.

Overall, older adults in our study proved to be less internal than the younger age groups (Blanchard-Fields & Robinson, 1987). At the outset this does not necessarily support the cognitive maturity assumption discussed above that describes youth to be more externally-regulated and mature thinkers to be more internally-regulated. However, if these results are examined more carefully, it is apparent that what is meant by internality merits further consideration. For example, across stressful contexts, younger individuals were more internal in their orientation than older adults with respect to the *cause* of the stressful situation. There were no age differences with regard to internal control over the *outcome* of the stressor. Consistent with this finding, Aldwin and Revenson (1985) found that older adults perceived themselves as less responsible for the occurrence of a stressful event; however, no age differences were evident in perceived responsibility for the management of the stressful event. Lachman (1986) also found that older adults maintained a sense of internality while acknowledging external sources of control.

In support of this finding, the data on behavioral predictions further demonstrated the differential dimensions of internality for younger and older individuals. For example, with respect to the coping strategy, self-blame, those older adults who perceived the cause of the stressful relationship situation as located internally or regarded it as something about themselves, more frequently endorsed self-blame as a coping strategy. By contrast internality as defined by controllability of outcome or seeing oneself as responsible for the outcome, was a better predictor of self-blame for adolescents. It appears that internality is a multidimensional construct.

Study 2. In a related study, we (Blanchard-Fields & Irion, in press) found a differential relation between internality and coping for different age groups that, again, supports the contention that internality is a multidimensional concept. Specifically, in a cross-sectional comparison of coping behaviors, 436 adolescents, young adults, adults, middle-aged adults, and older adults were administered Lazarus' *Ways of Coping* questionnaire (described in Study 1 and the Irion & Blanchard-Fields, 1987, study), Levenson's *Internality, Powerfulness of Others,* and *Chance Scales* (Levenson, 1981), and were asked to provide ratings of the appraised controllability of reported stressful situations in two contexts (threat and challenge). The subject sample was comprised of the same individuals described in the Irion and Blanchard-Fields' (1987) study described earlier. The procedure for administration of the *Ways of Coping* questionnaire was the same as in Study 1 substituting threat and challenge for relationship and achievement situations. Types of stressors that were reported included academic or work achievement situations, relationship conflicts, accidents/incidents, and health situations. Types of situations and their frequency in each category were quite comparable. The only exceptions were school-related situations more prominent with younger age groups, and job-related situations more prominent with older age groups. In addition, older adults reported more threats to their health. Levenson's controllability scale served as a measure of global control orientation. Internality measures the extent to which an individual feels personal control over his or her life situation. *Powerfulness of Others* assesses the extent to which life circumstances are felt to be controlled by external powerful others. Finally, *Chance* measures the extent to which life situations are attributed to chance or fate.

The purpose of this study was to determine relations between these global and situation specific measures of controllability and coping patterns among the various age groups. Results demonstrated that external regulation (e.g., high powerfulness of others and chance scores) was associated with the use of more emotion-focused strategies such as distancing, self-controlling, self-blame, escape-avoidance, and hostile reaction. Internality, on the other hand was associated with problem-focused coping (i.e., planful problem solving and confronting). Similarly, high situationally-specific controllability was associated with the use of problem-focused coping and planful problem solving. Low situationally-specific controllability was related to distancing, self-controlling, seeking social support, and hostile reaction. These findings lend support to previous research that examined the relation between controllability and coping (Anderson, 1977; Folkman & Lazarus, 1980; Parkes, 1984). In other words, more problem-focused coping is associated with controllability over the situation and more emotion-focused coping is associated with less control over the situation.

This study went beyond previous research in that it demonstrated that age moderates the relation between control orientation and coping. Thus, there were several Age by Controllability interactions in the prediction of coping behavior. For example, a global internal control orientation was positively related to escape-avoidance, hostile reaction, and self-blame for younger individuals, but negatively related to these coping strategies for older adults. Individuals in the older age groups who demonstrated an internal orientation were less likely to engage in these forms of coping behaviors. In other words, for older adults, internality was negatively related to the use of maladaptive and immature coping strategies. Perhaps, an internal control orientation has different meanings for youth as compared to middle-aged and older adults. Youthful individuals may equate internal control with self-blame in response to a stressor. Consequently, they deal with this blame by avoidance of the situation or by hostilely reacting toward the situation. On the other hand, the mature adult's conception of internal control involves perceiving the source of stress as located within the self-resulting in conscious, reflective appraisal. Again, the construct of internality appears to be multidimensional and related to adult developmental conceptions of maturity.

Finally, Study 2 (Blanchard-Fields & Irion, in press) also demonstrated a tendency for older adults to use more instrumental coping (e.g., planful problem-solving) in relation to external control as defined by a belief in powerful others, and more emotion-focused coping (e.g., distancing) in relation to external control as defined by chance. This suggests that locus of control is more differentiated for older adults. Perhaps if an outcome is thought of as determined by chance, older adults recognize that nothing can be done and choose to distance themselves from it. By contrast, externalization of control for younger individuals appears to result in a sense of "giving up control" (i.e., decreased instrumental coping) in relation to powerful others or hostile reaction in relation to chance.

Study 3. A final study examined (a) both age and social-cognitive maturity as potential developmental markers for predicting the use of coping mechanisms in adulthood, and (b) determined whether or not perceived controllability mediates the type of coping strategies selected by different age groups. Twenty adolescents, 20 young adults, and 20 middle-aged adults were administered Lazarus' *Ways of Coping* questionnaire (described in Study 1) and a social reasoning task. The coping questionnaire differed in this study in that it was assessed in terms of emotion-focused coping (i.e., attempts to relieve emotional stress) and problem-focused coping (i.e., attempts to directly solve the problem). In addition, each participant was asked to indicate which of the following appraisals listed ("could change or do something about it" and " must accept or get used to it") applied to the stressful situation they described.

The social reasoning task consisted of two ambiguously structured tasks ranging from high to low emotional saliency. Each task consisted of two divergent accounts of the same event sequence (see the description of the Blanchard-Fields, 1986 study above). The two tasks represented either a low level of emotional saliency or a high level of emotional saliency. Subjects were questioned as to how they perceived the discrepancies (see Blanchard-Fields & Irion, 1988). The scoring scheme assessed progression along dimensions of social-cognitive complexity.

In general, age differences were more apparent with the emotion-focused strategies than with the problem-focused strategies. Overall, the social reasoning task highest in emotional saliency was the best predictor of emotion-focused coping. This suggests that age, as an index for change, may not be the most important criterion for developmental differences in coping, in particular, emotion-focused coping. This is also congruent with research on emotional self-regulation and adult developmental change (Labouvie-Vief, 1984; Loevinger, 1980).

A further mediating variable of age differences in coping is suggested by the interaction effect found between coping style (emotion-focused and problem-focused), age group, and appraised controllability. These findings show that younger individuals endorsed more emotion-focused strategies (i.e., a defensive style of coping) irrespective of whether or not the stressful episode was appraised as controllable. In contrast, the appraised controllability of the stressful situation mediated whether or not more emotion-focused or problem-focused strategies were endorsed by older participants. Thus, the older adults endorsed more emotion-focused coping in noncontrollable situations and problem-focused coping in controllable situations. The literature suggests that, in general,

problem-focused strategies tend to be more effective in stressful
situations perceived as controllable, whereas emotion-focused coping
seems to be more effective for noncontrollable situations (Folkman &
Lazarus, 1980; Parkes, 1984).

Overall, the results of this study suggest that (a) dimensions of
developmental maturity such as social cognitive reasoning also serve
as important mediators of developmental differences in coping, and (b)
in contrast to youth, older adults demonstrated a more flexible
approach to coping contingent upon the appraised controllability of
the situation.

The Three Studies in Perspective

Overall, the findings of these three research projects suggest a
number of theoretical as well as methodological implications for
controllability and coping in older adult populations. Both Study 1
and Study 2 (Blanchard-Fields & Robinson, 1987; Blanchard-Fields &
Irion, in press) suggest that the relation between controllability and
coping reflect a similar cognitive-developmental process. On the one
hand, this is supported by the finding that a high level of internality was related to an emotion-focused strategy such as self-blame
for younger as opposed to older individuals (Blanchard-Fields &
Irion, in press). Similarly, it is supported by the Blanchard-
Fields and Robinson (1987) study demonstrating that internality and
self-blame were positively related for adolescents when internality
was defined in terms of the outcome of the stressor. Conversely, the
relation between internality and self-blame for older adults was
positive only when internality was defined in terms of the cause.
This suggests two implications.

First, just as externality has been assessed in terms of the two
dimensions of *Powerfulness of Others* and *Chance*, further research may
be necessary to examine in detail additional dimensions of internality
in order to specify developmental variations of more and less mature
appraisals. This notion is supported by several studies that have
differentiated (a) controllability in handling an event versus
controllability of the cause of an event (Gatz, Siegler, George &
Tyler, 1986); (b) responsibility for the cause of the event (blame)
versus responsibility for the outcome or solution (Karuza, Rabinowitz,
& Zevon, 1986); and (c) self-blame for actions causing the event
versus self-blame regarding one's own character (Krause, 1986).

Second, recent thinking suggests that reactions to perceived
sources of stress are mediated by internal control orientations which
are related to the self or ego (Folkman & Lazarus, 1980; Labouvie-
Vief, et al., 1987). Accordingly, there should be developmental
differences in the manner in which a stressor is appraised. The
allocation of blame, on the part of the youthful thinker, may be
split into either-or categories pitting internal causes, such as

personality traits, against external environmental factors. Over-attribution toward personal dispositional factors (i.e., self-blame) has been shown to be a potent source of social judgment bias (Doherty, 1981; Nisbett & Ross, 1980; Tversky & Kahneman, 1982).

Older adults were better able to differentiate cause from outcome (i.e., managing an event's outcome) and allocated blame only when they felt responsible for the cause. Again, this may indicate a more mature self-regulatory system in the sense of differentiating when self-blame is an appropriate conceptualization of the problem situation and when it is not. In this case the situation becomes more of a trigger for self-reflective, conscious thought processes for the older adult than it does for more youthful thinkers. This adaptive form of selective responding (differential coping) to situations perceived as internal or external on the part of older adults is further supported in the Blanchard-Fields and Irion (1988) study which demonstrated the ability of older adults to choose effectively between emotion- or problem-focused coping depending on the appraised controllability of the situation.

A final implication of these studies is the use of domain-specific as opposed to global measures of control orientation. For example, Blanchard-Fields and Robinson (1987) found age differences in locus of control when controllability was defined in the context of domain-specific measures. Domain-specific measures in conjunction with multidimensional conceptualizations of internality and exter-nality offer a more complete picture of when and how the older adult responds to stressful situations.

Controllability and Coping in an Applied Context

Currently, two of my associates are conducting studies examining controllability issues as well as coping and controllability relations in applied contexts. One study is examining the multidimensionality of internal control orientation in a nursing home setting (a disserta-tion currently in progress by Jane Irion) as it relates to adaptive functioning. Specifically, traditional global constructs of control orientation (i.e., internality, chance, and powerful others) were compared to more differentiated constructs of internality such as primary, secondary, and relinquished control (Rothbaum, Weisz, & Snyder, 1982) in their relationship to adjustment among nursing home residents. Primary control is associated with direct, instrumental action on the environment that influences outcomes. Secondary control is defined as the acceptance of existing realities which cannot be changed, while at the same time control is exerted over the psychological consequences of the stressor. Relinquishing control refers to more passive responses to stressful encounters, i.e., giving up or submitting to authority. One of the major goals of this study is to assess the relative predictive power of each of these control orientations (specific to the nursing home environment) for various psychological outcomes of the older adults. In addition, the differential use of primary and secondary control among these institutionalized adults is examined.

Participants included 70 nursing home residents from eight facilities. Primary, secondary, and relinquished control measures were administered in the form of a structured, open-ended interview (see Weisz, 1987). The specific domains of living assessed included meals/food, scheduling, privacy, and activities. In addition, a global measure of control orientation (Levenson's, 1981, *Scale of Internality, Chance, and Powerful Others*) was administered. Finally, outcome variables included measures of depression and well-being (Linn & Linn, 1984 and Kozma & Stones, 1980, respectively).

Preliminary findings suggest that perceptions of control differentially predict well-being and depression. Acceptance of the situation (secondary control) was related to lower levels of depression and higher levels of well-being. In contrast, relinquished control was related to higher levels of depression and lower levels of psychological well-being. The global measure of internality was not predictive of either depression or well-being. Nursing home residents used more secondary control than primary control, and used relinquished control least often. In general, secondary internality appears to be used more often and is more adaptive in the restrictive environment of a nursing home. Again, traditional, global measures of control orientation were not related to adjustment and neither global nor domain-specific control styles were adaptive for nursing home residents. The study points to the need to apply multiple dimensions of control orientation, particularly internality, to older population domains in order to gain a more complete picture of healthy adaptation in specific contexts (i.e., a nursing home).

The second study is investigating coping strategies and attributions of control of caregivers of victims of Alzheimer's Disease (a dissertation currently in progress by Audrey Sistler). Attributions of internality and controllability were found to be negatively correlated to escape-avoidance coping. Level of stress was positively correlated with escape-avoidance and distancing modes of coping. Open-ended interviews indicate the importance of family values and developmental maturity in the caregiving situation. Based on these preliminary results, both developmental maturity and attributions appear to be good predictors of coping strategies.

Conclusions

In sum, a clearer understanding of the role which controllability and the relation between controllability and coping play in the adaptive functioning of older adults can be gained by placing them in an adult developmental context. First, internality and externality are multidimensional constructs and must be examined in interaction with specific and varying situational contexts. Second, the developmental maturity of the individual will also interact with these constructs and contexts. Developmental maturity may index the ability on the part of the older individual in differentially applying various control processes in order to attain optimal adaptation.

References

Aldwin, C. M., & Revenson, T. A. (1985). Cohort differences in stress, coping, and appraisal. *The Gerontologist, 25*, (Special Issue), 66.

Anderson, C. R. (1977). Locus of control, coping behaviors, and performance in a stress setting: A longitudinal study. *Journal of Applied Psychology, 62*, 446-451.

Billings, A. G., & Moos, R. H. (1980). The role of coping responses and social resources in attenuating the stress of life events. *Journal of Behavioral Medicine, 4*, 139-157.

Blanchard-Fields, F. (1986). Reasoning on social dilemmas varying in emotional saliency: An adult developmental perspective. *Psychology and Aging, 1*, 325-333.

Blanchard-Fields, F., & Irion, J. (1988, in press). Coping strategies from the perspective of two developmental markers: Age and social reasoning. *Journal of Genetic Psychology, 149*.

Blanchard-Fields, F., & Irion, J. (in press). The relation between locus of control and coping in two contexts: Age as a moderator variable. *Psychology and Aging*.

Blanchard-Fields, F., & Robinson, S. (1987). Age differences in the relation between controllability and coping. *Journal of Gerontology, 42*, 497-501.

Cavanaugh, J., Kramer, D., Sinnott, J., Camp, C., & Markley, J. (1985). On missing links and such: Interfaces between cognitive research and everyday problem-solving. *Human Development, 28*, 146-168.

Commons, M. L., Richards, F. A., & Armon, C. (1984). *Beyond formal operations*. New York: Praeger.

Doherty, W. J. (1981). Cognitive processes in intimate conflict: I. extending attribution theory. *American Journal of Family Therapy, 9*, 3-13.

Felton, B., & Revenson, T. (1984). Coping with chronic illness: A study of illness controllability and the influence of coping strategies on psychological adjustment. *Journal of Consulting and Clinical Psychology, 52,* 343-353.

Folkman, S., & Lazarus, R. S. (1980). An analysis of coping in a middle-aged community sample. *Journal of Personality and Social Psychology, 21,* 219-239.

Gatz, M., & Siegler, I. C. (1981, August). *Locus of control: A retrospective.* Paper presented at the American Psychological Association Meeting, Los Angeles.

Gatz, M., Siegler, I. C., George, L. K., & Tyler, F. B. (1986). Attributional components of locus of control: Longitudinal, retrospective, and contemporaneous analyses. In M. M. Baltes & P. B. Baltes (Eds.), *The psychology of control and aging* (pp. 237-263). Hillsdale, NJ: Lawrence Erlbaum Associates.

Greenspan, S. I. (1979). *Intelligence and adaptation.* New York: International Universities Press.

Gutmann, D. L. (1970). Female ego styles and generational conflict. In J. M. Bardwick, E. Douvan, M. S. Horner, & D. L. Gutmann (Eds.), *Feminine personality and conflict* (pp. 61-78). Belmont, CA: Brooks-Cole.

Irion, J., & Blanchard-Fields, F. (1987). A cross-sectional comparison of adaptive coping in adulthood. *Journal of Gerontology, 42,* 502-504.

Karuza, J. Jr., Rabinowitz, V. C., & Zevon, M. A. (1986). Implications of control and responsibility on helping the aged. In M. M. Baltes & P. B. Baltes (Eds.), *The psychology of control and aging* (pp. 373-396). Hillsdale, NJ: Lawrence Erlbaum Associates.

Kozma, A., & Stones, M. J. (1980). The measurement of happiness: Development of the Memorial University of Newfoundland Scale of Happiness (MUNSH). *Journal of Gerontology, 35,* 906-912.

Kramer, D. A. (1983). Post-formal operations: A need for further conceptualization. *Human Development, 26,* 91-105.

Kramer, D. A., & Levine, C. (1987). *Cognitive development and conflict resolution.* Paper presented at the Third Beyond Formal Operations Symposium at Harvard University: Positive Development during Adolescence and Adulthood, June, Cambridge, MA.

Krause, N. (1986). Stress and coping: Reconceptualizing the role of locus of control beliefs. *Journal of Gerontology, 41,* 617-622.

Labouvie-Vief, G. (1984). Logic and self-regulation from youth to maturity: A model. In M. Commons, F. Richards & C. Armon (Eds.), *Beyond formal operations* (pp. 158-180). New York: Praeger.

Labouvie-Vief, G. (1985). Intelligence and cognition. In J. E. Birren & K. W. Schaie (Eds.), *Handbook of the psychology of aging* (pp. 500-530). New York: Van Nostrand-Reinhold.

Labouvie-Vief, G. (in press). Modes of knowledge and the organization of development. In M. L. Commons, C. Armon, F. A. Richards & J. Sinnott (Eds.), *Beyond formal operations: 2. The development of adolescent and adult thinking and perception.* New York: Praeger.

Labouvie-Vief, G., Hakim-Larson, J., & Hobart, C. J. (1987). Age, ego level, and the life-span development of coping and defense processes. *Psychology and Aging, 2,* 286-293.

Lachman, M.E. (1983). Perceptions of intellectual aging: Antecedent or consequence of intellectual functioning? *Developmental Psychology, 19,* 482-498.

Lachman, M. E. (1985). Personal efficacy in middle and old age: Differential and normative patterns of change. In G. H. Elder, Jr. (Ed.), *Life-course dynamics: Trajectories and transitions, 1968-1980* (pp. 188-213). Ithaca, NY: Cornell University Press.

Lachman, M. E. (1986). Locus of control in aging research: A case for multidimensional and domain-specific assessment. *Psychology and Aging, 1,* 34-40.

Levenson, H. (1981). Differentiating among internality, powerful others, and chance. In H. Lefcourt (Ed.), *Research with the locus of control construct, Volume 1* (pp. 15-63). New York: Academic Press.

Linn, M. W., & Linn, B. S. (1984). Self-Evaluation of Life Function (SELF) scale: A short comprehensive self-report of health for elderly adults. *Journal of Gerontology, 39,* 603-612.

Loevinger, J. (1980). *Ego development.* San Francisco: Jossey-Bass.

McCrae, R. R. (1982). Age differences in the use of coping mechanisms. *Journal of Gerontology, 37,* 454-460.

Nehrke, M. F., Hulicka, I. H., & Morganti, J. (1980). Age differences in life satisfaction, locus of control, and self-concept. *International Journal of Aging and Human Development, 11,* 25-33.

Nisbett, R. & Ross, L. (1980). *Human inference: Strategies and shortcomings of social judgment.* Englewood Cliffs, NJ: Prentice-Hall, Inc.

Parkes, K. R. (1984). Locus of control, cognitive appraisal, and coping in stressful episodes. *Journal of Personality and Social Psychology, 46,* 655-668.

Perry, W. G. (1970). *Forms of intellectual and ethical development in the college years.* New York: Holt, Rinehart, & Winston.

Pfeiffer, E. (1977). Psychopathology and social pathology. In J. E. Birren & K. W. Schaie (Eds.), *Handbook of the psychology of aging* (pp. 650-665). New York: Van Nostrand Reinhold.

Rothbaum, F., Weisz, J. R., & Snyder, S. S. (1982). Changing the world and changing the self: A two-process model of perceived control. *Journal of Personality and Social Psychology, 42,* 5-37.

Saltz, C., & Magruder-Habib, K. (1982, November). *Age as an indicator of depression and locus of control among non-psychiatric inpatients.* Paper presented at the meeting of the Gerontological Society of America, Boston, MA.

Seligman, M. E. P., Abramson, L. Y., Semmel, A., & von Baeyer, C. (1979). Depressive attributional style. *Journal of Abnormal Psychology, 88,* 242-247.

Siegler, I. C., & Gatz, M. (1985). Age patterns in locus of control. In E. Palmore, E. W. Busse, G. L. Maddox, J. B. Nowlin, & I. C. Siegler (Eds.), *Normal aging III* (pp. 259-267). Durham, NC: Duke University Press.

Sinnott, J. D. (1984). Postformal reasoning: The relativistic stage. In M. Commons, F. Richards, & C. Armon (Eds.), *Beyond formal operations* (pp. 298-325). New York: Praeger.

Stone, A. A. & Neale, J. M. (1984). New measure of daily coping: Development and preliminary results. *Journal of Personality and Social Psychology, 46,* 892-906.

Tversky, A.. & Kahneman, D. (1982). Causal schemas in judgments under uncertainty. In D. Kahneman, P. Slovic, & A. Tversky (Eds.), *Judgments under uncertainty: Heuristics and biases* (pp. 117-128). Cambridge: Cambridge University Press.

Vaillant, G.E. (1977). *Adaptation to life.* Boston: Little, Brown & Company.

Weisz, J. R. (1987). *Instructions for coding coping responses for primary, secondary, and relinquished control.* Unpublished manuscript.

White, C. B., & Janson, P. (1985, November). When does the absence of personal control lead to helplessness? In K. P. Riley & E. Kahana

(Chairs), *Learned helplessness: Putting theory to its proper use.* Symposium conducted at the annual meetings of the Gerontological Society of America, New Orleans.

Psychological Perspectives of Helplessness
and Control in the Elderly, P.S. Fry (ed.)
© Elsevier Science Publishers B.V. (North-Holland), 1989

Chapter Three

AUTONOMY, DESPAIR, AND GENERATIVITY IN ERIKSON'S THEORY

John A. MEACHAM
State University of New York at Buffalo

Abstract

The life-course perspective of Erik Erikson holds considerable promise as a conceptual framework within which to
understand helplessness and lack of control in aging.   In
this chapter, a notation system is introduced for representing the formal aspects of Erikson's theory, including
relationships between adjacent stages or crises.   The
notation system is employed as a tool to direct our
attention to particular features of Erikson's theory.   In a
narrow sense, helplessness and lack of control can be
understood as the experience and resolution of autonomy
versus shame and doubt in the second stage of Erikson's
theory and the subsequent modification of these ego
qualities across the life course.   To understand helplessness and lack of control in a broad sense, we must inquire
into the antecedents of despair.   The seventh stage of
generativity versus stagnation, especially caring for
children and grandchildren, is a crucial foundation for
successful resolution of the eighth crisis of ego integrity
versus despair.   The loss of feelings of autonomy and the
experience of helplessness in aging may derive from the
initial development of autonomy within a cultural context of
self-contained, competitive, and achievement-oriented
individualism.

It is fascinating that we, as a people, should cling so tenaciously to
our pipe dream of independence as we become increasingly dependent on
our interconnectedness.

Erikson, Erikson, and Kivnick, 1986, p. 328

Introduction

The choice of a conceptual framework within which to expand our
understanding of helplessness and lack of control in aging is not
easy. Loss of resources, increased vulnerability, incompetence, and
dependency have, unfortunately, long been a part of the stereotype of
aging (McTavish, 1971). Nevertheless, the reality of aging is that,
for individuals who are able to remain in good health, there are
impressive continuities across the life course in psychological and
interpersonal functioning, with few if any changes in remembering,
learning, intelligence, personality, and so forth (Meacham, 1983). It
would be desirable to have as a conceptual framework one that does not
contribute further to the negative stereotype of aging (Kalish,
1979). Instead, a framework is needed that provides an understanding
of helplessness and lack of control within the context of the
realities of normal aging.

One broad conceptual framework within which to understand the
realities of normal aging is the life course itself. From a life-
course perspective, stages of life such as childhood or adulthood or
aging cannot be studied and understood in isolation from each other,
first one and then the next, as the chapters in a text are sequenced.
Instead, each stage of life must be understood in the context of
developmental changes within all the others. For example, the
activities of childhood and adolescence reflect in large part
anticipation of and preparation for the tasks of work and family in
adulthood, and the construction of a meaningful existence in adulthood
and old age reflects in part a reworking of the goals and ideals of
youth. From a life-course perspective, the social context of the
family is not merely a backdrop for child development. Instead, the
development of each member of the family and of each generation of the
family must be understood in relation to developmental changes within
all the others. Not only do parents structure the development of
their children, but children structure the further development of
their parents (Gutmann, 1985; Kivnick, 1985). From a life-course
perspective, the cultural and historical context is not merely a
geographical variable, to be considered in a separate textbook chapter
on cross-cultural differences. Instead, this context is a temporal
variable, developing in its own right at the same time that families
and individual persons are developing within it (Baltes, 1987;
Meacham, 1984).

The work of Erikson (1959, 1963, 1982) is paradigmatic of the
life-course perspective, and so for this reason it holds considerable
promise as a conceptual framework within which to understand helplessness and lack of control in the context of the realities of normal
aging. On the basis of considerable psychoanalytic experience,
Erikson claims that ego development proceeds according to a sequence
of eight conflicts, crises, stages, or turning points, at each of
which the individual acquires new qualities that are essential to the

individual's experiencing, behaving, and unconscious motivation. This sequence of alternative basic attitudes includes, in infancy, childhood, and adolescence, basic trust versus mistrust, autonomy versus shame and doubt, initiative versus guilt, and industry versus inferiority and, in adulthood and aging, identity versus identity diffusion, intimacy versus isolation, generativity versus stagnation, and ego integrity versus despair. Recently, Erikson's theory has received renewed attention from both an empirical and a theoretical standpoint (e.g., Franz & White, 1985; Hassan & Bar-Yam, 1987; Logan, 1986; van Geert, 1986, 1987; Viney, 1987)

In addition to its life-course perspective and its basis in the experience and understanding of a master clinician, there are two further reasons for turning to Erikson's work as a conceptual framework within which to understand helplessness and lack of control. The third reason is that these terms are readily understood as variations on one of the sets of alternative basic attitudes within Erikson's theory. In the context of aging, one thinks perhaps most immediately of the eighth stage of ego integrity versus despair and, in particular, the associations to despair of disappointment, fear of death, and the feeling that there is insufficient time to start anew. Yet within Erikson's theory issues of helplessness and lack of control are most fundamental to and are resolved, for better or worse, not in the eighth stage of aging but rather in the second stage of autonomy versus shame and doubt in early childhood (and, to a lesser extent, the third stage of initiative versus guilt). Autonomy signifies free choice, self-determination, independence, self-reliance, willfulness, freedom from the influence or control of others. Lack of autonomy signifies influence or control by others, dependence on others, helplessness, and lack of self-control. Shame follows from the consciousness of being so exposed, vulnerable, and defenseless, and doubt follows from the fact of domination by the will of others (Erikson, 1963, p. 253). Thus, consistent with the life-course perspective, helplessness and lack of control in aging must be understood in the context of the life-long development of these attitudes from early childhood.

The fourth reason for turning to Erikson's theory as a conceptual framework for this chapter is that the corpus of his writings on late adulthood and aging has recently been much extended with the publication of *Vital Involvement in Old Age* (Erikson, Erikson, & Kivnick, 1986). This volume is a report on a series of interviews conducted with 29 individuals ranging in age from 75 to 95. All these individuals were parents of children who were participants in the Guidance Study initiated at Berkeley in 1928. Although the initial focus was not on the parents, the frequent and regular interviews with the children's families also provided considerable information on the adult development of the parents, information that has been drawn upon in providing an understanding of these 29 individuals as they are now involved in their own aging. I should make clear, at this point, that there are few if any insights in the present chapter that are not implicit, if not explicit, in this volume by Erikson et al. (1986). I hope merely, by some rearrangement of the material, to highlight those portions of the volume that touch most directly on issues related to helplessness and lack of control in aging.

Erikson et al. (1986) have organized the interview material according to the sequence of eight stages or crises, beginning with ego integrity versus despair and ending with trust versus mistrust. It is noteworthy that the number of pages devoted to two of these stages is roughly 50 percent greater than that allotted for any of the remaining six. The first of these is the second stage of autonomy versus shame and doubt. This fact serves to reinforce the assumption behind this chapter and presumably behind this volume that issues related to control are indeed central to an understanding of development in late adulthood and aging. The second stage to which a large number of pages has been devoted is the seventh, the crisis of generativity versus stagnation. Of course, in the context of Erikson's theory all seven preceding stages are necessary parts of the foundation for the last stage, and so one might argue successfully for any one of these as indispensable. Nevertheless, I will argue in the present chapter that, in addition to the second stage of autonomy versus shame and doubt, the stage most essential to understanding psychosocial development in late adulthood and aging is the seventh stage of generativity versus stagnation, the stage immediately preceding the final stage of ego integrity versus despair. In pursuing this argument, the course of discussion in the chapter will turn from a focus on individual development to interpersonal relations and subsequently to the cultural context of development. The chapter concludes with some concrete proposals for how our understanding of helplessness and lack of control in aging is expanded through considering these topics within the framework of Erikson's theory.

A Formal Analysis of Erikson's Theory

A Notation System

Erikson's psychosocial theory of ego development has provided an important framework for understanding late adulthood and aging in the context of the life course. In general, however, the research that has been derived from Erikson's writings has been focused primarily on the *intrastage* qualities, especially those of the fifth stage of identity and the relationships between features of this stage and other psychological constructs (e.g., Waterman, 1982). Still in need of further investigation, however, are the *interstage* or developmental relationships, that is, the transitions between one stage and the next. This latter task is an essential one if Erikson's theory is to be utilized as a life-course developmental theory and not merely as a description of isolated crises.

The purpose of this section is to introduce a notation system for representing the formal aspects of Erikson's theory in late adulthood and aging, including relationships between adjacent stages or crises and transitions from one stage to the next. This notation system can then be used as a tool for directing our attention to particular features of Erikson's theory, for comparing various interpretations of Erikson's theory (e.g., Hassan & Bar-Yam, 1987; Logan, 1986; van Geert, 1986, 1987), and for raising some researchable questions regarding Erikson's theory, in particular regarding the seventh stage or crisis, generativity, and the eighth stage, ego integrity.

The notation system introduced in this section has been described and introduced more fully in Meacham (1980), having been derived from earlier work by Van den Daele (1969, 1974, 1976) and Flavell (1972). Briefly, the letters A, B, C, etc. are taken to represent various social and psychological characteristics, with development proceeding through time from left to right. Sequences of characteristics can be described as simple or cumulative, depending on whether the individual is considered to display only one or several characteristics at a given point in time. For example, a person might be single or married, but not both at the same time (simple). When change occurs, it is a matter of substitution of a new characteristic for an old one. A simple sequence can be represented by A ----> B ----> C. On the other hand, a person might at one and the same point in life know how to play bridge, chess, and golf (cumulative). Change is a matter of characteristics being added to (or subtracted from) the set. A cumulative sequence can be represented by A ----> AB ----> ABC. In addition to simple or cumulative, sequences of characteristics can be described, orthogonally, as disjunctive, when the relationship between characteristics is said to be one of separateness or lack of overlap (both sequences already mentioned), or conjunctive, when some of the characteristics become included within or subordinate to others, as in Piaget's and Freud's theories (see Meacham, 1980, or Van den Daele, 1969, for details).

Some further examples will be helpful. The letters A, B, C, etc. can represent the stages of life, from infancy through young adulthood, middle age, young-old, and old-old; the consecutive stages of being single, married, and then single through widowhood or divorce; or the sequence from school to work to retirement. In all of these examples, the sequences are simple and disjunctive; they are disjunctive because being married does not, by definition, include being single, and being retired does not include working. The simple, disjunctive sequence also provides a representation of Havighurst's (1953) description of the developmental tasks that should be mastered in each major portion of the life course, if we let A, B, C, etc. represent sets of tasks (for example, the developmental tasks of later maturity include adjusting to retirement and reduced income, meeting social and civic obligations, etc.).

The simple, conjunctive sequence is illustrated by two major theories, those of Piaget (1960) and Freud (1933). Piaget describes the development of understanding of oneself and the world as an invariant sequence of four stages: sensorimotor, preoperational, concrete operational, and formal operational. The relationship between the stages is conjunctive because, as the child passes from one stage to the next, the higher-order logical structures incorporate and reorganize the structures of the earlier stages. These earlier characteristics can be represented by a lower-case letter to indicate that, although they are retained by the person in a transformed form, they are no longer directly observable in the person's behavior. The simple, conjunctive sequence is also illustrated by Freud's description of the sequence of personality development (oral, anal, phallic, latency, genital). Each stage in the sequence includes an integration of aspects of earlier stages. Although the theories of Piaget and Freud are not generally considered together, they are found to be quite similar, at least at this level of analysis of their formal aspects. The simple, conjunctive sequence can be represented by A ----> a'B ----> a'b'C and so forth, where the lower-case letters and the primes both indicate the relationship of conjunction, inclusion, or subordination.

The cumulative, disjunctive sequence is illustrated by the sequence of roles within the family of child, parent, and grandparent. As people grow older, they accumulate these roles, although at any particular moment a person might engage in only one. Finally, examples of cumulative, conjunctive sequences are Kohlberg's (1964) theory of stages of moral judgment and Freud's description of the unfolding of the structures of personality. In contrast to Piagetian stage research, research on moral judgment often reveals that a person who reasons according to the logic of a higher stage might, from time to time, reason according to the logic of lower stages. Thus Kohlberg's cumulative theory, although derived from Piaget's simple theory, permits a variety of within-person responses. The sequence of unfolding of structures of personality, with the ego developing out of the id in order to cope with reality, and the superego developing out of the ego in order to cope with adult and societal expectations, also illustrates the cumulative, conjunctive sequence. Such sequences can be represented by A ----> A'B ----> A'B'C and so forth, where the upper-case letters indicate that the sequence is cumulative, and the primes indicate the relationship of conjunction.

Erikson's Theory

These few examples provide a demonstration that the notation system can be useful as a tool for comparing and contrasting developmental theories and for directing our attention to particular features of those theories that might otherwise be neglected. But what description can be provided of the formal aspects of Erikson's psychosocial theory of ego development? Other writers, such as Van den Daele

(1974, p. 20), have commented on the difficulty of providing a formal description of Erikson's theory. This difficulty might reflect a lack of specificity in Erikson's writings on the nature of the interstage or between-stage relationships in his psychosocial theory. Wohlwill (1973, p. 194) compared several developmental theories in terms of both their horizontal structure, that is, the within-stage structure, and their vertical structure, the between-stage organization along some common dimension. Wohlwill describes Erikson's theory as similar to Piaget's in having a high degree of horizontal structure, but closer to Shirley's steps of motor development in infancy in its low degree of vertical structure.

At first, it would appear that Erikson's theory is a simple, disjunctive sequence, A ----> B ----> C, with A, B, C, etc. representing the successive stages or crises of trust, autonomy, initiative, industry, identity, etc. However, representation of Erikson's theory by such a sequence does not adequately represent Erikson's suggestions that (a) the resolutions to earlier crises are carried forward and affect the resolutions of later crises and (b) the themes of each of the eight crises exist in some form throughout the life course. These two points are explicit, for example, in the familiar eight by eight matrix provided by Erikson (1963, p. 273) as a guide to understanding his theory. Unfortunately, the matrix itself is difficult to understand. One interpretation of this matrix is that development is represented by movement from one cell to the next, so that a person might be in one of 64 different states. It seems more likely, however, that Erikson intended each of the rows to represent one of the stages, beginning with I (trust) at the bottom and ending with VIII (ego integrity) at the top. Thus development is represented by movement from one entire row, not cell, to the next. What, then, do the columns in the matrix represent? These are aspects of each of the eight crises that can be related to preceding and subsequent crises. Within each row, cells above the diagonal represent the integration of aspects of earlier, completed crises with each current crisis and its resolution; cells below the diagonal represent aspects of earlier crises that prepare the way for later crises and their resolution (Erikson, 1963, p. 270; 1982, p. 29).

Thus a more appropriate representation of Erikson's theory is as a simple, conjunctive sequence, Abcdefgh ----> a'Bcdefgh ----> a'b'Cdefgh, where A, B, C, etc. represent the current crises. To be more precise, each lower-case letter could be provided with an upper-case subscript indicating the current dominant crisis, in order to distinguish, for example, trust during the crisis of identity, a' sub E, from trust during the crisis of intimacy, a' sub F, and to represent the continual integration of the products of earlier crises within the dynamics of contemporary crises. Such subscripts do not appear to be required at present, however. The utility of the notation system can be further illustrated by calling attention to the resemblances, at this formal level, between Erikson's theory and Levinson's (1978) description of periods in the development of a group of adult men, descriptions such as "leaving the family" and "getting into the adult world." Levinson (1978, p. 321) provides explicit statements regarding the interstage relationships: "Each period is 'interpenetrated' with the others. The current period is predominant, but the others are present in it. It is *not* the case that a period begins, runs its independent course, and ends, to be followed by another period that has its own separate character." Levinson's theory can be represented similarly to Erikson's, as a simple, conjunctive sequence, Abcd ----> a'Bcd ----> a'b'Cd, and so forth.

This representation of Erikson's theory as a simple, conjunctive sequence is still not adequate, however, for it rests upon the assumption that each successive crisis can result in only a successful resolution or outcome. Erikson's theory is commonly interpreted, however, as one in which the outcomes of each crisis might be successful or unsuccessful, for example, trust versus mistrust, identity versus identity diffusion, etc. Thus an improved description of the formal aspects of Erikson's theory would be one in which the primes are replaced by the superscripts + and - in order to indicate whether resolution of a particular crisis had been successful or not: a+b-c+Defgh. A partial representation of Erikson's theory of psychosocial development as a simple, conjunctive sequence is shown in Figure 1. For simplicity, the four childhood stages or crises of trust, autonomy, initiative, and industry are not shown.

Inspection of Figure 1 leads to two general comments. First, by late adulthood there are 2 (outcomes) to the 8th (stages), or 256, possible types of individuals, with each type representing a unique developmental sequence. *A priori*, the likelihood for resolving the eighth crisis in the direction of ego integrity is equal to that of resolving it in the direction of despair: in Figure 1, there are eight odd-numbered outcomes in favor of ego integrity, and eight even-numbered outcomes in favor of despair. It seems reasonable, however, that the likelihood for some of these outcomes would be very low or even zero, for example, outcome 15 (e-f-g-h+), while for others the likelihood would be high. At each stage, the interstage transitional probabilities, which must sum to one, could be derived from theoretical considerations and then tested empirically. This would certainly be an important step in the more complete utilization of Erikson's theory as a life-course developmental theory. Some steps in this direction are taken in the remainder of this chapter, in which the following questions are raised: Which of the 16 outcomes in Figure 1 are more likely? Is there reason to believe that the likelihood is greater for resolving the eighth crisis in favor of ego integrity or in favor of despair? What are the antecedents of successful and unsuccessful resolutions of the eighth stage? In other words, what is the relationship between the nature of resolutions of the earlier stages, for example, autonomy and generativity, and the outcome of the final stage?

Figure 1

The Four Adult Stages:

identity (E), intimacy (F), generativity (G), and ego integrity (H)

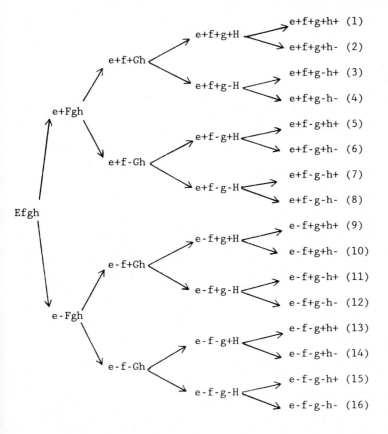

A second general comment is that Figure 1 reminds us, as does Erikson's eight by eight matrix discussed above, of the need to distinguish individuals who might appear to display characteristics of depression or "despair" because they have not yet entered and experienced the eighth crisis (H) and so have merely not yet achieved ego integrity from those individuals who have experienced this final crisis and have failed to attain a successful resolution. In the notation system, the distinction is between h during an earlier crisis such as generativity, e+f+Gh, and h- as a resolution of the eighth crisis, e+f+g+h-. A similar problem has existed in the investigation of adolescence, where many researchers have failed to distinguish individuals whose identity is "diffuse" because they have not yet experienced the identity crisis (E) from individuals who have experienced this crisis but have failed to attain a successful resolution. The failure to make such a distinction reflects the contemporary emphasis given to the intrastage typology of Erikson's theory rather than, as in this chapter, the interstage developmental dynamics. Clearly, making such distinctions is essential if researchers hope to establish relationships between outcomes of Erikson's stages and other psychological constructs.

Interstage Relationships

The representation of Erikson's theory in Figure 1 serves to make explicit several assumptions, and so to raise several questions, regarding interstage relationships and transitions in late adulthood and aging. First, this simple, conjunctive sequence is consistent with what appears to be a common assumption that one must always be in one of the eight stages or crises described by Erikson. That is, it has not been thought necessary to introduce, between crises, a non-crisis stage, such as e+f+g+h between generativity and ego integrity. Nevertheless, at the conclusion of Figure 1 are 16 such non-crisis stages, in which the crisis of generativity has been resolved either successfully or unsuccessfully. Should we conceive of this eighth crisis as one that is susceptible to resolution, or is it perhaps the case that a positive resolution of this crisis is nevertheless unstable, threatened with dissolving into a repeat of the crisis or into the unsuccessful resolution of despair unless one strives to maintain the resolution of ego integrity? Whether such intermediate, non-crisis stages and a final, non-crisis stage should be important parts of a representation of Erikson's theory will likely depend on what is meant by resolution of a crisis, a question to be discussed subsequently in this chapter.

Second, implied in the representation in Figure 1 is that one can *experience* an ensuing crisis without having successfully resolved a preceding crisis, as in e+f+g-H. This seems implied by the assumption of the preceding paragraph and is also consistent with what appears accepted among researchers, for example, that one might resolve the first crisis in the direction of mistrust and yet still experience an identity crisis. Third, and most important, is the implication that one can *resolve* a crisis, that is, progress developmentally, without having resolved a preceding crisis successfully. For example, an individual might progress from stagnation, that is, an unsuccessful resolution of the seventh crisis, to either a successful or unsuccessful resolution of the crisis of ego integrity versus despair (see Figure 1, outcomes 3 and 4, 7 and 8, etc.).

Some evidence against the simple, conjunctive sequence of Figure 1 and against the notion of successful crisis resolution following unsuccessful resolution of earlier crises is provided by research with young adults indicating that levels of intimacy, the sixth stage, are associated with the degree of resolution of prior crises. On the basis of interviews, Orlofsky (1978) placed college males into one of five intimacy statuses. These scores were then compared with scores on a measure of outcomes of the five earlier stages. Those men scoring highest on intimacy also scored highest on the earlier stages (see also Orlofsky, Marcia, & Lesser, 1973). Similar results were obtained by Kacerguis and Adams (1980), who measured intimacy status of both male and female college students. For both sexes, high levels of intimacy status were associated with high levels of identity achievement. Waterman (1982, p. 353) summarizes several additional studies demonstrating positive correlations between scores on early-stage measures and the nature of resolution of the identity crisis.

These two studies suggest, then, that failure to successfully resolve an earlier crisis can be an impediment to resolving later crises successfully, so that we might expect that whether the eighth crisis is resolved in the direction of ego integrity or despair will depend on the nature of resolutions of the crises of identity, intimacy, and generativity. Certainly through longitudinal research the probabilities for each of the numerous developmental outcomes in Figure 1 could be established, including the extent to which these outcomes are conditional upon the nature of the resolution of earlier crises and even upon other developmental achievements, such as the acquisition of formal operations (Berzonsky & Barclay, 1981). Such empirical efforts might establish that the probabilities for some paths, such as a successful resolution following an unsuccessful resolution of a preceding crisis, as in outcome 3 (e+f+g-h+), are so low that Figure 1 could be simplified to only a few major sequences (or to even the single, topmost outcome).

Epigenesis

Erikson, in discussing interstage relationships, makes reference to the concept of epigenesis, in one instance quoting extensively and approvingly from the embryologist Stockard (Erikson, 1982, p. 27). Unfortunately, what is properly meant by the concept of epigenesis, especially as this concept is transferred from embryology into the social sciences and psychology, is a subject of considerable debate [see, for example, the exchange between Kitchener (1978, 1980) and Lerner (1980)]. Kitchener (1980) has even questioned whether it is appropriate to borrow such terms or models from biology and attempt to use them in developmental psychology. Such debates over the concept are acknowledged by Erikson, for he prefaces a recent discussion of epigenesis with "whatever its status today" (Erikson, 1982, p. 26). The following quotation from this discussion should serve as an indication of what Erikson intends by the term, regardless of what others have interpreted epigenesis to mean: "If the organ misses its time of ascendance, it is not only doomed as an entity, it endangers . . . the whole hierarchy of organs" (Erikson, 1982, p. 27). Erikson repeats an example provided by Stockard, that the full development of the eye depends on this development taking place at the proper time, for the subsequent times are the times for the development of other parts of the organism.

What are the implications of this conception of epigenesis for the psychosocial theory of ego development? The sequence of stages "is indeed an epigenetic sequence in which no stage and no strength must have missed its early rudiments, its 'natural' crisis, and its potential renewal in all later stages" (Erikson, 1982, p. 78). Not only is there a normal order to the eight stages or crises (the diagonal in the eight by eight matrix), but for Erikson epigenesis also implies the vertical linkages represented in the eight by eight matrix, so that *"the whole ensemble depends on the proper development in the proper sequence of each item* (Erikson, 1982, p. 29). Elsewhere, Erikson (1963) briefly states as the basic claim "only that psychosocial development proceeds by critical steps" (Erikson, 1963, p. 270).

Nevertheless, there remain important questions about what is meant by epigenesis and intrastage relationships in the context of Erikson's theory. First, as Kitchener (1978, 1980) points out, the concept of epigenesis in biology is one that gives the environment, in contrast to the genes, relatively little causal role. Yet one of Erikson's contributions to psychoanalytic theory was precisely to call attention to the importance of interpersonal and cultural factors. Erikson briefly alludes to this difficulty in his use of the term epigenesis (note also his use of quotation marks around the word natural in the quotation in the preceding paragraph), but does not resolve the difficulty, other than to assert that the stages of life are not only "linked" to bodily processes but also are independent on psychological and social processes (Erikson, 1982, p. 59).

Second, it remains unclear whether the notion of epigenesis should be taken to mean that the crises must be experienced in order, whether they must be resolved (successfully or unsuccessfully) in order, or whether they must be resolved successfully in order. There is no simple answer to this question, and indeed much of the remainder of this chapter will be concerned with exploring these and other possibilities. Nevertheless, it can be helpful at this point to consider briefly what Erikson has said. On the one hand, Erikson suggests that the eight crises must be resolved successfully in order, if we understand the word "proper" to mean suitable, appropriate, fitting, and correct: "They all depend on the *proper* development in the *proper* sequence of each item. . . . Each comes to its ascendance, meets its crisis, and finds its *lasting solution* during the stage indicated" (Erikson, 1963, p. 271, emphasis added).

On the other hand, two pages later, Erikson denies that what is acquired is "secured once and for all . . . impervious to new inner conflicts and to changing conditions" (pp. 273-274), implying that unsuccessful resolutions might be made successful and successful resolutions might become unsuccessful at a later time. Elsewhere, Erikson describes some of his older informants as "struggling to bring lifelong dystonic [negative] tendencies into balance with acknowledged psychosocial strengths. For some, too, weaknesses continue to outweigh strengths in ways that remain quite painful" (Erikson et al., 1986, p. 72). Statements such as these imply that the crises do not need to be resolved successfully in order for development to proceed to the next stage or crisis. This will be taken as an assumption for much of the remainder of the chapter; discussion of the possible developmental sequences, if we assume that crises must be resolved successfully, will be postponed until a later section of the chapter.

Foreclosure Upon Despair

Despite the promise of an earlier section, that the number of sequences and outcomes might be fewer than 256, other considerations threaten to increase the number of sequences and outcomes. Foremost among these is the possibility of foreclosure, that is, the tentative commitment to a set of beliefs, values, or goals prior to the experiencing of that crisis, that is, prior to the questioning, the consideration of alternatives, the attempts to make a choice among these, and the commitment that are associated with the period of crisis. The notion of foreclosure has been developed most fully in connection with the fifth stage of identity, in which foreclosure often implies a commitment that reflects merely the wishes of one's parents, teachers, or other significant adults. There has been considerable description of the nature of the foreclosed identity status (e.g., Marcia, 1980), but there has been relatively little discussion of the point in development at which this particular state emerges, and how this state is different from the usual course of development. Elsewhere, I have argued for the reasonableness of understanding the foreclosed identity not in the context of the identity crisis, for the individual has not yet experienced this crisis, but rather in terms of the preceding stage of industry with its nascent themes of work, cooperation, and occupation (Meacham and Santilli, 1982).

In extending the notion of foreclosure to crises other than that of identity versus identity diffusion, we are faced with an issue of whether foreclosure is with respect to only the successful outcome of the crisis or whether an individual may foreclose on the unsuccessful outcome as well. Certainly in the literature on adolescent identity, the term foreclosure has been intended to mean a tentative commitment to only the successful resolution, that is, adolescents who have foreclosed appear in many respects to be similar to those who have experienced the crisis and are now identity achievers. There does not appear to be a discussion, within that literature, of the possibility of foreclosure upon identity diffusion--one is already in the state of identity diffusion at the time at which one forecloses. But this discussion in the adolescent literature reflects the failure, as noted above, to distinguish individuals whose identity is "diffuse" (e) because they have not yet experienced the identity crisis (E) from individuals who have experienced this crisis but have failed to attain a successful resolution (e-). This issue of how to conceptualize foreclosure for the stages other than identity is further complicated by the question of what is meant by the resolution of a crisis, whether a choice of the positive or the negative characteristics of each crisis or some other manner of crisis resolution. This question will be discussed, but not entirely resolved, further along in this chapter. In the face of these unanswered questions, then, I will tentatively adopt the stance that foreclosure can be with respect to either the successful or the unsuccessful outcome of each stage or crisis.

✓ In the context of the eighth stage, foreclosures upon either of the outcomes, ego integrity or despair, seem reasonable possibilities. Erikson et al. (1986, p. 70) briefly mention the possibility of "pseudo-integration," the construction of an apparently satisfactory overview of the life cycle that nevertheless does not fulfill the criteria for a successful resolution. Let us represent these foreclosed outcomes with parentheses--e+f+g+h(+), for foreclosure upon ego integrity, and e+f+g+h(-), for foreclosure upon despair--for these foreclosures are unstable. These foreclosures threaten to dissolve, whenever these tentative commitments are *challenged*, into (a) whatever state characterized the individual prior to the tentative commitment of foreclosure. Again, the question of whether there can be inter-mediate, non-crisis stages is raised. This remains an open question, and so it seems parsimonious to struggle forward in this analysis without introducing a new assumption that the answer to the question is yes. Instead, therefore, let's assume that a collapse of fore-closure upon ego integrity or despair will lead to a return to the immediately preceding stage or crisis of generativity versus stagna-tion (e+f+Gh).

(b) Second, these tentative, unstable commitments might dissolve into each other, that is, foreclosure upon ego integrity may in the face of challenge dissolve into foreclosure upon despair, and vice versa. (c) Third, the foreclosures may dissolve into the stage-appropriate crisis (e+f+g+H). These various possible sequences are portrayed in Figure 2. Despite the additional developmental sequences that have been introduced beyond those of Figure 1 as well as the possible developmental delays during the period of foreclosure and during the second experience and resolution of the preceding stage of generativity versus stagnation (G), no new outcomes have been introduced. All these new sequences terminate in outcomes that are identical to outcomes 1 through 4 in Figure 1. What is significant is that, while the focus was initially upon the eighth stage of ego integrity versus despair, the occurrence of foreclosure prior to this crisis opens the possibility for repeated recycling, perhaps for many years or decades (broken lines in Figure 2), through the immediately preceding crisis of generativity versus stagnation.

Figure 2

Foreclosure Upon Ego Integrity [h(+)] and Despair [h(-)]

(Broken lines indicate movement from right to left)

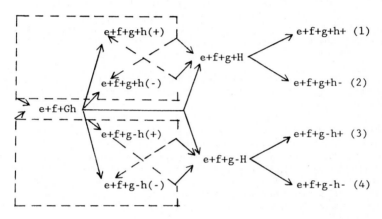

Now that the consequences of foreclosure at the eighth stage have been considered, I will turn briefly to the antecedents of such foreclosures. We might, for example, interpret Waterman's (1982, p. 351) suggestion that foreclosed adolescents have unusually close relationships with their parents as evidence that dynamics in the resolution of the first crisis of trust versus mistrust can predispose individuals towards foreclosure at the fifth stage. In terms of the sequences portrayed in Figure 1, a normal resolution of the seventh crisis of generativity versus stagnation would lead directly to the eighth crisis (H), by definition bypassing the possibility of foreclosure upon despair. Thus, just as the antecedents of the foreclosed identity were sought not in the identity crisis per se but in preceding crises such as trust (Waterman, 1982) or industry (Meacham & Santilli, 1982), so the antecedents of foreclosure upon despair must be sought not in the eighth crisis but instead in preceding crises, for example, autonomy, identity, intimacy, and generativity, and the antecedents of foreclosure upon generativity or stagnation must be sought as well in the preceding crises of, for example, autonomy, identity, and intimacy. Certainly there are various sequences within the theory, as portrayed in Figure 1, that might increase the likelihood of foreclosing upon despair, namely, all the sequences with unsuccessful outcomes of earlier crises (sequences 2 through 16).

Foreclosure Upon Generativity

In order to understand more fully the possible antecedents of foreclosure upon despair as well as the antecedents of despair as a resolution of the eighth crisis, let us now consider the immediately preceding crisis of generativity. A quick comparison of Figure 3 with Figure 2 will show that foreclosure upon either generativity or stagnation leads to quite different developmental sequences and outcomes than does foreclosure in the last stage, for the simple reason that the seventh stage is followed by another stage while the eighth stage, being the last, is not. There are several developmental sequences that can follow from foreclosure upon generativity or stagnation. In order to keep the presentation as simple as possible, these sequences will be described primarily for the possibility of foreclosure upon generativity; the description of foreclosure upon stagnation would be parallel.

Assuming, again, that it would not be parsimonious at this point to introduce a non-crisis stage such as e+f+g(+)h, then foreclosure upon generativity will be represented by e+f+g(+)H, as in Figure 3. In this case, the crisis of generativity versus stagnation has not yet been experienced. The individual has moved from experiencing and resolving the sixth crisis of intimacy versus isolation (F) to the eighth crisis of ego integrity versus despair(H).

The possibilities for further movement parallel those discussed earlier in the case of foreclosure upon ego integrity and despair: (a) The foreclosure might dissolve into the immediately preceding stage, that is, the stage or crisis of intimacy versus isolation (e+Fgh). (b) Foreclosure upon generativity might dissolve, when challenged, into foreclosure upon stagnation (and vice versa). (See broken lines in Figure 3.)

There are more interesting possibilities: (c) The current crisis of ego integrity versus despair might not be susceptible to resolution without the individual first resolving the preceding stage at which foreclosure has taken place (see Figure 3, top, e+f+Gh). This sequence differs in an important way from the sequence outlined in the case of foreclosure upon ego integrity, for which there was no current crisis (Figure 2). In the present case of foreclosure upon generativity, however, the individual at the same time *experiences* the crisis of ego integrity versus despair (H). This sequence would still be consistent with Erikson's hypothesized ordering of the crises, if we take the major point to be not that the crises be experienced in order but rather that they be *resolved* in a normal order. To be concrete: an individual who, upon resolution of the crisis of intimacy,

forecloses at the stage of generativity might *experience* in sequence
the crises of intimacy versus isolation, ego integrity versus despair,
generativity versus stagnation, and, again, ego integrity versus
despair. But the sequence of crisis *resolutions* will be as Erikson
hypothesized--intimacy versus isolation, generativity versus stagnation, and ego integrity versus despair. No new outcomes have been
introduced; the outcomes at the top of Figure 3 are identical to
outcomes 1 through 4 in Figure 1. The main point to be taken from
this discussion of the top of Figure 3 is the repetition of the
experience of the crisis of ego integrity and despair and, for
purposes of the present chapter, the possibility of several repeti-
tions (broken lines in Figure 3) of the negative aspects of this
crisis. That is, foreclosure upon generativity or stagnation might
manifest itself in symptoms of depression and despair seemingly
characteristic not of the seventh but of the eighth stage.

(d) The individual who has foreclosed at the seventh stage of
generativity versus stagnation and so is experiencing the eighth
crisis of ego integrity versus despair might, on the other hand, be
able to resolve this last crisis in a straight-forward fashion, as
shown in the middle part of Figure 3. Two new outcomes have been
introduced (17 and 18), both characterized by the inclusion of
whatever ego qualities are associated with the foreclosure upon
generativity, qualities that furthermore have been carried forward and
integrated within the resolution of the last crisis of ego integrity
versus despair. For individuals who have followed either of these
sequences, their personality structure during late adulthood and old
age would be described in terms of the resolutions of the crises of
identity, intimacy, and ego integrity, but *without* the special
qualities associated with generativity, for that crisis has been
neither experienced nor resolved. This would not be consistent with
Erikson's theory, that is, to have a later crisis resolved before an
earlier one has been experienced or resolved.

(e) A further developmental sequence is shown at the bottom of
Figure 3. In this case, the individual who has foreclosed upon
generativity experiences and furthermore resolves the crisis of ego
integrity versus despair, either successfully or unsuccessfully, and
subsequently experiences and presumably resolves the crisis of
generativity versus stagnation. The outcomes of these sequences are
in some respects like those of the normal sequence (outcomes 1 through
4), but in contrast to Erikson's claim of a normal order of crisis
resolution the sequence of resolutions for the final two stages is
reversed. These four new outcomes are numbered 19 through 22 in
Figure 3. The necessity for distinguishing these four as separate
outcomes follows from the fact that, in Erikson's theory, the
resolutions to earlier crises are carried forward and affect the
resolutions of later crises. Thus if the crisis of ego integrity is
resolved prior to that of generativity, it is resolved without the
possibility of building upon or integrating those ego qualities that

Figure 3

Foreclosure Upon Generativity [g(+)] and Stagnation [g(-)]

(Omitted from the figure are unsuccessful resolutions of identity
and intimacy, the normal outcomes following successful
resolution of intimacy versus isolation, and sequences
following from foreclosure upon stagnation)

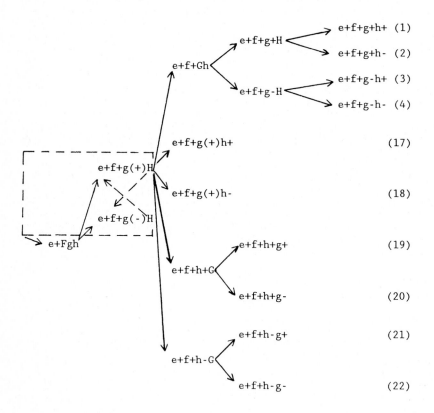

should have emerged relating to generativity; further, the crisis of
generativity will be resolved in the context of whatever qualities
are carried forward from the crisis of ego integrity, a crisis that
might have been resolved in the unsuccessful direction of despair.
This sequence, as the preceding one, would not be consistent with
Erikson's theory, for a later crisis has been resolved before an
earlier one has been resolved (and, further, the earlier one is then
resolved after the later one).

What is a Crisis Resolution?

All of the discussion to this point in the chapter, including Figures 1, 2, and 3, has been based on the common assumption that individuals can continue to progress developmentally without having successfully resolved a particular crisis. Nevertheless, as noted earlier, Erikson can be interpreted as saying that individuals do *not* move forward without "properly" or successfully resolving each crisis in turn, so that a simple, conjunctive model such as the top sequence in Figure 1 (outcome 1) becomes a complete representation of the theory. On such a narrow view, the number of possible sequences and outcomes is severely restricted. Many of the sequences and outcomes shown in Figures 1 and 3 must be extended or interrupted and revised, to be consistent with this view that in the case of *unsuccessful* crisis resolution development is stalled until the contemporary crisis is re-experienced and resolved successfully (Figure 4, outcomes 2', 3', and 4'). Similarly, sequences and outcomes 5 through 16 in Figure 1 would need to be interrupted and revised so as to yield a sequence of crisis resolutions consistent with that of sequence and outcome 1 at the top of Figure 1. Similarly, in the case of *foreclosure*, development is stalled until the contemporary crisis is experienced and resolved successfully (outcomes 17' through 22'). Outcomes 2' through 22' are then the same as outcome 1. Despite the collapsing of the number of possible sequences and outcomes, the result is not trivial, for the implication is that large numbers of individuals might be characterized, for substantial portions of the life course, in terms of unsuccessful resolutions of the late adult crises, namely, stagnation and despair, or in terms of foreclosure upon either the positive (generativity, ego integrity) or the negative (stagnation, despair) aspects of these crises.

Figure 4

Extended and Revised Sequences,
Assuming Normal Order of Crisis Resolution

e+f+g+h- ----> e+f+g+H ----> e+f+g+h+   (2')

e+f+g-H [or e+f+g-h?] ----> e+f+Gh ----> e+f+g+H ----> e+f+g+h+

(3'and 4')

e+f+g(+)H [or e+f+g(+)h?] ----> e+f+Gh ----> e+f+g+H ----> e+f+g+h+

(17' through 22')

Should all of the other sequences and outcomes be rejected? In particular, should we reject those sequences (middle and lower parts of Figure 3) that imply an ordering of stages or crises that is different from Erikson's proposed normal sequence? This implication of different orders is not new, for it follows from data gathered by Douvan and Adelson (1966) and more recently by Hodgson and Fischer (1979) and Fischer (1981) suggesting that for some women the crisis of intimacy precedes the crisis of identity. If inversions of stage or crisis order are possible in adolescence and young adulthood, then we should be open to their possibility in late adulthood and aging as well. What to do about these inconsistencies with Erikson's claim of a normal sequence is in part an empirical question, one that awaits longitudinal investigation and careful assessment of the experiencing and the resolving of crises as well as of whether individuals have indeed resolved crises or have merely foreclosed.

The problem is also a conceptual one, depending on how we conceive of crises and their resolution. According to Erikson, a resolution is not merely a choice by the individual of the positive characteristics of each stage over the negative. Instead, "What the individual acquires at a given stage is a certain *ratio* between the positive and the negative which, if the *balance* is *toward* the positive, will help him to meet later crises with a better chance for unimpaired total development" (Erikson, 1959, p. 61; emphasis added). Erikson (1963) later remarked, in a footnote to his classic chapter on the "eight ages of man," that some researchers, in making achievement scales out of his stages, "blithely omit all the 'negative' senses (basic mistrust, etc.) which are and remain the dynamic counterpoint of the 'positive' ones throughout life" (p. 273). Perhaps it was to emphasize this point that, in contrast to earlier publications in which alternative attitudes were joined by "versus" (Erikson, 1963, 1982), in the most recent publication "versus" has been replaced with "and" (Erikson et al., 1986).

What are the implications of these statements for the analysis, up to this point in the chapter, of the formal aspects of Erikson's theory? One interpretation of the earlier analyses--an interpretation that should be *rejected*--is that in the notation system + represents the positive characteristics of each stage and a - the negative characteristics. Such an inappropriate interpretation, however, would be consistent with how the notion of foreclosure has been employed in the literature on adolescent identity development, namely, that foreclosed adolescents appear more similar to identity achieving adolescents than to identity diffuse adolescents, with the implication that one cannot foreclose on identity diffusion.

But the present notation system is entirely consistent with Erikson's view that successful resolution is an appropriate balance of positive and negative characteristics, if we let + represent such an appropriate balance and - represent an imbalance of *either* the positive over the negative characteristics *or* the negative over the positive. That is, the relationship between + and -, on the one hand, and successful and unsuccessful resolution, on the other, is not changed. But the nature of an unsuccessful resolution is now more clearly specified as *not* a choice of the negative characteristics of a stage as opposed to the positive, but rather an imbalance in the relationship between the negative and the positive characteristics. The tentative commitments of foreclosure, occurring prior to the stage-appropriate crisis, might be upon an appropriate balance or upon such an imbalance between the positive and the negative characteristics.

A Balance Between Positive and Negative

It remains, however, not entirely clear what is meant by a ratio between positive and negative with, at the same time, the balance being towards the positive, especially when one considers problems of assessment of whether a particular crisis has been resolved successfully or not. For example, suppose we employ a traditional procedure in which older adults are presented with ten pairs of statements, one statement in each pair expressing a positive attitude corresponding to ego integrity and the other statement expressing a negative attitude corresponding to despair, and ask these adults to choose the one statement in each pair with which they are most in agreement. Would evidence of an appropriate balance towards the positive, of a successful resolution of the eighth crisis, be the choice of six or seven positive statements, out of ten, and four or three negative statements? Would evidence of an inappropriate balance be the choice of eight or more positive statements, or of five or more negative statements? Perhaps.

But such an assessment procedure would not yet distinguish individuals who had experienced and successfully resolved this eighth crisis of ego integrity versus despair from those who might have foreclosed upon an appropriate or inappropriate balance or who might have merely chosen statements at random. One step towards an improved assessment procedure has been taken by Keller (1978), who advanced an interpretation of the resolution of crises in terms of the construction of dialectical syntheses between opposing issues and attitudes. Keller's research procedure permitted older people to either choose one of two opposing statements, or to choose both (the latter would not be permitted in a procedure based on the traditional positive versus negative interpretation). For example, given the two statements "There have been many good things in life; there have been many bad things in life," one person responded: "Both are true, but from bad things we often learn much leading to good. And if all things were pleasant, that might lead to complacency, or we wouldn't experience good as such anymore." Keller's data provided better support for various predictions derived from Erikson's theory when responses such as this one, affirming both the positive and the negative in a synthesis of the two, were scored as evidence for ego

integrity than when traditional scoring procedures were followed. If
one were to follow Keller's argument that a successful resolution is a
dialectical synthesis, then in the present notation system a + could
represent such a synthesis and a - could represent a choice of either
the positive thesis or the negative antithesis.

Of course, by any interpretation a crisis resolution emphasizing
the negative characteristics of isolation, stagnation, and despair
would hardly be considered a successful resolution. Yet now it can be
seen that any crisis resolution--or, indeed, any interpretation of
late adulthood and aging--emphasizing only the positive characteristics of intimacy, generativity, and ego integrity and so neglecting
the negative aspects cannot be considered to be successful. Erikson
et al. (1986) characterize as maladaptive the "tendency to overdo and
to overdevelop the syntonic [positive] predisposition in an attempt to
let the dystonic [negative] wither away" (p. 40) and further provide
brief descriptions of such positive imbalances for each of the four
adult stages: fanaticism, promiscuity, overextension, and presumption
(p. 45).

The positive imbalance for the second stage of autonomy is
shameless willfulness, and is illustrated by the case of a woman in
her eighties, crippled with arthritis and unable to walk without
assistance, long characterized by determination, who denies her
disability and insists that she will not use a wheelchair. Apparently
because the wheelchair was an unacceptable symbol of helplessness, she
is now in a state of real helplessness (Erikson et al., 1986, p.
198). In the case of this woman, we might say that the lack of a
successful resolution of a childhood crisis, in terms of an appropriate balance between autonomy versus shame and doubt, has
predisposed her towards despair in old age. In other cases, living
independently can be an important symbol of autonomy, one that can
conflict with realistic needs to obtain advice and assistance from
families, friends, and social service agencies.

Summary of Erikson's Theory

Before turning to some concrete proposals for how our understanding of
helplessness and lack of control in aging is expanded through
considering these topics within the framework of Erikson's theory, I
will first provide a summary evaluation of Erikson's theory as a
result of the preceding analysis of its formal characteristics. If we
are to make further use of Erikson's theory as a conceptual framework,
then we must be thoroughly familiar with the range of possible
developmental sequences and outcomes implied by the theory as well as
with the theory's strengths and weaknesses. Still unresolved at this
point in the analysis is the issue of how strict a constraint on
development is implied by Erikson's statements that the sequence of
stages and crises is epigenetic, that psychosocial development
proceeds by critical steps. Is the constraint on development (a) that

successfully resolving a crisis depends on successfully resolving the preceding crisis (Figure 1, outcome 1; Figure 4)? (b) that resolving a crisis (successfully or unsuccessfully) depends on resolving the previous crisis (successfully or unsuccessfully) (Figures 1 and 2)? (c) that the crises must be experienced in order, but may be resolved out of order?   (d) that the crises may be experienced out of order, but must be resolved (successfully or unsuccessfully) in a normal order (Figure 3, top)? or (e) that the crises may be experienced out of order, but must be resolved successfully in order (Figure 4, where g+ must precede h+)? Or (f) are there no constraints on the order of experiencing or resolving crises (Figure 3, middle and bottom)? The choice among these and other interpretations of the epigenetic, normal sequence of development likely will depend on what we mean by experiencing a crisis and by resolving a crisis.

A second, major unresolved issue concerns the need for more clear criteria for linking evidence, whether from interviews or from questionnaire data, to particular states or stages hypothesized as constructs within the theory. Consider, for example, a woman in her early nineties, afflicted with arthritis. Although she is able to walk, she is afraid of falling, and so she rarely goes out of her home in order to avoid the potential embarrassment, the threat to her self-image that might follow from falling. This restriction of social and behavioral functioning by a physical disability that need not necessarily be so limiting is interpreted in terms of an imbalance in the resolution of the crisis of autonomy versus shame and doubt, that is, social appropriateness and consciousness of her image has become too important for this woman (Erikson et al., 1986, p. 194).

At issue is not this interpretation of current functioning in terms of autonomy versus shame and doubt, but rather the locating of this psychological dynamic within the framework of the theory. Does this example represent: (a) a childhood foreclosure upon autonomy, that is, a failure to experience the crisis of autonomy versus shame and doubt [b(+)]? (b) a failure to resolve this crisis of autonomy versus shame and doubt [b]? (c) an unsuccessful resolution of this crisis, unsuccessful in the sense that the imbalance was too much towards the positive [b-]? In the case of either (a), (b), or (c), has development stopped at this point in childhood, or has development nevertheless proceeded through subsequent stages or crises and their resolutions? Or does the example represent (d) a contemporary experience or re-experience of the crisis of autonomy versus shame and doubt, perhaps because of an earlier foreclosure or failure to resolve the crisis or to resolve the crisis successfully [B]? or (e) merely a reworking of the products of the earlier crisis in the context of a contemporary crisis, such as ego integrity versus despair [b+ sub H, or cell VIII 2 in Erikson's matrix]? Similar questions can be raised regarding men and women who see their children's creative and productive accomplishments as an expression of their own hitherto unexpressed creativity and productivity (Erikson et al., 1986, p. 82).

Erikson (Erikson et al., 1986) suggests that an overemphasis on the syntonic, as in the case of the woman in the preceding paragraph, "could eventually be recorrected by readaptation, spontaneous or therapeutically induced" (p. 41). Similarly, the suggestion is made that after decades in which a particular balance has been precarious there may be a "reevaluating and recasting of earlier experiences" (Erikson et al., 1986, p. 111). Erikson et al. (1986) provide numerous examples of individuals who might be said to have foreclosed upon or unsuccessfully resolved earlier crises, but who now in late adulthood are apparently making progress towards more successful resolutions of these earlier crises. For example, a salesman who for decades had felt inadequate and inferior achieves a new sense of mastery and *industry* following financial success in a new line of work (Erikson et al., 1986, p. 156). A lifelong frustrated musician is able to construct a new *identity* for himself based on the musical accomplishments of his children (Erikson et al., 1986, p. 145). A married couple is able to achieve *intimacy* despite serious marital difficulties forty years ago (Erikson et al., 1986, p. 112). Many individuals who had difficulty with parenthood nevertheless are able to make progress towards *generativity* through the experience of having grandchildren (Erikson et al., 1986, p. 93). These examples imply that alternative (d) in the preceding paragraph is a reasonable one, but it remains unclear how to square the notions of recasting and readaptation or "the principle of reexperiencing" (Erikson et al., 1986, p. 40) with that of epigenesis.

A number of other questions about Erikson's theory that have arisen or were implied in the course of this analysis can be briefly mentioned: (a) Must one always be in one of the stages or crises, or is it reasonable to introduce intermediate non-crisis stages? In the discussion of foreclosure, it was deemed more parsimonious to assume that one is always in a stage or crisis, but there seems no a priori reason for having assumed this. In Figure 4, possible non-crisis stages such as e+f+g-h or e+f+g(+)h are shown in brackets. (b) Might not the consequence of unsuccessful resolutions of crises be a strong disposition towards further unsuccessful resolutions, e.g., a+b+c-d-e--f-g-? If so, then the 16 potential outcomes of Figure 1 would be reduced in number to only five, namely, outcome 1 (all successful resolutions) and outcomes 2, 4, 8, and 16 (with from one to four unsuccessful resolutions of the adult crises). (c) Similarly, might not the consequence of foreclosure be a strong disposition towards foreclosure upon subsequent stages, e.g., e(+)f(+)g(+)h(+), so that the ego structure becomes increasingly unstable and likely to collapse in the face of even a modest challenge? (d) Can an individual be in two or three crises at one and the same time? The assumption that the answer is no led to the sequences in Figures 3 and 4 being as they are; again, there seems no a priori reason why the answer should be no, so that Figures 3 and 4 might be revised to include a stage such as, for example, e+f+GH.

Implications for Helplessness and Lack of Control

The formal analysis of Erikson's psychosocial theory of ego development in the preceding section was intended to call attention to
particular features of the theory that have potential for expanding
our understanding of helplessness and lack of control, in particular,
the interstage or developmental relationships, and to briefly outline
the strengths of the theory, in particular, its breadth of scope, and
its weaknesses, in particular, the need for clarity on what is meant
by experiencing a crisis and by resolving a crisis. It is now
possible to turn more directly to the issues of helplessness and lack
of control and to point to several conclusions that follow directly
from an understanding of Erikson's theory and from the formal
analysis.

Autonomy

In a narrow sense, helplessness and lack of control in aging can be
understood as the experience and resolution of autonomy versus shame
and doubt in the second stage of childhood and the subsequent
modification of these ego qualities across the life course. The
construction of a sense of autonomy and independence follows initially
from the sense of confidence in the environment and in one's own body
that are products of the first crisis of infancy, trust versus
mistrust (Erikson et al., 1986, p. 228). Subsequently the autonomy of
the two-year-old is modified to become "a family-tolerated autonomy, a
healthy school-age autonomy, a young-adulthood autonomy, and a
generative adult and an old-age determination" (Erikson et al., 1986,
p. 40). In old age, individuals must struggle to maintain this
willfulness and independence in the face of increased weakening of the
body, as well as damage through disease and accidents. How older
individuals respond to these physical changes reflects the sense of
autonomy and self-determination developed over the life course. Two
women, both in their eighties, provide examples of continued self-
determination while adjusting to physical abilities by choosing to
become involved in those activities that are still possible. The
first, in poor health and unable to maintain her rural home alone,
moved to an urban area, established a garden, and began writing short
stories for publication; the second, suffering numerous disabilities
including blindness, nevertheless remains informed about world events,
strives to engage others in conversation, and takes the initiative in
household chores (Erikson et al., 1986, p. 191-193). Although the
circumstances of these two women might realistically induce feelings
of shame, doubt, and helplessness, nevertheless their ability to
maintain a balance between these feelings and a sense of autonomy has
been instrumental in limiting the impact of their physical disabilities.

In contrast, for several individuals relatively minor physical disabilities have led to severe restrictions on psychological and interpersonal functioning. Two examples, illustrating an imbalance of autonomy over shame and doubt, have been noted earlier, the woman in her eighties crippled with arthritis yet unable to accept a wheelchair (Erikson et al., 1986, p. 198) and the woman in her nineties who rarely leaves her home so as to avoid the embarrassment that might follow from falling (p. 194). Neither of these have been able to integrate the potential feelings of shame and embarrassment with the self-image of autonomy, independence, and self-reliance that have been personally important and have been seen as socially desirable during many earlier decades of the life course, so that requiring or receiving assistance of any kind represents a failure of their sense of autonomy. Especially among the men, the individualism of youth and the self-sufficiency of middle age are associated with stubbornness in response to their children's offers of assistance (Erikson et al., 1986, p. 207).

For several individuals, regarding assistance from others as facilitating one's own independence rather than threatening it has been important in achieving a balance between maintaining feelings of autonomy while acknowledging realistic helplessness and embarrassment (Erikson et al., 1986, p. 203). For example, one man is comfortable, independent, and self-reliant living in an isolated rural setting, for he knows that in an emergency his son can be at his side in only three hours (Erikson et al., p. 206). A second example is provided by a man whose failing vision and slowed reflexes made driving hazardous, threatening him with feelings of helplessness and embarrassment. The dangerous situation was resolved by his giving the car to his daughter, an action that not only enhanced his feelings of autonomy through his initiative but also showed generative concern for his daughter (Erikson et al., 1986, p. 195). Erikson provides an excellent example of the interweaving of issues across stages (and across generations) in his observation that being able to accept care from others not only enhances one's own independence but, if the care is accepted in a way that is itself caring, can enhance feelings of generativity in those who are giving the care (Erikson et al., 1986, p. 74). For other individuals, providing assistance to others, clearly an expression of generativity, can be at the same time an expression of continued self-determination, independence, and autonomy.

Despair

To understand helplessness and lack of control in the broadest possible terms, we must turn to the eighth stage of ego integrity versus despair. Feelings of integrity and despair are, ideally, brought into balance through a review of all the earlier psychosocial conflicts or crises and an acceptance of the life one has lived. Imbalance towards despair brings disappointment, cynicism, fear of death, the feeling that there is insufficient time to start anew, helplessness, and hopelessness. Yet Erikson is quite clear in asserting that these dystonic or negative feelings cannot be denied or excluded, but instead must be integrated within any resolution of the eighth and final crisis, for feelings of despair and even defeat are a part of the struggle for balance within each of the preceding seven stages (see, for example, Erikson et al., 1986, p. 72, 288). Thus in the broadest terms we can seek the antecedents of helplessness and lack of control in aging by inquiring into the antecedents, among each of the preceding stages, of despair in aging.

The preceding formal analysis of Erikson's theory suggests the following developmental sequences and events as antecedents of despair: (a) Foreclosure upon either ego integrity or despair prior to the eighth crisis with its associated life review can lead to a delay in the achievement of ego integrity as well as more time spent in foreclosure upon despair. As shown in Figure 2, the unstable commitments of foreclosure upon ego integrity are likely, when challenged, to dissolve into foreclosure upon despair. Further, there might be repeated recycling through the outcome of despair (Figure 2, broken lines).

(b) Foreclosure upon either generativity or stagnation, prior to the seventh crisis, leads immediately to an experience of the crisis of ego integrity versus despair (Figure 3, left side). It is possible that more time will be spent in this crisis of ego integrity versus despair than would normally be the case, not only because the crisis is experienced out of order and without benefit of those ego qualities normally carried forward from the seventh stage of generativity versus stagnation, but also because the crisis might be experienced early in chronological years and the individual might lack certain experiences and challenges essential to resolution of the crisis. (c) Foreclosure upon either generativity or stagnation might markedly increase the time spent in the crisis of generativity versus despair, if there is extended recycling between these foreclosures of the seventh stage (Figure 3, broken lines). (d) Even when a foreclosure upon generativity or stagnation is promptly resolved, there might be a repetition of the crisis of ego integrity versus despair (Figure 3, top). Experiencing this eighth crisis twice rather than once implies not only more time spent in the crisis of ego integrity versus despair and a doubling of the opportunity for resolving it in the direction of ego integrity, but also a doubling of the risk for resolving the crisis in the direction of despair. (e) Foreclosure upon generativity or stagnation, rather than proper resolution of the seventh stage, might increase the likelihood of resolving the eighth crisis in the direction of despair, for the eighth crisis might have to be resolved without the benefit of those ego qualities that are normally carried forward from the seventh stage (Figure 3, outcomes 18, 21, and 22).

(f) Finally, and perhaps most important, is the possibility that the eighth crisis of ego integrity versus despair can't be resolved

successfully in the direction of ego integrity, or will be resolved
unsuccessfully in the direction of despair, unless all seven of the
preceding crises have been resolved successfully. Either these seven
crises must be resolved successfully in their normal order (consistent
with only the top sequence in Figure 1 and with the sequences shown in
Figure 4), or during the eighth crisis of ego integrity versus despair
earlier crises not yet successfully resolved must be successfully
resolved through some process of reworking, recasting, readaptation,
and so forth. The antecedents of despair might be found in any and
all of the preceding seven stages, including the first crisis of
infancy, trust versus mistrust, an antecedent Erikson explicitly
discusses in relationship to ego integrity and despair (e.g., Erikson,
1963, p. 269; Erikson et al., 1986, p. 218, 228). Erikson (1982, p.
63) also notes, for example, that many of the overt symptoms of
despair that older people present in psychotherapy are, in fact,
reflections of their continuing sense of stagnation. So the formal
analysis of possible developmental sequences that has been carried out
in this chapter for the seventh and eighth stages of generativity and
of ego integrity, including the possibilities for and consequences of
foreclosure, might be carried out for each of the remaining six
stages. Yet the implication of the majority of points listed in the
preceding paragraphs is that the antecedents of increased time spent
in the crisis of ego integrity versus despair and increased risk of
resolving this crisis in the direction of despair lie not in the
eighth stage per se but in the immediately preceding stage of
generativity versus stagnation.

Generativity

It is significant that in both the preceding sections, concerned with
autonomy and with despair in relation to helplessness and lack of
control in aging, we have been led to the seventh stage of generativity versus stagnation. Generativity is primarily a concern for the
next generation, but also includes productivity and creativity;
stagnation is associated with personal impoverishment, frustration,
pseudo-intimacy, self-absorption, and self-indulgence. Resolution of
the seventh crisis in the direction of generativity depends, of
course, upon the outcomes of all the earlier crises. Nevertheless,
two developmental sequences placing individuals at higher risk for
resolving the crisis in the direction of stagnation (and so, presumably, placing the individual at higher risk for resolving the subsequent
crisis in the direction of despair) follow from the formal analysis of
Erikson's theory carried out earlier in this chapter. (a) Foreclosure
upon either generativity or stagnation might lead to recycling
through these two foreclosures and so perhaps increased time spent in
foreclosure upon stagnation (Figure 3, broken lines). (b) Surprisingly, more time spent in the crisis of generativity versus stagnation
might follow from foreclosure upon the *subsequent* stage of ego
integrity versus despair, for one outcome of the collapse of these
fragile foreclosures is an immediate return to the preceding crisis of

generativity versus stagnation (Figure 2, broken lines), so that there might be two or more experiences of this seventh crisis.

The significance of the crisis of generativity versus stagnation for the achievement of ego integrity has already been noted, by reference to the number of pages this seventh stage commands in *Vital Involvement in Old Age* (Erikson et al., 1986). For many of the individuals interviewed, generativity is expressed as a choice of caring for the long-term well-being of children and grandchildren over caring for oneself (Erikson et al., 1986, p. 84). The importance of ego qualities carried forward from this seventh stage for resolution of the eighth and final stage, and in particular as a counterbalance to the threat of despair in old age, is extreme for several of these individuals. A sad, desperate woman in her late eighties, in poor health, alone, with a feeling of guilt from past actions, nevertheless continues to endure the pain of her present life rather than commit suicide, because she is concerned with the possible impact upon her grandchildren, fearing that they would not understand, would become upset, or would no longer respect her (Erikson et al., 1986, p. 95). A man in his nineties, who feels that he was not successful in caring for his own family and who now is ready to die, nevertheless is kept alive by his feelings of responsibility to care for his sister-in-law (Erikson et al., 1986, p. 97). Indeed, many of these individuals are involved in caretaking for siblings or cousins or for other older people in the community and furthermore express an enduring concern for country and for humankind (Erikson et al., 1986, pp. 97-100). Not all of these individuals are successful at warding off despair through their generative involvement. A woman whose early involvement in painting and drawing was interrupted by raising three children and the need to involve herself in her husband's business, both activities towards which she was ambivalent, now feels that it is too late in life to resume her earlier creative involvement, so that she experiences feelings of stagnation and despair (Erikson et al., 1986, p. 85).

A major portion of *Vital Involvement in Old Age* (Erikson et al., 1986) is devoted to an interpretation of the life of Dr. Isak Borg, the protagonist in the film *Wild Strawberries* directed by Ingmar Bergmann, as an example of an almost completed life history. Although the life history is quite complex and many issues remain not entirely resolved--indeed, there is hope that their resolution will take a new course--nevertheless a quick gloss of Dr. Borg's life history is that in old age he is independent and strong-willed, yet unable to construct a satisfactory meaning for his life course and to resolve the eighth crisis of ego integrity versus despair. To the extent there has been any expression of generativity it has been in caring for his medical career (and himself) and only to the slightest extent in caring for family and community. The way is prepared for his crisis of generativity versus stagnation, indeed the likely resolution in the direction of stagnation is previewed, in the earlier stages: Dr. Borg lacks competence and industry in his roles as husband, father, and father-in-law (Erikson et al., 1986, p. 279), these roles

are not part of his identity (p. 280), and his interpersonal relationships have been lacking in true intimacy (p. 285).

Autonomy and Generativity in Cultural Context

Have we arrived at a paradoxical conclusion in our understanding of
helplessness and lack of control? For some individuals, coping with
the circumstances of aging is a matter of maintaining and asserting
autonomy, independence, and self-reliance; for others, however, the
assertion of autonomy becomes a major obstacle to receiving assistance
and so maintaining one's independence. The discussion of autonomy and
of despair led in several cases to issues involved in the seventh
stage of generativity versus isolation, yet in many respects the
notions of autonomy, independence, and self-reliance appear at first
to be in stark contrast to those of generativity, caring, and
interdependence. How can these paradoxes be resolved, so that
autonomy is reconciled with generativity?

A hint towards the resolution of these paradoxes is to be found
in Erikson's observation that the individuals who were interviewed
have lived within a culture that places a high value on individuality,
self-reliance, and independence (Erikson et al., 1986, p. 217), on
independence rather than interdependence (p. 301). The fact that
these notions of autonomy, individualism, and independence take on
particular meanings in different cultural contexts is made clear by
Sampson (1977, 1988), who distinguishes two radically different
notions of individualism: self-contained individualism and ensembled
individualism. In the case of self-contained individualism, the North
American cultural ideal reflected in and legitimized by American
psychology, the individual is expected to strive for self-sufficiency
and to not be dependent upon others for fulfillment in his or her life
goals. The resolution of the crisis of autonomy versus shame and
doubt is given a particular cultural twist, an emphasis upon the
self-contained nature of the autonomy, which in turn becomes the
foundation for the construction of a unidimensional identity focused
on production, competition, and achievement within the workplace but
quite unsuited to life following retirement from work (Meacham,
1983). The responsibility for coping with and adjustment to the
circumstances of aging also falls, within the cultural context of
self-contained individualism, primarily upon the individual, so that
those who are unable to cope on their own are embarrassed, are
ashamed, and have failed; to have to depend upon others for assistance
is merely to aggravate the failure in light of the cultural ideal. In
striking agreement with Erikson, Sampson (1988) observes that
"self-contained individualism actually thwarts achieving the very core
values it purports to realize" (p. 20), for the cost to an individual
of receiving assistance is to have his or her self-reliance and
independence be undermined. Thus the cultural emphasis on self-contained autonomy from childhood through middle adulthood might ensure,

for many individuals, the loss of feelings of autonomy and so the experience of helplessness and lack of control in aging.

In ensembled individualism, which Sampson (1988) argues is the more prevalent worldwide cultural context, individuals define themselves in relationship to others, to family and society, so that they can both provide and receive assistance without having to experience or interpret this as threatening to a sense of personal freedom, independence, or autonomy. The notion of interdependence at the basis of ensembled individualism is, of course, entirely consistent with the mutual assistance and caring, both between and within generations, contained within Erikson's concept of generativity. Erikson helps to complete the picture of autonomy and independence in the cultural context of ensembled individualism by reminding us that the development of autonomy in the two-year-old child depends on the support, encouragement, and security provided by the family (Erikson et al., 1986, p. 205). The notion of self-contained individualism is thus an illusion at its developmental base as well as being an illusion in practice for, as Erikson reminds us, we all need advice and assistance throughout the life course (Erikson et al., 1986, p. 202).

Understanding Erikson's theory as consistent with the notion of ensembled individualism, rather than self-contained individualism, is essential in order to protect the theory from Lichtman's (1987) critique of stage theories as mere attempts to legitimize the individualistic achievement, competition, desire, consumption, and sense of self required by capitalism. Lichtman's principal target is Levinson's (1978) description of adult development, like Erikson's a simple, conjunctive stage sequence. Among many provocative points, Lichtman (1987) argues that it is profoundly important to capitalism that "one does not deny the failure of one's now spent life but regards it as the necessary preliminary for the success of one's children. They are to reap the benefit of disaster" (p. 137). Such rationalization, along with the acceptance of despair, defeat, and death, is clearly reminiscent of Erikson's argument for the necessity of basing ego integrity upon the prior stage of generativity and his argument that feelings of despair and defeat must not be excluded from a successful resolution of the eighth crisis of ego integrity versus despair. Yet identity is not, for Erikson, an independent, self-sufficient, self-contained identity. Instead, identity is confirmed only in relation to other people, in one's choice of roles to play in the family and in society, and in the meaning that one has for others. As Erikson (1982) puts it: "Nobody can quite 'know' who he or she 'is' until promising partners in work and love have been encountered and tested" (p. 72). Still, Franz and White (1985) and Hassan and Bar-Yam (1987) have argued for elaborations upon Erikson's theory so as to give greater emphasis to interpersonal relations, connectedness, and interdependence.

Generativity and interdependence are thus the foundation for the initial development of autonomy as well as for the maintenance of autonomy over the life course. This thesis is consistent with the view that we must reject individual cognition and consciousness as a basis for individual and societal development in favor of interpersonal relations, communication, and cooperation as that basis (Meacham and Emont, in press). Arguments in support of this view have been made by a number of writers. Vygotsky (1978), for example, emphasized that all cognitive abilities appear first in social interaction, and only subsequently at the intrapsychological level. Similarly, Habermas (1984) rejects intrasubjectivity as the starting point in understanding the individual and society, arguing instead for basing these in intersubjectivity, in the community of subjects in dialogue. Harre (1984) argues that the primary reality is the array of persons in conversation, with the psychological realities of human minds brought into being only as secondary realities. What is needed in order to further our understanding of helplessness and lack of control in aging is to locate the basis for autonomy, individualism, and independence not within the mind of the individual, but within interpersonal relations.

Conclusions

Erikson (1963) remarks in passing that "a chart is only a tool to think with" (p. 270). In this spirit, the formal analysis of Erikson's theory and the accompanying figures of this chapter are not an end in themselves, but merely a tool for discovering and bringing attention to some aspects of Erikson's writings that can expand our understanding of helplessness and lack of control in aging. If nothing else, I hope to have shown that the potential dynamics of his theory are complex and subtle and, more importantly, that there is much that can be gained from his writings towards our understanding of these topics. Although the focus of this chapter has been upon theory, nevertheless the theory has been constructed on the experience and understanding of a master clinician, so that the conclusions derived from considering the theory should not be too far removed from clinical practice and from research possibilities.

The discussion in the present chapter has led to the following conclusions: (1) In seeking to understand helplessness and lack of control in aging, it is essential to adopt a life-course perspective. Helplessness and lack of control cannot be understood by considering merely the plight of older people. One must consider the lifelong development of these attitudes, beginning in early childhood with the stage or crisis of autonomy versus shame and doubt. (2) Any conception of autonomy, independence, and self-control in old age must include, in appropriate balance, the dystonic or negative aspects of shame, doubt, helplessness, and lack of control as a normal part of life-course development. (3) The essence of autonomy, independence, and self-control is to be found not within the illusion of a self-contained, competitive, and achieving individual, but within a framework of interdependence and generative concern. (4) The achievement of ego integrity in late adulthood and aging must involve coming to terms with despair, helplessness, and lack of control, not a rejecting of these. (5) The essence of ego integrity and the avoidance of despair is to be found not within one's self, but within the faith and hope that derive from trusting relationships with others. (6) Many apparent symptoms of helplessness, lack of control, depression, and despair in aging might have their roots not in the eighth stage of ego integrity versus despair, but in unresolved issues associated with any of the earlier stages but in particular the crises of autonomy versus shame and doubt and of generativity versus stagnation.

References

Baltes, P. B. (1987). Theoretical propositions of life-span developmental psychology: On the dynamics between growth and decline. *Developmental Psychology, 23*, 611-626.

Berzonsky, M. D., & Barclay, C. R. (1981). Formal reasoning and identity formation: A reconceptualization. In J. A. Meacham & N. R. Santilli (Eds.), *Social development in youth: Structure and content* (pp. 64-76). Basel: Karger.

Douvan, E., & Adelson, J. (1966). *The adolescent experience.* New York: Wiley & Sons.

Erikson, E. H. (1959). Identity and the life cycle. *Psychological Issues, 1*(1, Whole No. 1), 50-100.

Erikson, E. H. (1963). *Childhood and society* (2nd ed.). New York: Norton.

Erikson, E. H. (1982). *The life cycle completed.* New York: Norton.

Erikson, E. H., Erikson, J. M., & Kivnick, H. Q. (1986). *Vital involvement in old age.* New York: Norton.

Fischer, J. L. (1981). Transitions in relationship style from adolescence to young adulthood. *Journal of Youth and Adolescence, 10*, 11-24.

Flavell, J. H. (1972). An analysis of cognitive-developmental sequences. *Genetic Psychology Monographs, 86*, 279-350.

Franz, C. E., & White, K. M. (1985). Individuation and attachment in personality development: Extending Erikson's theory. *Journal of Personality, 53*, 224-256.

Freud, S. (1933). *New introductory lectures on psycho-analysis.* New York: Norton.

Gutmann, D. L. (1985). The parental imperative revisited: Towards a developmental psychology of adulthood and later life. In J. A. Meacham (Ed.), *Family and individual development* (pp. 31-60). Basel: Karger.

Habermas, J. (1984). *The theory of communicative action* (Vol. 1. Reason and the rationalization of society). Boston: Beacon Press.

Harre, R. (1984). *Personal being.* Cambridge, MA: Harvard University Press.

Hassan, A. B., & Bar-Yam, M. (1987). Interpersonal development across the life span: Communion and its interaction with agency in psychosocial development. In J. A. Meacham (Ed.), *Interpersonal relations: Family, peers, friends.* Basel: Karger.

Havighurst, R. J. (1953). *Human development and education.* New York: David McKay.

Hodgson, J. W., & Fischer, J. L. (1979). Sex differences in identity and intimacy development in college youth. *Journal of Youth and Adolescence, 8,* 37-50.

Kacerguis, M. A., & Adams, G. R. (1980). Erikson's stage resolution: The relationship between identity and intimacy. *Journal of Youth and Adolescence, 9,* 117-126.

Kalish, R. A. (1979). The new ageism and the failure models: A polemic. *The Gerontologist, 19,* 398-402.

Keller, A. (1978). *Ego integrity, perspective-taking, and cautiousness.* Unpublished doctoral dissertation, State University of New York at Buffalo.

Kitchener, R. F. (1978). Epigenesis: The role of biological models in developmental psychology. *Human Development, 21,* 141-160.

Kitchener, R. F. (1980). Predetermined versus probabilistic epigenesis: A reply to Lerner. *Human Development, 23,* 73-76.

Kivnick, H. Q. (1985). Intergenerational relations: Personal meaning in the life cycle. In J. A. Meacham (Ed.), *Family and individual development* (pp. 93-102). Basel: Karger.

Kohlberg, L. (1964). Development of moral character and moral ideology. In M. L. Hoffman & L. W. Hoffman (Eds.), *Review of child development research* (pp. 383-432). New York: Russell Sage Foundation.

Lerner, R. M. (1980). Concepts of epigenesis: Descriptive and explanatory issues. A critique of Kitchener's comments. *Human Development, 23,* 63-72.

Levinson, D. T. (1978). *The seasons of a man's life.* New York: Ballantine Books.

Lichtman, R. (1987). The illusion of maturation in an age of decline. In J. M. Broughton (Ed.), *Critical theories of psychological development* (pp. 127-148). New York: Plenum Press.

Logan, R. D. (1986). A reconceptualization of Erikson's theory: The repetition of existential and instrumental themes. *Human Development, 29,* 125-136.

Marcia, J. E. (1980). Identity in adolescence. In J. Adelson (Ed.), *Handbook of adolescent psychology* (pp. 159-187). New York: Wiley & Sons.

McTavish, D. G. (1971). Perceptions of old people: A review of research methodologies and findings. *The Gerontologist, 11,* 90-101.

Meacham, J. A. (1980). Formal aspects of theories of development. *Experimental Aging Research, 6,* 475-487.

Meacham, J. A. (1983). Aging, work, and youth: New words for a new age of old age. In B. Bain (Ed.), *The sociogenesis of language and human conduct* (pp. 153-162). New York: Plenum Press.

Meacham, J. A. (1984). The individual as consumer and producer of historical change. In K. A. McCluskey & H. W. Reese (Eds.), *Life-span developmental psychology: Historical and generational effects* (pp. 47-71). New York: Academic Press.

Meacham, J. A., & Emont, N. C. (in press). The interpersonal basis of everyday problem-solving. In J. D. Sinnott (Ed.), *Everyday problem-solving: Theory and application.* New York: Praeger.

Meacham, J. A., & Santilli, N. R. (1982). Interstage relationships in Erikson's theory: Identity and intimacy. *Child Development, 53,* 1461-1467.

Orlofsky, J. L. (1978). The relationship between intimacy status and antecedent personality components. *Adolescence, 13,* 419-441.

Orlofsky, J. L., Marcia, J. E., & Lesser, I. M. (1973). Ego identity and the intimacy vs. isolation crisis of young adulthood. *Journal of Personality and Social Psychology, 27,* 211-219.

Piaget, J. (1960). *Psychology of intelligence.* Totawa, NJ: Littlefield, Adams.

Sampson, E. E. (1977). Psychology and the American ideal. *Journal of Personality and Social Psychology, 35,* 767-782.

Sampson, E. E. (1988). The debate on individualism: Indigenous psychologies of the individual and their role in personal and societal functioning. *American Psychologist, 43,* 15-22.

Van den Daele, L. D. (1969). Qualitative models in developmental analysis. *Developmental Psychology, 1,* 303-310.

Van den Daele, L. D. (1974). Infrastructure and transition in developmental analysis. *Human Development, 17,* 1-23.

Van den Daele, L. D. (1976). Formal models of development. In K. F. Riegel & J. A. Meacham (Eds.), *The developing individual in a changing world* (Vol. 1) (pp. 69-78). The Hague: Mouton.

van Geert, P. (1986). The structure of developmental theories. In P. van Geert (Ed.), *Theory building in developmental psychology* (pp. 51-102). Amsterdam: North-Holland.

van Geert, P. (1987). The structure of Erikson's model of the eight ages: A generative approach. *Human Development, 30,* 236-254.

Viney, L. L. (1987). A sociophenomenological approach to life-span development complementing Erikson's sociodynamic approach. *Human Development, 30,* 125-136.

Vygotsky, L. S. (1978). *Mind in society.* Cambridge: Harvard University Press.

Waterman, A. S. (1982). Identity development from adolescence to adulthood: An extension of theory and a review of research. *Developmental Psychology, 18,* 341-358.

Wohlwill, J. F. (1973). *The study of behavioral development.* New York: Academic Press.

Psychological Perspectives of Helplessness and Control in the Elderly, P.S. Fry (ed.)
© *Elsevier Science Publishers B.V. (North-Holland), 1989*

Chapter Four

ACTION-THEORETICAL APPROACHES TO THE DEVELOPMENT OF CONTROL ORIENTATIONS IN THE AGED

Friedrich E. HEIL and Günter KRAMPEN
University of Trier, FRG

Abstract

The chapter presents a short review of recent findings on the development of control orientations in adulthood and old age. The authors contend that older adults in general do not experience a lower level of control than younger adults. But there is a need to identify different developmental patterns of control orientations and the relation of these to one's psychological well-being. An action-theoretical approach to human development is proposed. Within this perspective which emphasizes the individuals' own contributions to their development, person and personality variables are specified in terms of self-related cognitions, emotions and actions. Certain conceptual differentiations of special relevance to development in old age are discussed. For example, the concepts of situational ambiguity and action frequency are considered to explain differences in the behavior of active and disengaged older people. The findings confirm that there are significant relationships between action frequency, control orientation, and life satisfaction. Long-term antecedents of control orientations are discussed in terms of the need for older persons to reconceptualize their lives in ways which take account of age-related differences in control orientations and the role of emotional evaluations of one's own development, psychological well-being, and activity.

Introduction

In addition to the established topics of biological, social and intellectual aging processes, the development of subjective control orientations and other self-related cognitions in old age has recently come into the focus of gerontological research (e.g., Baltes & Baltes, 1986). This can be seen as a consequence of the increasing attention cognitive theories of personality and development have received in the last decades. These theories--like the social-cognitive approaches of learned helplessness, self-efficacy, expectancy-value theory, attribution theory etc.--postulate, that control orientations are relevant predictors of behavior and experience. One of the attractions for psychological gerontology lies in the assumed plasticity of individual control perceptions in the life-course in general and, particularly, in adulthood and old age. Cognitive theories on psychological aging focused first on the subjective experience and evaluation of growing old, analyzing person variables like the subjective age, life satisfaction, subjective state of health etc. in the elderly (see e.g., Thomae, 1971, 1976). Recent approaches focus on social-cognitive variables like reinforcement values or goal evaluations, expectations, efficacy beliefs, cognitive plans and (re-)constructions etc. to predict the above mentioned subjective evaluations of a person's own aging process. More or less generalized control expectancies are of central importance in the set of social-cognitive variables. These expectancies involve prospective beliefs about the controllability and self-determination of subjectively relevant reinforcers and events in one's own life (internality) versus prospective beliefs about the degree to which such reinforcers and events depend on other (powerful) people, situation forces, chance factors etc.--in sum, factors which are not under control of the individual, at least under conditions of weak control (externality).

Following a short review of the more recent literature on the development of control beliefs in adulthood and old age which relate new findings to the ambiguous construct of wisdom, we will concentrate on the heuristic value and utility of an action-theoretical founded approach to human development in general, and its implications for psychological gerontology. A general outline of such a research program in developmental psychology, which emphasizes individuals' own contributions to their development, will be given. This will be done by specifying a heuristic of development-related person and personality variables in terms of self-related cognitions, emotions and actions. A special emphasis will be put on the following three topics: (1) situational ambiguity as a predictor of behavior and experience in old age, (2) frequencies of actions in old age and their relevance for changes in control orientations, and (3) the developmental antecedents of control beliefs in the elderly after retirement.

Internality and Externality of Control Orientations: Multidimensional Perception of Events in Old Age as an Aspect of Wisdom?

Recent literature reviews on the development of control orientations in adulthood (Krampen, 1987a; Lachman, 1986) verify that the findings produced with the help of the "classical" bipolar, uni-dimensional measurement approach to generalized locus of control (in the tradition of the ROT-IE; Rotter, 1966) are very inconsistent. In addition to a medium (correlative) stability of generalized control beliefs in adulthood and old age (with an average value of $r = .55$), some findings indicate increasing externality, while others indicate decreasing externality with age and some did not find any relation between locus of control and age at all. Such inconsistencies have led to the conceptualization of control orientations as a multi-facet construct and the development and application of multidimensional and/or domain-specific measures of control orientations in various research domains (see e.g., Krampen, 1982, 1987b). First of all, the results of such studies on locus of control and aging (for an overview see Krampen, 1987a; Lachman, 1986) confirm the medium correlative stability of different aspects of general and domain-specific control beliefs in adulthood and old age. It is interesting to note that these results do not point to differences in developmental stability or plasticity of control orientations in different age groups after childhood (including adolescence, early, middle and late adulthood). Secondly, the findings demonstrate that the development of control perceptions is different not only for different domains of life, but also that there is a general trend which in unselected samples points to (1) weak increases of externality, *and* (2) weak increases of internality or stability of internality in locus of control.

These inconsistent findings led Kuhl (1986) to the hypothesis that we can differentiate at least two patterns of aging in this domain of variables. The first pattern is characterized by a decrease in externality or stability of control orientations which is related to an active life, high life satisfaction, action-orientation and general well-being in old age. By contrast, the second pattern is characterized by an increase in externality which is related to low life satisfaction, depressive mood, learned and/or functional helplessness, and state-orientation in old age. The latter pattern of aging may be connected to a stereotype of wisdom in some older adults. According to Kuhl (1986) this stereotype involves focusing on state-orientations, social acceptance, and reflective, conservative, "wise" attitudes. Obviously, this type of wisdom seems to be related to some "hidden costs", e.g., to depressive symptoms, feelings of personal helplessness, and low future orientations.

The Hidden Costs of Wisdom

Within the context of the foregoing findings, the hidden costs of wisdom may be specified as an increase in the multidimensionality of factors which an individual considers as determinants of reinforcers and events in general. Indeed, this multifactorial perception of the determination of events and the consideration of many such internal/controllable as well as external/not controllable factors in expectations may be a relevant aspect of a reflective, state-oriented,

"wise" attitude.   In other words, these factors reflect the stereotypes of wisdom.

     The perception of a rather uni- versus multifactorial determina-
tion of events and of one's own development is the central content
of McKinney's (1981) dimensional personality construct of "agent
versus patient engagement style."   It also represents the central
content of Hoff and Hohner's (1986) typology of personality.   In
McKinney's terminology, the extremes of an agent versus patient
engagement style are defined as extreme internality versus externality
in self-perception, locating multifactorial perceptions of the
determination of one's own development in the middle area of this
continuum.   In contrast, Hoff and Hohner (1986) differentiate between
different types of control awareness.   The authors postulate a
normative developmental model of control awareness, the range of which
stretches from a fatalistic control awareness (no control at all) at
one end of the continuum to a unideterministic type of control
awareness (either internal or external).   It is followed by an
additive deterministic control awareness which is both internal and
external.   Finally at the end of the continuum is the interactionistic
type of control awareness characterized not only by a person's
consideration of many internal and external factors, but of their
dynamic interaction as well.

     Empirical evidence for the hidden costs of additive control
perceptions and expectancies comes from a study by Krampen, von Eye
and Brandtstädter (1987), in which the psychodiagnostic relevance of
configurations of high versus low internality (I), high versus low
powerful others control (P) and high versus low chance control (C) was
investigated.   Before and after a two-year interval, 1268 West German
adults (age range: 30 to 62 years; response rate at second testing: 81
percent) responded to three different instruments: (1) the IPC-Scales
measuring the three aspects of generalized locus of control (Krampen,
1981; Levenson, 1972), (2) a German multidimensional personality trait
inventory, and (3) a life satisfaction scale.   The results confirm
that the observed frequencies of all eight IPC-configurations are
relevant for psychodiagnostic purposes and that the IPC-scores as well
as the IPC-configurations show a medium degree of stability over two
years.   Central for the present argumentation is the fact that all
eight IPC-configurations can be discriminated from each other using
the personality traits and the life satisfaction measure.   While
persons with low scores in all three IPC-scales can be best described
with reference to the personality variables of mental health and high
life satisfaction, persons with high scores in internality, powerful
others, and chance control show many psychological deviations
including psychosomatic symptoms, depression, neuroticism, and low
life satisfaction (Krampen et al., 1987).   These findings illustrate
empirically the hidden psychological costs of multifactorial perceptions of the determination of life events and one's own development.
In other words, the hidden costs of at least an additive control
orientation, or even the costs of an interactionistic control

awareness, as postulated by Hoff and Hohner (1986), are demonstrated empirically.   Cross-sequential data from the same sample of adults concerning perceptions and expectations of control over personal development also confirm the developmental trend described before: longitudinally there is an increase of internality as well as an increase in externality in developmentrelated control perceptions (Brandtstädter, Krampen & Baltes-Götz, 1988).

In short, recent results on the development of control orientations show that older adults in general do not experience a lower level of control than younger adults.   These studies do, however, confirm the relationship between perceptions of control and one's psychological well-being.   Regardless of age (at least in adolescence and adulthood) there is a medium degree of stability in control orientations, which leaves enough latitude for plasticity of psychological aging in this domain of variables.   Within a differential gerontological approach to self-related cognitions we need to identify the antecedent variables of different developmental patterns and their psychological "costs" and "benefits."

In the section which follows we will go beyond the pure description of the development of control orientations to search for interpretations within an action-theoretical frame of reference for aging and human development.

Action-Theoretical Perspectives for the Development of Control Orientations in Old Age

From an action-theoretical perspective, individual development is conceptualized as a "central target area of personal action and control" (Brandtstädter, Krampen & Heil, 1986, p. 266).   Based on an "organismic" or "contextual" understanding of developmental psychology, an action-theoretical approach emphasizes the individuals' own contributions to their development, or to their context perceptions and their development-related cognitions, emotions, and actions within a given life-situation or context (cf. Brandtstädter, 1984; Brandtstädter et al., 1986; Chapman, 1984; Lerner & Busch-Rossnagel, 1981). However, for a better understanding of the essentials of such an approach to human development it seems necessary to elaborate on the relationship between action-theory and personality variables.

In order to bridge the gap between action-theory and constructs of personality theory Krampen (1987b, in press) proposed an *action-theoretical model of personality (AMP)*.   AMP (see Figure 1) is conceived as a further development and differentiation of Rotter's social learning theory of personality (Rotter, 1954, 1982).   By presenting a heuristic of self-related cognitions, the AMP helps to identify particular personality variables which are possible predictors of actions, action intentions, and life experiences.   Most social-cognitive   approaches   to   personality   emphasize   situation-

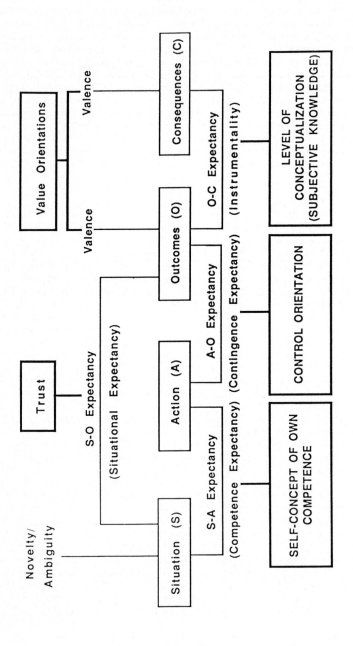

Figure 1. Heuristics of an Action-Theoretical Model of Personality (AMP; from Krampen, 1988)

specific person variables, which are derived from more or less differentiated expectancy-value models (e.g., Feather, 1982; Krampen, 1987b). The inner part of Figure 1 contains such a differentiated expectancy-value model, postulating various relations between situation-specific aspects of valences and expectancies on one side and behavior and experience on the other. The outer part of Figure 1 refers to generalizations of these situation-specific person variables, i.e., personality variables. Within the expanded framework of the inner and outer parts of the personality model described in Figure 1, it can be seen that personality variables such as self-concept of one's own competence, control orientations, level of conceptualization, trust, and value orientations are central constituents of the action-theoretical model of personality.

An Action-Theoretical Approach to Development

Getting back to developmental psychology, it now seems necessary to specify the variables of an action-theoretical approach to human development and to explicate their interrelations. In an earlier publication (Brandtstädter, Krampen & Heil, 1986), we presented a heuristic of the conceptual and functional linkages of development-related variables. Our objective was to distinguish between (1) development-related actions and control efforts, (2) affective-emotional evaluations of personal development and aging, and (3) the cognitive-motivational antecedents of these development-related actions and emotions. It should be noted that cognitive-motivational antecedents include self-related cognitions such as subjective perceptions and expectancies related to personal development and aging; personal goals and values related to development and aging; and subjective potentials for control over developmental outcomes. Thus, in an action-theoretical perspective of human development, control orientations are of both descriptive and predictive relevance. First, control beliefs are considered to be relevant predictors of development-related actions and emotions. Second, it is assumed that control perceptions are of at least medium plasticity; they change under the influence of life experience, context variables, etc.

As is evident from the action-theoretical model of personality (AMP) described in Figure 1, the conceptual and functional linkages of development-related actions, emotions, and cognitions can be further specified (see Figure 2). The time continuum of life course respectively, is split into the *personal past* and the *personal future* suggesting that the psychological conception of time and of one's own development is different from the physical conception of time. The actual psychological living situation lies somewhere between the personal past and the personal future and involves retrospective as well as prospective development-related evaluations and cognitions.

Our model of development suggests that life satisfaction and the satisfaction with one's own past development stem from retrospective

F. E. Heil & G. Krampen

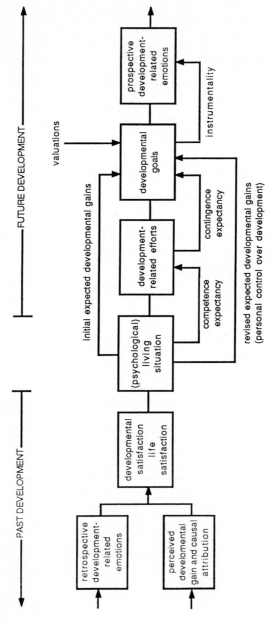

Figure 2. Heuristics of development-related cognitive, behavioral and emotional variables for the past and the future.

development-related emotions (like pride, happiness, anger, resignation) and the perceived developmental gain (i.e., the approach to or distance from personal developmental goals), which is attributed to internal and external factors. In this aspect our heuristic refers to the influential approaches of attribution theory and the model of learned helplessness. Prospectively-oriented developmental efforts and actions (e.g., self-corrective behaviors) as well as prospective development-related emotions (like optimism, hopelessness, anxiety, depressive mood) are assumed to be a function of several aspects of valences and expectancies. With regard to anticipated developmental events or anticipated approach or avoidance respectively, of subjectively evaluated developmental goals, we differentiate between initially expected developmental gains (i.e., gains not assuming changes in life-style and behavior) and revised expected developmental gains assuming development-related efforts and changes in life-style. Such development-related actions are based on subjective competence and control expectancies, as well as on personal goals and their instrumentalities for (anticipated) affective-emotional evaluations of personal development and aging.

Taken together, Figures 1 and 2 form a system of development-related and personality variables. Within this system of self-related cognitions, emotions and actions are integrated with concepts from motivation and personality psychology as well as from developmental psychology. This can be seen as a first step towards a differentiated action-theoretical model of development in adulthood and old age.

Situational Ambiguity and Control Orientations in Old Age

In the section which follows we will specify this general approach to adult development by focusing on some theoretical and conceptual differentiations of special relevance to personality development after retirement. The concepts of *subjective novelty* and *ambiguity of the living situation* will be discussed first.

Differential developmental patterns in late adulthood are described in the controversial models of disengagement theory (e.g., Cummings & Henry, 1961) and of the activity theory of aging (e.g., Havighurst, 1968; Knapp, 1977). An implication of these different approaches which has been overlooked until recently refers to the type of life-situations and experiences which are relevant for disengaged and active old people. Disengagement implies that people act primarily in well-known, subjectively well-defined, and nonambiguous situations. In contrast, the active elderly seem to be able to act and collect experiences also in subjectively new, ambiguous, and more or less ill-defined situations. For these situations adequate and complete cognitive representations (or cognitive maps), including specific expectancies and action goals have to be developed yet.

Perceived situational novelty and ambiguity have been included as a core concept in the social learning theory of personality (Rotter, 1954, 1982). It is postulated that individual behavior and experience in well-defined and known situations (so-called "strong" situations) can be predicted best by situation-specific and action-specific goals and expectancies. In this model personality variables with a relatively high stability over situations and time do not contribute substantially to the prediction of behavior in such "strong" situations. By contrast, in "weak" situations (i.e., situations that are subjectively ill-defined, novel, or ambiguous) it is assumed that the predictive value of personality variables will be high and the predictive value of situation-specific person variables will be low. The individual has no adequate cognitive structures at his disposal to deal with such situations. Thus, behavior and experience of disengaged older adults can be analyzed in terms of situation-specific person variables, whereas the behavior of active older adults can be understood in terms of generalized or domain-specific personality variables. Of crucial importance is the meaning and representation of the "psychological situation," a concept which has been overlooked for a long time in developmental psychology (see e.g., Steitz, 1982).

Action-Frequency and Control Experience in Old Age

A comparably specific approach to the development of control orientations is described by Skinner (1985). She argues that individuals influence the amount of control they subjectively experience by means of their own actions or, more precisely, their action frequencies. The application of simple probability theory leads Skinner to the conclusion that the frequency/probability of an action contributes substantially to the subjective control experience by directly affecting the probability of confirmations and disconfirmations of action-outcome expectancies. Skinner (1985) shows that there is a lot of empirical evidence in favour of systematic individual differences in the probability of actions. With respect to the elderly and retired we may again find the two extreme groups of activists and disengaged. Disengagement in older adults is linked to lower action frequency in new and ambiguous situations. On the other hand there are more (habitual) action-automatisms and experiences in well-defined situations confirming existing situation-action expectancies (i.e., competence) and action-outcome expectancies (i.e., control orientations). As a result the disengaged elderly have fewer opportunities to acquire new experiences. The avoidance of new action contexts and ambiguous situations can finally lead--in its generalization--to an increase in externality (i.e., powerful others and chance control) on the part of the older adults and a corresponding decrease in internality. The decrease in internality can also be explained in terms of the older adults' tendency to avoid novel and ambiguous situations requiring novel action-related responses. As a result, their repertoire of actions is restricted to fewer, habitual ones. By contrast, activists will have many opportunities to acquire new situation-action and action-outcome experiences by means of their own actions and by virtue of a higher frequency of participation activities. Their freedom of action is greater because they engage not only in habitual behavior but in action-autonomisms too.

A Research Demonstration

The results of one of our studies confirm our hypothesis that there are significant relations between action frequency, control orientation and life satisfaction. Before going into details, however, a short overview of this study will be given.

Subjects for our pilot study were 20 selected non-institutionalized, elderly males (M = 71.5, SD = 4.21 years; age range: 66 to 81 years) who had been retired for at least two years. The sample consisted of two subgroups: 10 men who were socially engaged in activities in the community and the church (e.g., organizing meetings, club activities, visiting/community services etc.) comprised the "activists" group in the study; the other 10 men in our sample were not engaged in similar activities, and were leading a rather passive and retired life. They comprised the "disengaged" group in the study. It is worth noting that these two subsamples were matched for (a) age (M = 71.6 and M = 71.3 years respectively), (b) education, (c) former occupation (mainly white collar workers), (d) marital status (14 married, 4 widowed, and 2 divorced), (e) mental health (no history of psychiatric or psychological treatment), and (f) physical well-being (6 men had received one hospital treatment in the last two years; 9 men received outpatient treatment only).

Data were gathered by structured interviews and questionnaires including (1) a slightly modified version of the *IPC-Scales* (Krampen, 1981; Levenson, 1972), (2) a *Daily Living Activities Inventory* (NAA; Oswald & Fleischmann, 1986), (3) the *Hopelessness-Scale* (H-Scale; Beck, Weissman, Lester & Trexler, 1974; Krampen, 1979), (4) the *Beck Depression Inventory* (BDI; Beck & Beck, 1972; Kammer, 1983), (5) a *Life Satisfaction Scale* (LZ, Löhr & Walter, 1974), and (6) retrospective ratings of the degree of self-determination and learning in four developmental phases. In the present sample the internal consistency of all scales exceeds $r(tt)$ = .67. The variables (3), (4) and (5) refer to generalized development-related emotions and evaluations; variable (2) refers to a special aspect of development-related actions in everyday life; variable (1) refers to aspects of generalized locus of control; and variable (6) refers to potential developmental antecedents of control orientations in old age with reference to the theoretical approach of Seve (1972) discussed later.

As mentioned before, the results of this study confirm Skinner's hypotheses of significant relations between action frequency and the development of control orientations. First, as expected, the "activists" have higher scores in the *Daily Living Activities*

Inventory than the "disengaged" (*t* (18) = 3.43, *p* < .01). Second, the amount of daily activities is correlated substantially (*p* < .05) with internality (*r* = .47), powerful others control (*r* = -.45), and chance control (*r* = -.61). Third, multiple regression analyses confirm the high predictive value of generalized control orientations and daily living activities for the dependent variables of actual, and retro-spectively- as well as prospectively-oriented generalized emotional evaluations of one's own development (i.e., life satisfaction, depression, and hopelessness). The results of these regression analyses are presented in Table 1.

As seen in Table 1, frequency of daily activities, high intern-ality, and low chance control are good predictors of life satisfac-tion. By comparison, low internality and high externality are good predictors of depression and high externality and few daily activities are good predictors of hopelessness. Action frequency and the amount of control subjectively perceived--which is, in part, influenced by one's own actions--are relatively good predictor variables for the development-related affective evaluations under investigation. This pattern of results confirms Skinner's (1985) hypothesis in a sample of elderly. Consequently, it seems necessary to consider the relevance of action frequency when analyzing the development of control orientations in old age.

Control Experiences in the Life Course and Control Orientations in the Aged

As discussed earlier, we postulate that novelty and ambiguity of life situations, and various development-related action orientations and emotions as well as action frequency are core concepts within an action-theoretical perspective for adult development and aging. In addition to considering some of the short-term antecedents and correlates of control orientations of older adults, we contend that long-term factors must also be considered in studies of life span development and perceptions of the self. We maintain that individuals learn control orientations through their own actions but the orienta-tions themselves are influenced by the individual's life experiences, life events, context variables etc. Derived from cross-sectional, longitudinal, retrospective and cross-sequential data, to date, most of the results refer to the development of control beliefs in childhood and adolescence (for an overview see e.g., Gilmore, 1978; Krampen, 1987a). There are fewer results which refer to the develop-mental antecedents of control orientations in early and middle adulthood (see e.g., Hoff & Hohner, 1986) and no results for old age.

If we want to investigate the long-term antecedents of control orientations in the aged, we have to consider the whole life course. This approach may help to identify some of the antecedents of differential developments in the retired and aged (i.e., why some retired become activists and others become disengaged). Seve's (1972)

Table 1. Results of the Multiple Regression Analyses (N = 20)[a]

Predictor	Life Satisfaction (LZ)			Depression (BDI)			Hopelessness		
	r_{crit}	beta	Struct.	r_{crit}	beta	Struct.	r_{crit}	beta	Struct.
Daily Activities Inventory (NAA)	.48*	.09	.74	-.32	-.27	-.45	-.47*	-.08	-.70
Internality (I)	.50*	.40	.77	-.51*	-.52	-.72	-.27	-.12	-.40
Powerful Others Externality (P)	-.28	.05	-.43	.38	.13	.54	.46*	.16	.69
Chance Control (C)	-.46*	-.35	-.71	.47*	.47	.66	.59*	.43	.88
Multiple Correlation (R)	.67*			.71*			.65*		
Multiple Determination (R²)	.45			.50			.42		

*p < .05

[a] r_{crit} = predictor-criterion correlation, beta = beta weight, Struct. = regression-factor-structure coefficient

dialectical theory of personality and personality development presents a broad, action-oriented conceptual frame of reference for such investigations. Against a marxistic background, Seve argues that personality development must be analyzed in terms of the structure of actions/activities which an individual performs in his or her life course (time structure). It is assumed that an individual biography can be characterized by normative changes in the structure of central activities. In order to characterize central features of activity structure in the four main life phases, Seve (1972) proposed the bipolar concepts of (1) self-determination *versus* determination by others, and (2) learning of new competencies and skills *versus* application of learned competencies and skills. In a given social and historical context it is argued that (a) childhood and family socialization represent a rather self-determined phase of learning; (b) activity structure in adolescence and early adulthood is more frequently determined by other people and characterized by learning new competencies and skills, i.e., in school and occupational education; (c) activities during middle adulthood and being on the job are more frequently determined by other people and require the application of learned skills; and (d) old age, i.e., the time after retirement, finally, can be seen as a rather self-determined phase of application of learned skills and competencies.

The first empirical investigation of this theory (M. Krampen, 1982) led to inconsistent results. University students and 24 older adults ($M = 75.5$ years) had to rate the degree of self-determination and the degree of learning for various typical activities in childhood, adolescence/early adulthood, middle adulthood and old age. The students' ratings were in agreement with the pattern described by Seve (1972). The ratings of the old, however, did not support Seve's hypotheses. Of course, it must be considered that the students (young adults) had to interpret all four developmental phases and the main activities related to these phases notwithstanding the fact that they had experienced only the first two phases in their real lives. Hence, it can be argued that the ratings may reflect the students' social stereotypes about the different life phases derived from their naive understanding of developmental theories (Heckhausen, Dixon & Baltes, in press). In contrast, the judgments of the elderly may reflect effects of social desirability because they had to rate their own experiences and biography retrospectively. The results of our own study with 10 active and 10 disengaged retired men confirm these interpretations and relate the core concepts of Seve's (1972) theory to the degree of perceived control in old age.

As found in our study of the 20 older adults, there are substantial correlations ($p < .05$) between the three aspects of locus of control and the ratings of self-determination in the four developmental phases described by Seve (1972). Internality is correlated positively with remembered self-determination in adolescence/early adulthood and education ($r = .48$), middle adulthood/being on the job ($r = .52$) and old age/retirement ($r = .62$). Similar but negative correlations exist between powerful others and chance control, on the one hand, and between the amount of self-determination and the last two developmental phases on the other hand. The degree of learning new skills and competencies is correlated only with internality (r = .51, p < .01) and chance control (r = -.59, p < .01) for the last developmental phase. Thus, high internality and low externality are related significantly to ratings of high self-determination in the biography, and to the opinion that one learns new skills also after retirement. The results comparing the two subgroups are even more interesting. Activists rate the degree of self-determination for adolescence, adulthood and old age, as well as the degree of learning in old age significantly higher than do the disengaged (t (18) > 2.19, p < .05).

Seve's (1972) hypothesis about the time structuring of main activity patterns in the life course was tested by means of a prediction analysis of cross classification (Von Eye & Krampen, 1987). This analysis led to a nonsignificant result (*Del* = .07, z = 0.948, p = .086) indicating that there is little agreement between Seve's description of the developmental phases and the ratings of the 20 old men in our study. However, analyzing the two subgroups separately leads to different results: the (combined) ratings of the 10 dis-engaged men conform very well to Seve's descriptions. Prediction analysis of the data of this subsample results in *Del* = .34 (z = 3.234, p < .001), indicating that there are 34 percent fewer predic-tion errors when we apply Seve's hypothesis to our data. In contrast, the results for our activist group are totally contrary to what Seve's hypothesis postulates (*Del* = -.20, z = -1.302, p = .452). The ratings of the active men diverge from the proposed description of the life course in terms of activities and time structures.

In sum, our results show that the degree of experienced and remembered self-determination (and learning new skills) in different developmental phases is correlated with the amount of subjectively perceived control in old age. However, Seve's descriptions of the life course fit only with the descriptive profiles provided by the group of the passive, disengaged elderly. Together with the findings of M. Krampen (1982), who got the same pattern of results in a sample of university students but not in an unselected sample of aged, the results of our pilot study with 20 older adults confirm our hypothesis that reduced subjectively perceived control in old age is related to a stereotype of human development and the aging process. This stereo-type includes a normative scheduling of the life course into several developmental phases with typical, socially valuated activity structures. According to this stereotype the final developmental phase may be one of disengagement, reflexivity, "wisdom" and pass-ivity. It is important to note that active elderly persons do not conceive their lives in such categories. They remember other types of time and activity structures as experienced during their lives. Of course, it must be admitted that the findings of our exploratory study of reminiscence are based on retrospective data having a rather

weak methodological foundation. However, if we want to study the life
course in its total life span, there are few methodological alternatives. Within a differential gerontology framework which emphasizes
the relativity and plasticity of psychological aging (Baltes & Baltes,
1977), our results, at least, show some different ways in which older
persons reconceptualize their lives. These different ways are
strongly related to differences in control orientations, emotional
evaluations of one's own development, psychological well-being, and
activity in the aged.

Conclusions

Our theoretical perspective for an explicit action-theoretical
approach to human development and aging shows that control orientations are by no means simply descriptive, developmental variables.
They are, in addition, predictive variables for action intentions,
actions and activities as well as affective evaluations of a person's
own developmental processes. Control orientations are strongly
related to psychological well-being, daily and social activities,
depression, hopelessness, and life satisfaction of older persons. The
concept of a differential gerontology, which focuses on interindividual differences in developmental and aging processes seems most
appropriate for this research context. The results of our exploratory
study show that the proposed action-theoretical approach to development and personality is able to describe developmental processes and
to predict behavior and experiences not only for active elderly
persons, but also for disengaged and passive elderly persons. Thus,
the model represents an integrative framework for the hitherto
contradictory approaches of disengagement theory and activity theory
to aging. Our heuristic of retrospectively- and prospectively-
oriented development-related cognitions, emotions and actions implies
hypotheses about the variables which must be considered in the
analyses of active and disengaged aging processes.

In order to optimize research on developments in old age our
action-theoretical approach points to the need for studying particular
variables such as action frequency, the degree of experienced and/or
remembered self-determination throughout the life course, factors of
situational ambiguity and novelty, as well as development-related
cognitions, perceptions, emotions and efforts in the aged. Moreover,
it is assumed that these variables should be core concepts in
application (prevention and treatment) too. Optimizing psychological
aging processes and well-being in the aged implies optimizing the
opportunities for control experiences.

These ideas and findings presented in this chapter may suggest
some ideas or concepts which should necessarily be included in such an
optimizing process. Without going into detail, it seems first
necessary to shut off a misleading and disadvantaging social stereotype of aging which denominates reflexive, state-oriented, passive

attitudes as "wise." Pursuing this stereotype may promote social acceptance, but it is related to subjective feelings of powerlessness, resignation, depression and dissatisfaction. As far as it concerns the frequency of actions in various living contexts, older persons may need assistance in acquiring more diversified life experiences. Additionally, they should be encouraged to collect experiences not only in well-known, but also in new and ambiguous action situations. A guided subjective reconception of the life course, finally, may help in the determination of central activities and possibly suggest alternatives for a more self-determined way of life in old age. Bearing in mind the heterogeneous patterns of aging, however, it should be evident that there are many possible implications for treatment and prevention which definitely need further elaboration.

References

Baltes, M. M., & Baltes, P. B. (1977). The ecopsychological relativity and plasticity of psychological aging. *Zeitschrift für Experimentelle und Angewandte Psychologie, 24,* 179-197.

Baltes, M. M., & Baltes, P. B. (Eds.) (1986). *The psychology of control and aging.* Hillsdale, NJ: Lawrence Erlbaum Associates.

Beck, A. T., & Beck, R. W. (1972). Screening depressed patients in family practice: A rapid technique. *Postgraduate Medicine, 52,* 81-85.

Beck, A. T., Weissman, A., Lester, D., & Trexler, L. (1974). The measurement of pessimism: The hopelessness scale. *Journal of Consulting & Clinical Psychology, 42,* 861-865.

Brandtstädter, J. (1984). Personal and social control over development. In P. B. Baltes & O. G. Brim Jr. (Eds.), *Life-span development and behavior Vol. 6* (pp. 1-32). New York: Academic Press.

Brandtstädter, J., Krampen, G., & Baltes-Götz, B. (1988). Kontrollüberzeugungen im Kontext persönlicher Entwicklung. In G. Krampen (Ed.), *Diagnostik von Attributionen und Kontrollüberzeugungen.* (in press) Göttingen, FRG: Hogrefe.

Brandtstädter, J., Krampen, G., & Heil, F. E. (1986). Personal control and emotional evaluation of development in partnership relations during adulthood. In M. M. Baltes & P. B. Baltes (Eds.), *The psychology of control and aging* (pp. 265-296). Hillsdale, NJ: Lawrence Erlbaum Associates.

Chapman, M. (Ed.) (1984). Intentional action as a paradigm for developmental psychology: A symposium. *Human Development, 27,* 113-144.

Cummings, E., & Henry, W. E. (Eds.) (1961). *Growing old: The process of disengagement.* New York: Basic Books.

Feather, N. T. (Ed.) (1982). *Expectations and actions.* Hillsdale, NJ: Lawrence Erlbaum Associates.

Gilmore, T. M. (1978). Locus of control as a mediator of adaptive behaviour in children and adolescents. *Canadian Psychological Review, 19,* 1-26.

Havighurst, R. J. (1968). Personality and patterns of aging. *The Gerontologist, 8,* 20-23.

Heckhausen, J., Dixon, R. A., & Baltes, P. B. (in press). Gains and losses in development throughout adulthood as perceived by different adult age groups. *Developmental Psychology.*

Hoff, E. H., & Hohner, H. U. (1986). Occupational careers, work, and control. In M. M. Baltes & P. B. Baltes (Eds.), *The psychology of control and aging* (pp. 345-371). Hillsdale, NJ: Lawrence Erlbaum Associates.

Kammer, D. (1983). Eine Untersuchung der psychometrischen Eigenschaften des deutschen Beck-Depressionsinventars (BDI). *Diagnostica, 29,* 48-60.

Knapp, M. R. (1977). The activity theory of aging. *The Gerontologist, 17,* 553-559.

Krampen, G. (1979). Hoffnungslosigkeit bei stationären Patienten. *Medizinische Psychologie, 5,* 39-49.

Krampen, G. (1981). *IPC-Fragebogen zu Kontrollüberzeugungen.* Göttingen, FRG: Hogrefe.

Krampen, G. (1982). *Differentialpsychologie der Kontrollüberzeugungen.* Göttingen, FRG: Hogrefe.

Krampen, G. (1987a). Entwicklung von Kontrollüberzeugungen: Thesen zum Forschungsstand und Perspektiven. *Zeitschrift für Entwicklungspsychologie und Pädagogische Psychologie, 19,* 195-227.

Krampen, G. (1987b). *Handlungstheoretische Persönlichkeitspsychologie.* Göttingen, FRG: Hogrefe.

Krampen, G. (1988). Toward an action-theoretical model of personality. *European Journal of Personality, 2,* 39-55.

Krampen, G., von Eye, A., & Brandtstädter, J. (1987). Konfigurationstypen generalisierter Kontrollüberzeugungen. *Zeitschrift für Differentielle und Diagnostische Psychologie, 8,* 111-119.

Krampen, M. (1982). Zur Einschätzung von Unabhängigkeit und Lerngewinn in Tätigkeiten des eigenen Lebens durch alternde Menschen. *Zeitschrift für Gerontologie, 15,* 46-49.

Kuhl, J. (1986). Aging and models of control: The hidden costs of wisdom. In M. M. Baltes & P. B. Baltes (Eds.), *The psychology of control and aging* (pp. 1-33). Hillsdale, NJ: Lawrence Erlbaum Associates.

Lachman, M. E. (1986). Locus of control in aging research. *Psychology and Aging, 1,* 34-40.

Lerner, R. M., & Busch-Rossnagel, N. A. (Eds.) (1981). *Individuals as producers of their development.* New York: Academic Press.

Levenson, H. (1972). Distinctions within the concept of internal-external control. *Proceedings of the 80th Annual Convention of the APA, 7,* 261-262.

Löhr, G., & Walter, A. (1974). Die LZ-Skala. Zur Erfassung der subjektiven Lebenszufriedenheit im Alter. *Diagnostica, 20,* 83-91.

McKinney, J.P. (1981). The construct of engagement style. In H. M. Lefcourt (Ed.), *Research within the locus of control construct Vol. 1* (pp. 359-383). New York: Academic Press.

Oswald, W. D., & Fleischmann, U. M. (1986). *Nürnberger-Alters-Inventar (NAI).* Nürnberg, FRG: Universität Erlangen-Nürnberg.

Rotter, J. B. (1954). *Social learning and clinical psychology.* Englewood-Cliffs, NJ: Prentice-Hall.

Rotter, J. B. (1966). Generalized expectancies for internal versus external control of reinforcement. *Psychological Monographs, 80* (1, no. 609).

Rotter, J. B. (1982). *The development and application of social learning theory.* New York: Praeger.

Seve, L. (1972). *Marxismus und Theorie der Persönlichkeit.* Frankfurt/Main, FRG: Verlag Marxistische Blätter.

Skinner, E. A. (1985). Action, control judgments, and the structure of control experience. *Psychological Review, 92,* 39-58.

Steitz, J. A. (1982). Locus of control as a life-span developmental process. *International Journal of Behavioral Development, 5,* 199-316.

Thomae, H. (1971). Die Bedeutung einer kognitiven Persönlichkeitstheorie für die Theorie des Alterns. *Zeitschrift für Gerontologie,* *4*, 8-18.

Thomae, H. (1976). *Patterns of aging: Findings from the Bonn longitudinal study of aging.* Basel, Switzerland: Karger.

von Eye, A., & Krampen, G. (1987). BASIC programs for prediction analysis of cross classification. *Educational & Psychological Measurement, 47,* 141-143.

Psychological Perspectives of Helplessness
and Control in the Elderly, P.S. Fry (ed.)
© *Elsevier Science Publishers B.V. (North-Holland), 1989*

Chapter Five

PERSON-ENVIRONMENT TRANSACTIONS RELEVANT TO CONTROL AND HELPLESSNESS IN INSTITUTIONAL SETTINGS

Eva KAHANA
Case Western Reserve University

Boaz KAHANA
Cleveland State University

Kathy RILEY
Cleveland State University

Abstract

This chapter presents a review of prevalent conceptualization about the impact of long term care institutionalization on personal control and well-being of the elderly. Alternative formulations which focus on learned helplessness, environmentally-induced deficits and dependency are presented in accounting for adverse psychosocial influences on residents. In an effort to extend existing formulations to also account for potentially favorable post-institutional outcomes a congruence model of personal and environmental control and dependency is presented and integrated with existing models. Physical environmental features, institutional policies and staff attitudes are proposed as salient influences which are mediated through staff behaviors to exert their effects on residents. It is proposed that congruence between patient needs and staff behavior along dimensions of control and dependency are major determinants of well-being and competence of frail elderly after institutionalization. Lack of congruence between these factors may be diminished through coping efforts of residents in environments where staff response is contingent on resident behaviors. Secondary dependency may represent a useful coping response in such environments. Where there is no contingency between staff responses and resident behaviors lack of person-environment fit cannot be altered by successful coping efforts. Consequently adverse post-institutional outcomes are likely to ensue resulting in learned helplessness, depression and other environmentally induced deficits. A brief review of intervention strategies based on alternative conceptualizations of control is provided and direction for future research in the area of person-environment transactions relevant to control and helplessness is noted.

Introduction

Long term care institutions serve the oldest and frailest segment of
the population, a group for whom issues of dependency, loss of control
and helplessness are particularly salient concerns. As such, the
institutionalized elderly represent a unique population for understanding person-environment transactions which relate to issues of
control and helplessness. Ideally the institution may be expected
to serve both prosthetic and therapeutic functions which should
enhance resident well-being (Lawton, 1980). In reality, however, much
of the literature on the impact of institutionalization documents the
negative effects of institutional life which serve to contribute to
greater dependency, helplessness and loss of control among institutionalized elders (Avorn & Langer, 1982; Barton, Baltes, Orzech, 1980;
Gubrium, 1975; Solomon, 1982; Vladek, 1980). Institutions have thus
been considered to have iatrogenic effects, and treatment programs in
institutional facilities are often directed at reducing these adverse
environmental influences (Langer & Rodin, 1976; Schulz & Hanusa,
1978).

Adverse outcomes among institutionalized aged have been attributed to institutional policies, environmental features and staff
behaviors, all of which inappropriately reduce patient control and
choices and reinforce dependency (Barton, 1982; Brody, 1977; Fish,
1986; White & Janson, 1986). At the same time we note evidence from
recent research that positive psychosocial outcomes are also possible
under conditions of institutional living (Kahana, Kahana, & Young,
1985). A critical challenge presented to gerontologists is the need
to identify the mechanisms responsible for such post-institutional
outcomes. A major aim of this chapter is to provide a better
understanding of the linkages which exist between institutional
characteristics, personal predispositions and coping efforts and
adverse personal outcomes for institutionalized elders.

The first section of this chapter is devoted to prevalent
conceptualizations and research regarding the development of adverse
psychosocial outcomes among institutionalized aged. Special emphasis
is placed on the most widely used conceptualization related to
development of learned helplessness. The second section of the
chapter presents a congruence model for understanding adverse as well
as positive post-institutional outcomes. This model is offered in an
effort to reconsider the often contradictory and disparate expectations about the role of personal and of institutional control in
psychosocial well-being of institutionalized elderly. The final
portion of the chapter outlines treatment approaches which have
utilized concepts of control and dependency in an effort to improve
mental health of the institutionalized aged.

Personal Control and Institutional Living

Institutionalization generally occurs as a function of disabilities combined with insufficient social supports to maintain the frail older person in the community (Shanas, 1979). Thus, the typical older person entering an institution is likely to be a widowed woman over the age of 80 with problems in activities of daily living (Branch & Jette, 1982). It is noteworthy that most older persons fear the prospect of institutionalization and enter long term care facilities against their wishes (Johnson & Grant, 1985). Because the decision to enter is generally made by others (or by others in consultation with the older person) (Kahana, Kahana & Young, 1985), the very occurrence of institutionalization often represents a major loss of personal control which precedes any loss of control brought about by institutional living. In addition, entry to an institution may define the older person as being incompetent and unable to exert personal choice, control, or independent behavior (Avorn & Langer, 1982).

Adverse effects have been frequently attributed to relocation to institutional settings (Kasl, 1972; Pastalan, 1983). Since these negative effects are not observed subsequent to voluntary residential moves (Lawton, 1980; Wittels & Botwinick, 1974) it is possible that lack of control may, in fact, be a major component of relocation stress involving institutional placements. It is presumed that certain institutional influences operate to diminish personal control, reinforce dependency and exaggerate rather than ameliorate manifestations of behavioral deficits among frail elders (Baltes & Baltes, 1986; Langer & Rodin, 1976; Solomon, 1982). Major underlying assumptions in developing this argument relate to defining the environment as a co-determining factor of biological decline and belief in the plasticity rather than trait-like stability of behavior (Baltes & Werner-Wahl, 1987). In an effort to elucidate control-relevant institutional influences, we will turn to a review of prevalent conceptualizations about the impact of institutionalization on the elderly.

The institution presents an ideal context for exploring the development of dependency and helplessness in late life. It provides an observable, definable and relatively constant social setting where both residents' personal characteristics and specific features of the physical and social environment may be readily delineated. Since residents are typically limited in opportunities to modify the environment or to leave the setting, analyses of person-environment transactions would most clearly portray the impact of the institution on psychosocial functioning and well-being of residents.

In an effort to go beyond explanatory models which focus primarily on adverse post-institutional outcomes a conceptual model is proposed here which allows for consideration of personal predispositions, environmental features, and post-institutional outcomes related to issues of control. In order to develop a clearer understanding of environmental impact on the institutionalized aged, we must go beyond the prevalent approach of viewing the institution as exerting a unitary influence on its inhabitants. Instead, it is useful to define specific aspects of the personal environment and link these aspects to specific personal outcomes. In terms of specific mechanisms for transmitting institutional influences, we have identified the behavior of nursing home staff as a critical mediator of social influences that have an impact on institutionalized aged. Physical environmental features, institutional policies and staff attitudes are seen as important influences which are mediated through staff behaviors to exert their effect on residents. It is suggested that congruence between patient needs and behavior of caregiver staff are major determinants of well-being and competence of the frail elderly after institutionalization. Where incongruence between institutional policies or influences and resident needs arise, residents will engage in diverse efforts to cope with such incongruence. In settings where environmental responses (i.e. staff behaviors) are contingent upon residents' behavior, such coping efforts will succeed in diminishing adverse outcomes. In contrast, in non-contingent environments residents' coping efforts will have no impact on staff behavior, and learned helplessness, depression and excess disability are likely to develop in the residents.

The concept of control plays a central role in the proposed model and is a relevant characteristic of both the person and the environment. Consideration of the older adult's preferences for personal control and self determination is critical in determining the amount and kind of environmental supplies and assistance that are necessary for optimal post-institutional outcomes. It is important to place such personal needs for control in the context of institutional control, which may be construed as a homogenizing force to insure conformity of residents to the policies and norms of the institution.

The proposed congruence model will be developed in greater detail after a review of prevalent conceptualizations about control-relevant institutional influences.

Prevalent Conceptualizations Regarding Control and Institutionalization

Learned Helplessness and Institutionalization

The concept of learned helplessness has served as a useful explanatory construct and has received a great deal of attention in recent years in considering the impact of institutionalization on the elderly. The concept of "helplessness" conjures up many common images, including the enfeebled, apathetic, powerless older person. This term may help conceptualize the behaviors seen in the institutionalized elderly. The "learned" component of learned helplessness is intriguing because it implies that institutional policies and care-givers may "teach" the older adult to be helpless. On an optimistic note, it further implies that helplessness may be unlearned. Thus, the learned helplessness paradigm is appealing from a humanistic, as well as theoretical/scientific viewpoint, as we try to understand the cognitive, behavioral, and emotional deficits so often observed in the institutionalized elderly.

The concept of learned helplessness has been put forth in two separate forms which may or may not be linked in research efforts (Costello, 1986; Kennelly, Hayslip, & Richardson, 1985; Pinder, 1983; Seligman, 1975). Concerned gerontologists employ the concept as an appealing interpretive tool in their research and commentary on the life situations of frail elderly persons in institutional settings. Generally, the concept of helplessness is used as an explanation of observed decline in the psychosocial well-being of these individuals. Yet there is little empirical research documenting the actual development of learned helplessness among older adults residing in long term care facilities (Avorn & Langer, 1982; Taylor, 1979; White & Janson, 1986).

In contrast to this generalized definition and use of learned helplessness, there is a carefully articulated theoretical formulation advanced by Seligman and his colleagues (Abramson, Seligman & Teasdale, 1978; Seligman, 1975) that refers to a specific set of behaviors brought about when an individual is exposed to uncontrollable events with the expectation that they will continue to be uncontrollable. This formulation hypothesizes an association between learned helplessness and depression. The helplessness model of depression proposes that four distinct deficits derive from learned helplessness: deficits in motivation, cognition, self-esteem and affect. Experimental research, generally involving young persons in laboratory settings, has substantiated some of the basic tenets of Seligman's theory. In addition some studies have documented the development and behavioral manifestations of learned helplessness in "natural" or community samples of young and older adults (Hochhauser, 1981; Huesmann, 1978; Kennelly et al., 1985; Priddy, Teitelman, Kivlighan & Fubermann, 1982).

In this chapter we will discuss Seligman's definition of learned helplessness, and how this term has both potential positive and negative implications when applied to the elderly. In addition, we will discuss the interactionist model that we have been using to understand the behaviors of institutionalized older persons. Our aim is to help develop a bridge between an elegant and appealing theory and the everyday usage of the term "helplessness", in the context of understanding post-institutional outcomes of the aged.

There are a number of valid and useful ways of examining environmental conditions in institutions and psychosocial outcomes of the elderly that do not invoke Seligman's conceptualization of learned helplessness. These include the constructs of control, perceived choice, depression, and dependency. Each of these constructs has produced an independent area of research, but these constructs may also be seen as components of the learned helplessness paradigm. An examination of the ways in which learned helplessness has been used in gerontological work indicates that at least one unfortunate outcome of the use of this term is the perpetuation of the stereotype of the elderly (especially those in institutions) as depressed, apathetic, and overly dependent (Solomon, 1982). Integration of Seligman's framework with the congruence model suggested here permits considera-tion of positive as well as negative post-institutional outcomes for residents.

An extensive search of relevant literature conducted in 1988 revealed that there has been fairly substantial interest over the past 10 years in applying the concept of learned helplessness to geron-tological concerns. However, only a minority of published articles focused on Seligman's full paradigm (Hochhauser, 1981; Kennelly, et al., 1985; Priddy et al., 1982; Solomon, 1982), while the majority invoke learned helplessness as a corollary to, or comment on studies of related issues in the aged, such as depression or lack of control in institutional settings (Avorn & Langer, 1982; Schulz & Hanusa, 1978; White & Janson, 1986). Furthermore, a number of research dissertations have included the helplessness concept in their studies of depressed or institutionalized older adults (Barton, 1982; Fish, 1986; Maiden, 1981; Patrick, 1985).

The logical appeal of the term learned helplessness and the documented interest in this framework indicate that it may be quite useful to the researcher or practitioner who wants to explore person-environment transactions, especially in the case of the institutional-ized elderly individual. However, the involved nature of the learned helplessness paradigm and its reformulations have made the operationa-lization and application of this theory to research somewhat problema-tic. Detailed reviews of the learned helplessness paradigm have been published (Abramson, et al. 1978; Huesmann, 1978). However, three issues are particularly relevant to our discussion. The first relates to the manifestations of helplessness in depression; the second, to the attributions made by individuals; the third area concerns the non-contingent or uncontrollable events that have been at the base of learned helplessness theory. While it is generally known that depression is the most common affective disorder among the aged, if we are going to invoke learned helplessness as an explanatory construct, then we should also work to identify the specific conditions and components of depression as outlined in the theory. These include demonstrating uncontrollable events or non-contingency between personal and environmental response, as well as the motivational, cognitive, affective, and self-esteem deficits of the helpless individual. This is not to suggest that a learned helplessness model of depression is the preferred way of conceptualizing depression in the aged, but it may provide a very useful method of linking environ-

mental conditions and staff behavior to the behaviors of institutionalized older adults.

Recent Modifications of Learned Helplessness Paradigm

A major refinement in Seligman's original theory is the emphasis
placed on the conclusions reached by the helpless individual under
conditions of non-contingency. Of greatest relevance here is the
distinction between personal versus universal attributional style.
Personal helplessness exists when the individual believes that he or
she has failed to achieve control because of an internal fault or
deficit.   In contrast, universal helplessness involves the attributional conclusion that everyone in the same situation would also fail
to demonstrate control over the outcome. Felton & Kahana (1974) have
demonstrated that external locus of control was related to positive
well-being among the residents of a home for the aged. This finding
is consistent with Seligman's parallel hypothesis that personal
attributions regarding lack or loss of control (an internal locus of
control) are likely to lead to greater deficits in self-esteem and
more intense depressive affect in the helpless individual than a
universal attribution.

An additional demonstration that an institutionalized older
person is experiencing learned helplessness would be the identification of non-contingent conditions in the environment. Seligman and a
host of other researchers have created non-contingent conditions in
laboratory settings and then proceeded to measure the deficits
associated with learned helplessness (Huesmann, 1978; Kennelly, et
al., 1985). It is in this area that gerontological research has been
most limited by failing to demonstrate empirically that non-contingent
conditions actually exist for the elderly (see Baltes, Horn, Barton,
Orzech, & Lago, 1983; Solomon, 1982; White & Janson, 1986). Rather
than assuming that institutional environments are characterized by
non-contingencies and lack of individual control, researchers need to
demonstrate that such conditions exist and produce the expected
effects.

Finally, the modified concepts of learned helplessness and non-
contingency require that the individual realize and learn to expect
that the behaviors available to him or her will have no impact on
achieving a highly desirable outcome, or in preventing one that is
highly aversive. Thus, in the case of the institutionalized older
person, it be must demonstrated that he or she feels unable to
influence events. Furthermore, these events must be meaningful and
relevant in order for learned helplessness to ensue. Thus, the loss
of control over events such as meal time, bedtime, and recreational
activities will lead to helplessness only if they are highly valued by
the individual.

Applications in Gerontology

The degree to which published gerontological studies include each of the components of the formal learned helplessness theory is varied. This diversity is even more pronounced in the unpublished dissertations. For the most part, the process of aging itself, accompanied by many life events and losses, has been described as leading to learned helplessness and its accompanying behavioral deficits (Avorn, 1983). In addition, institutions have been characterized as highly constraining environments which deprive elderly residents of control over most aspects of their lives (Baltes & Baltes, 1986; White and Janson, 1986). Learned helplessness is then presumed to result in increased frailty for these aged persons (Pinder, 1983; Solomon, 1982). This notion, however, does not receive empirical support in so far that internal locus of control does not appear to decline with age during the adult life span (Lao, 1974; Ryckman & Malikoski, 1975; Kuypers, 1972). In one of the few published studies to experimentally produce learned helplessness in older adults, Avorn & Langer (1982) concluded that depression and helplessness may be responsible for frequently observed cognitive deficits among institutionalized adults. Other researchers have linked the negative effects of forced relocation and the concomitant loss of control to learned helplessness and mortality among the elderly. Solomon (1982) has identified characteristics of health care settings that are likely to lead to learned helplessness, including stereotyping by staff, the effects of unequal personal exchange, and the adoption of the sick role by some older adults.

Although the scenarios postulated by such authors as Solomon (1982) and others are logical, they do not demonstrate that learned helplessness actually exists in older individuals who have been relocated, hospitalized, or institutionalized. While it is not difficult to demonstrate the lack or loss of control inherent in negative life events such as widowhood or institutionalization (Langer & Rodin, 1976; Schulz, 1976) these situations can be distinguished from the non-contingent conditions that lead to helplessness. Furthermore, as the concept of Person-Environment Fit indicates, (Kahana, 1982) it is most likely that the match or mismatch of individual expectations for control of the environment and the actual availability of environmental resources will determine whether or not negative psychosocial outcomes will occur in the institutionalized elderly.

The "Environmentally Induced Deficits" Paradigm

Thus far, we have been discussing learned helplessness as a means of studying person-environment transactions and the psychological condition of older persons in institutions. An alternative approach is one that the authors have called the "environmentally-induced deficits" model.

When institutional policies or staff exert influences which are aimed to facilitate efficient management of residents through promoting resident dependency and institutional control, then we may find "environmentally-induced deficits" in individual residents. These deficits are likely to be manifested in low self-esteem, morale, or other psychosocial outcomes. One specific outcome may be the development of "excess disability". This term was defined by Kahn (1975) and further developed by Brody and her colleagues (1977). Simply put, excess disability refers to a level of functioning that fails to reach the level indicated by actual physical or cognitive impairments. Relevant behaviors would include those found on activities of daily living scales and other related measures. In related work, Avorn and Langer (1982) have described "induced disability" in nursing homes, in which they demonstrated task performance and self-esteem deficits among residents who were given unnecessary assistance with a problem-solving task. In the same study, residents who were given encouragement but no assistance, demonstrated better task performance than the "helped" group.

The common link between the models of learned helplessness and environmentally-induced deficits described thus far is one that will be developed in detail in this chapter -- that is, when the individual needs, preferences, and wishes of the institutionalized aged are ignored, denied, or refuted, negative outcomes are likely to develop. The source of this lack of environmental responsiveness may include negative stereotyping of the elderly by staff (Solomon, 1982), impatience of staff in overseeing an older person's slow performance of instrumental activities and highly constraining institutional policies (Fish, 1986; White & Janson, 1986). Even more basically, the message of incompetence that often accompanies institutionalization itself (Avorn & Langer, 1982) may be associated with negative outcomes, for example, excess disability, learned helplessness, environmentally-induced deficits, or induced disability. The environmentally-induced deficits model may be viewed as a variant of the learned helplessness paradigm and in spite of its promise and salience has not been fully developed in gerontological inquiry.

Dependency in an Institutional Setting

In seeking to understand the dependency of institutionalized aged, it has been generally assumed that dependency-inducing staff behaviors are responsible for diminished levels of patient functioning (Baltes, 1982; Solomon, 1982). Yet, dependence on others for care is a central and inherent characteristic of the institutionalized older person (Kalish, 1969).

There has been an ongoing controversy among gerontologists and social scientists about the impact of diverse institutional features and of staff behaviors on dependency of the aged. According to some experts, staff behavior aimed at meeting dependency needs of residents is both necessary and desirable (Goldfarb, 1969). Others argue that dependency-inducing staff behaviors make management of patients easier but are likely to create greater dependency and induce learned helplessness in patients (Solomon, 1982; Raps, Peterson, Jones, & Seligman, 1982).

An important advance in considering the alternative functions of dependency in an institutional context is reflected in recent work of Baltes & Reisenzein (1986) and White & Janson (1986). Moving beyond consideration of dependency needs as predisposing factors or dependency only as a deleterious outcome of institutionalization, these authors consider the potential adaptive value of dependent responses and consider dependency as a useful secondary control mechanism in institutional settings. They argue and cite research to demonstrate that dependent behaviors are likely to result in contingent reinforcement, attention and interactive behaviors from staff in institutional settings. In this latter view dependency may be construed as a useful and proactive coping mechanism rather than a personal predisposition or an environmentally-induced deficit. This orientation is a very significant innovation in the direction of viewing frail elderly as potent actors rather than simply as passive reactors to environmental influences.

Proposed Congruence Based Conceptual Model

Stemming from an ecological framework, a congruence model of personal dependency needs and staff behavior is proposed which would permit integration of the previously suggested diverse models. In this model, we adopt an interactionist approach to understanding the relationship between dependency and well-being among institutionalized older persons. We attempt to move beyond the relatively simplistic assertion that institutionalization creates dependency, and we consider not only environmental conditions, but also the initial needs and preferences of the individual with regard to dependency. In this view, positive outcomes would be most likely when behaviors of significant staff are congruent with dependency needs of particular residents. Such expectations are consistent with Clark's (1969) suggestion that greater autonomy may be generated for the elderly when their dependency needs are met first. Accordingly, poor person-environment (P-E) fit between staff behavior and resident needs regarding independence or dependency may account for the development of a variety of negative outcomes. Conversely a good fit should lead to positive outcomes.

The congruence model has its roots in Lewin's (1951) theory that behavior is a function of the relationship between the person and his/her environment and in Murray's (1938) need-press model of human behavior. It is also consistent with Piaget's (1950) concepts of the child's continual adaptation to the environment during growth and development (e.g., assimilation and accommodation). In Murray's model it is assumed that environmental press provides a situational counterpart to internalized needs and environmental press may facilitate or hinder the gratification of needs. The model suggest that consideration of the fit between personal needs or preferences and environmental demands or supplies improves prediction of outcomes beyond that possible by consideration of only personal or environmental factors. Furthermore, personal and environmental characteristics are to be considered along commensurate dimensions (Kahana, 1975).

According to the congruence model, individuals are most likely to seek and be found in environments that are congruent with their needs. Dissonance between press and need is seen as leading to modification of the press or to the individual's leaving the field in free choice situations. When such a choice is unavailable and the individual must function in a dissonant milieu, stress and discomfort follow (Stern, 1970). The concept of congruence or person-environment fit has been suggested as a fruitful theoretical scheme for understanding the impact of environments on the well-being of older people (French, Rodgers & Cobb, 1974; Kahana, 1975).

For older people, whose adaptive capacities may be diminished, person-environment fit is especially important. As outlined by Lawton (1980) in his environmental docility hypothesis, the importance of the environment is likely to be magnified for vulnerable individuals. Furthermore, older persons have far fewer options than do younger persons for leaving or changing their environments in situations where lack of fit produces stress. Whenever there is a lack of congruence between the individual's needs and the environment, various adaptive strategies are called upon to increase this fit (see the section on coping below). A detailed exposition of the concept of person-environment fit is provided in French et al., 1974; Kahana, 1982; Kahana, Liang & Felton, 1980. The conceptual models reviewed are depicted in Figure 1.

Elements of the Congruence Model of Control

Based on the larger conceptual model outlined above, a specific conceptualization is proposed here. In order to integrate the proposed model with existing formulations about learned helplessness Figure 2 depicts how congruence operates under alternative environmental conditions of environmental non-contingency and under conditions of contingent environmental control. It is suggested by our model that environmental influences on personal well-being are likely to be mediated through behavioral indications displayed by significant others. Accordingly, it is hypothesized that both institutional policies and staff attitudes are likely to be translated through staff behaviors and through environmental ecology into significant environmental influences which impact on the elderly patient. Specifically, it is proposed that institutional policies and physical

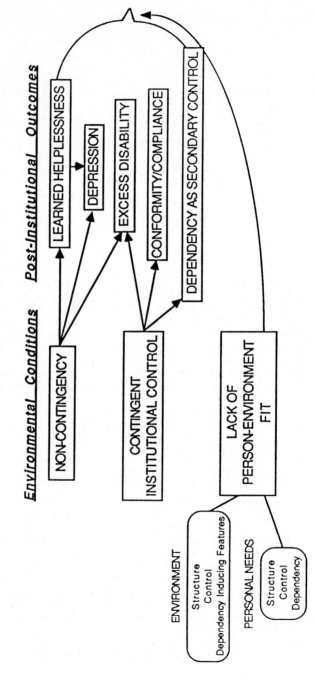

FIGURE 1
MODELS OF INSTITUTIONAL INFLUENCES RELEVANT TO
CONTROL DERIVED FROM LITERATURE

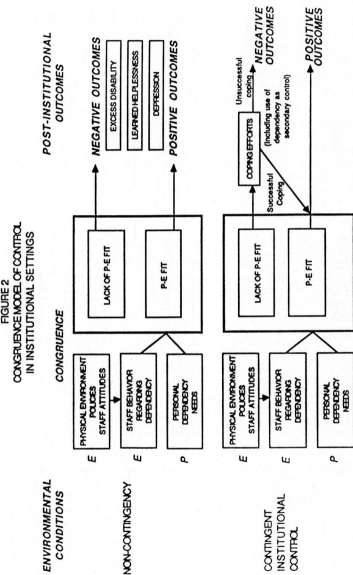

FIGURE 2
CONGRUENCE MODEL OF CONTROL
IN INSTITUTIONAL SETTINGS

environmental features that permit choice and autonomy for residents are likely to translate into independence-inducing behaviors on the part of the staff. Conversely, institutional policies and environmental features which limit patient freedom and choices are likely to translate into dependency-inducing or "caretaking" staff behaviors. Similarly, staff attitudes which reflect beliefs about elderly clients as dependent, or requiring clear structure and extensive services are likely to result in dependency-inducing behaviors.

It is important to note that in the proposed model no value judgments are attached to dependency/versus independence-inducing environmental and staff factors. Either may be expected to result in positive or negative patient outcomes depending on their interaction with patient characteristics (Brody, 1973).

Personal satisfaction with care, better mental health and a sense of competence are all expected to result from the fit between patient-dependency needs and characteristics of the social environment. Thus it is proposed that the competence of frail older adults may be best maintained or enhanced when their dependency needs are met. Alternatively, those with strong preferences for retaining a sense of autonomy may benefit when provided with choices and opportunities to control their environment and attend to their own needs. In this sense the proposed model allows us to reconcile alternative expectations about the value of meeting dependency needs versus fostering independence in long term care facilities for the frail elderly (Clark, 1969). Furthermore, our model is consistent with Brody's (1973) observation that neither dependence nor independence should be negatively evaluated as characteristics of the aged.

To the extent that congruence exists it is anticipated that clients will not develop excess disability as shown by manifesting dependent behavior and lack of competence in activities of daily living. When an incongruence between personal dependency needs and staff responses occurs due to staff doing too little or too much for a given client, competence is expected to diminish and an increase in instrumental dependency is anticipated. These expectations fit in with the general tenets of learned helplessness theory (Seligman, 1975).

In addition to considering outcomes as simple functions of P-E fit we also propose consideration of the role of personal coping efforts in enhancing lack of P-E fit. In contingent environments where coping efforts and personal responses of residents have an impact on staff behaviors, such environmental opportunities for enhancing P-E fit exist. In contrast, in non-contingent environments where there is no environmental response to resident behaviors, coping efforts would likely cease and learned helplessness and depression would develop. Dependency as a form of secondary control may serve useful functions in environments characterized by contingent environmental control and it may reduce stress posed by lack of P-E fit.

The remainder of this chapter will focus on the components of the person-environment fit model (Kahana, 1982) by delineating specific aspects of the individual's needs and preferences as they relate to control and independence/dependence (person variables), as well as those aspects of the environment that serve to meet these needs (environment variables). These environmental influences have been defined as institutional policies, the physical environment and the social environment, including both staff attitudes and behavior. Efforts to cope with lack of P-E fit will be noted. Post-institutional outcomes will be related to congruence/incongruence between individual needs and environmental responses.

Person Variables Related to Dependency

One important source of dependency among institutionalized elderly is based on disabilities which arise from residents' physical and or mental impairments. Such dependency may be referred to as functional dependency, and includes needs for assistance with activities of daily living such as dressing, eating or toileting.

Emotional need for dependency represents another dimension of dependency which may be viewed as an important feature of personality throughout the life span. Differentiation, separation and autonomy have traditionally been seen by developmental theorists as hallmarks of psychological development (Giele, 1980). Gould's (1972) characterization of the unique features of later life refer to older persons' freedom to act as truly autonomous individuals during this life stage. Cohler (1983) argues that fulfillment of needs for autonomy represents an important aspect of late life psychological development. In a study of elderly residents of San Francisco, Clark (1969) found that the elderly place a great premium on maintaining a sense of independence and such values of independence and self-reliance are deeply ingrained in the American culture (Clark, 1969).

On the other hand, evidence for a "dependency model" of social interaction in late life comes from studies of personality change versus continuity, indicating a more passive orientation by the aged than by younger persons (Riley & Foner, 1968). Typologies such as the "passive-dependent" personalities of the Kansas City studies of adult life (Neugarten, 1964) and the "rocking chair men" of Reichard, Livson and Peterson's study (1962) represent prototypes of dependent adaptation to aging. Accordingly, Baltes, et al. (1983) argue that dependence is not only a conspicuous characteristic of early childhood but also of old age. This notion supports work by Havighurst (1973) which suggests that older adults exhibit great needs for succorance. According to many researchers, increased dependency reflects increased frailty and vulnerability of the aged (Exton-Smith & Evans, 1977; Kalish, 1969). Conversely, some mental health professionals and researchers consider dependency in later life to be a healthy and desirable state (Berezin, 1963).

Recent work of Baltes & Werner-Wahl (1987) draws a useful distinction between two different forms of dependency. One type of dependency reflects adverse outcomes and helplessness while another may comprise a proactive coping modality (i.e., getting others to provide help), allowing the older person to conserve limited energies for selective activities. Both excessive needs for autonomy or dependency have been viewed as problematic (Brody, 1973). When the older person enters an institutional facility, environmental demands and opportunities come into play that may either meet dependency or autonomy needs or present obstacles to the fulfillment of such needs. The significant factor is the environment's potential for meeting the resident's autonomy or dependency needs.

Environmental Variables Related to Dependency

Goffman's (1961) framework of the total institution has long served as the classic theoretical underpinning of research focusing on social environments in institutional settings. This approach has yielded a useful and sensible conceptual framework, but has proven to be forbiddingly difficult to operationalize. One great problem has been posed by the lack of guidelines for categorizing the institutional milieu into measurable units or elements. A second problem relates to treating the institution and its staff in a unitary fashion, assuming that a general set of staff norms uniformly affect all residents. Smaller units of analysis allow for less global and more readily quantifiable data on elements of the institutional milieu which lead to development of learned helplessness or other adverse outcomes for elders.

Lawton (1980) has provided a more pragmatic classification scheme of environments which is useful for consideration of the impact of environments on social behavior. The *personal environment* refers to specific "significant others" surrounding or available to the older person. The *group environment* refers to social phenomena exerted by the environment which transcend individual characteristics of personal or physical attributes of the milieu. These include social norms, reference groups, or group pressures for conformity. Thus, individual staff members are defined as the significant others surrounding the resident. Furthermore, institutional norms and policies (comprising Lawton's group environment) may be considered as they impact on both significant staff and the dependence or independence of the individual residents.

Group Environment: Policies

Previous research (Lawton, 1980) has generally focused on the impact of institutional policies on resident well-being with only minimal attention directed at the impact of institutional policies on staff attitudes and behaviors (Kahana & Kiyak, 1984). But institutional norms and policies constitute environmental influences which are likely to affect both staff behavior and resident outcomes. Institutional policies, as part of the social environment, have been considered as potential predictors of the degree of intimacy or distance between staff and residents. These policies can regulate the degree of contact and the type of interactions occurring among residents and also between staff and residents (Lieberman & Tobin, 1983).

In settings where options and freedom of choice are limited, residents have been found to have lower levels of self-esteem and psychosocial well-being than in those settings which are not so limited (Moos & Lemke, 1984). Similarly, Lieberman (1974) found better post-institutional adjustments among elderly residents in institutions whose policies gave residents a sense of control and autonomy. Greater latitude of choice has been shown to increase life satisfaction (Hulicka, Morganti & Cataldo, 1975; Langer & Rodin, 1976), and to improve the psychological and physical status of residents (Langer & Rodin, 1976; Schulz, 1976). Harel (1981) found that allowing nursing home residents to have more opportunities to exercise choice and responsibilities is important in determining morale, life satisfaction, and satisfaction with treatment offered to them. It may be anticipated that dependency-inducing policies (e.g., not permitting residents to make their own beds) would likely affect staff behavior (i.e., staff would assume caretaking function) and contribute to resident dependency.

Moos and Igra (1980) developed the *Multiphasic Environmental Assessment Procedure* (MEAP) and used it to determine environmental effects on residents' perceptions of seven characteristics of institutional social environments. Included among these characteristics was "independence," which demonstrated significant and positive correlations with five dimensions of the policy and programmatic resources of the institution as measured by the MEAP. The independence factor in the MEAP measures the degree to which residents are encouraged to exercise responsibility and self-direction. These variables accounted for the largest proportion of variance with respect to resident independence and resident influence. Moos and Igra (1980) pointed out that the policy and program factors are probably most amenable to change. This research demonstrates influences of institutional policies on resident control and dependency.

Marlowe (1973) found that institutionalized elderly showed improvements in functioning in those environments which encouraged

autonomy and resident control over their lives, offered less succorance (did not foster dependency by doing things which individuals
could do for themselves), and did not expect docility or passivity.
Segal and Moyles (1979) examined the effects of management style on
the development of institutional dependency. They studied facilities
described either as *client-centered* (placing responsibility for
decision-making on the resident) or *management-centered* (stressing
structure and following rules). Three measures of dependency were
employed: (1) resident's perception of obligation to seek approval for
routine daily activities; (2) resident's apathy, manifested in the
wish to remain indefinitely in the institution; and (3) resident's
perception of obstacles to leaving the institution. These researchers
found that, in the management-centered facilities, the three measures
of dependency were interrelated, whereas in the client-centered
facilities they were not. They concluded that a strongly interrelated
pattern of dependency is produced in settings that emphasize a
controlling management-centered environment. This corresponds, albeit
indirectly, to the observation of Moos and Igra (1980) that policy
choice is related to residents' independence.

Although research generally supports the positive functions of
independence-supporting policies in institutions, Lawton and Nahemow
(1973) acknowledge the need for an interactional framework suggesting
that environments for the elderly should encourage the exercise of
skills without over-taxing patients' tolerance for stress. There have
been only limited efforts to test a congruence model in regard to
institutional policies and resident dependency needs. One study by
Kahana, Liang & Felton (1980) demonstrated that fit between institutional characteristics (including policies) along control dimensions
and personal preferences for control were better predictors of
resident morale than either person or environmental characteristics
alone.

Physical Environment

Although the importance of the physical environment in shaping
behaviors of participants is increasingly recognized (Lawton, 1980)
specific studies investigating the role of physical environmental
features in influencing both institutional staff and residents have
been limited. Byerts (1973) has called attention to architectural
features which can increase functional independence of residents.
Thus, barriers and hazards such as steps, slippery surfaces, and poor
lighting provide useful examples of environmental features which limit
independent activities of functionally impaired or vulnerable aged.
On the other hand, provision of prostheses through color coding,
ramps, grab bars, clearly demarcated spaces, and reachable light
switches, would likely foster independent behaviors in residents. The
use of orienting devices such as clocks and calendars also has been
demonstrated to foster autonomous behavior by institutionalized
elderly (Lawton, 1980). The architectural design of the home in terms

of placing dining areas close to or at a distance from residents' rooms is also likely to impact both on staff behavior and resident independence-dependence. Where the physical environment requires that staff provide assistance to residents, more dependency-inducing behaviors are likely to result. Thus, the physical setting may exert its influence on resident behaviors so as to promote independence or dependence.

Personal Environment

For the majority of institutionalized elderly, staff comprise the most consistent and important interpersonal contact (Gottesman & Bourestom, 1974). Thus Lawton's (1980) concept of personal environment referring to significant others surrounding the older person largely applies to staff influences.

The importance of staff attitudes and staff behavior for determining quality of care in institutions has been almost universally acknowledged (Baltes & Baltes, 1986; Lawton, 1980). Thus, it is generally assumed that positive staff attitudes and behavior reflect high quality of care and thereby improve patient satisfaction and outcomes. However, the nature of the implied linkages has not been subjected to specific empirical research and is largely implicit.

Researchers have generally relied on aggregate measures of attitudes or behaviors of different levels of staff (eg. professional, para-professional staff) or they have attempted to develop modal indices of staff behavior (for overview, see Kahana & Kiyak, 1984). Accordingly, quality of care in a given facility is generally defined by prevailing norms of staff/patient relationships, staff turnover or staff education. Yet, both common wisdom and more qualitative studies reveal that not all residents in a given facility share the same social environment. Those hospitalized patients who are cared for by a kindly and empathetic nurse may have an entirely different view of their hospital stay than would persons cared for by a discontented or uncaring individual. The "personal" social environment of a resident in an institution is most likely to be defined by the actions of those staff members caring for that individual (Felton & Kahana, 1974). Thus, in examining post-institutional outcomes such as excess disability or learned helplessness, the older individual's personal social environment must be examined if we are to understand fully the role of the institution in the development of negative psychosocial or emotional outcomes.

Staff Attitudes. Negative attitudes of service providers toward elderly clients have frequently been noted in the gerontological literature (Davis, 1968, Schwartz, 1974; Tuckman & Lorge, 1954). Such negative attitudes have been assumed, but not yet proven, to be responsible for the poor quality of care often received by institutionalized elders. A review of the gerontological literature, however, reveals inconsistent findings about the determinants and sequelae of attitudes toward the elderly.

Gerontologists working in the area of staff attitudes and behavior have generally hypothesized a dynamic interaction between staff attitudes and behaviors. Research by Kahana and Kiyak (1984) lends partial support to the link between implicit staff attitude and staff behavior. There is little available research, however, to tell us whether this dynamic interaction between staff attitudes and their behavioral manifestations affects the client's competence or well-being. The staff members' perceptions about residents' competence or dependency which are inconsistent with the perceptions of the residents themselves represent one important source of problems. A study by Noelker (1975) found a significant discrepancy between the beliefs of staff and residents regarding resident dependency. Whereas residents generally portrayed an independent self-image, staff typically viewed them as dependent. It may be anticipated that residents' self-concepts are likely to change more quickly in the course of institutional living than are the staff members' beliefs about the residents.

Staff Behavior. The importance of staff behaviors as determinants of quality of care has been widely recognized in the field of social gerontology (Baltes & Reisenzein, 1986; Kahana, 1975; Tobin and Lieberman, 1976). Documentation of adverse effects of staff neglect or coercive staff behaviors has come largely from qualitative studies often employing participant observation (Goffman, 1961; Gubrium, 1975; Henry, 1968). These studies have emphasized dehumanizing and even malevolent interactions between caretakers and residents, and have called attention to depersonalizing aspects of institutional living (Kahana and Coe, 1969). Staff behavior has often been portrayed as being aimed at efficient patient management rather than consideration of patients' needs and preferences or restoration to higher levels of functioning (Gottesman and Bourestom, 1974). On the other hand, it may be argued that qualitative observations tend to highlight atypical behaviors while placing less stress on routine or normative interactions. One noteworthy attempt to develop behavioral criteria for quality of care is a study by Gottesman and Bourestom (1974). In their study, a remarkable absence of meaningful interaction between staff and residents was generally observed and considered to be responsible for resident apathy and helplessness.

It has been suggested that learned helplessness is one of many negative effects of staff attitudes and behaviors that convey the message to institutionalized elderly persons that they have little or no control over response outcomes (Solomon, 1982). Raps, Peterson, Jones and Seligman (1982) accepted the assumption that hospitals force patients to relinquish control over many daily functions (see Taylor, 1979), and subsequently documented increases in cognitive and emotional deficits. Such impairments were interpreted to reflect learned helplessness among patients who were hospitalized. Raps et

al. (1982) argue that behavioral deficits are likely to be manifestations of helplessness and environmentally-induced dependency.

Additional research in this area has been conducted by M. Baltes
and her collaborators (Baltes, Horn, Barton, Orzech & Lago, 1983;
Baltes, & Reinsenzein, 1986; Barton, Baltes & Orzech, 1980) focusing
on staff behavior in nursing homes. These studies identified
dependence versus independence-inducing staff behavior as the critical
variable affecting the life styles of residents. Findings suggested
that behavior of nursing home residents may be modified and that
behavior is generally responsive to environmental inputs and contacts.
Their research has been conducted largely in a learning theory
framework wherein elderly patients were defined as responding to
various environmental contingencies generated by the staff and other
residents.

In one observational study of transactions between residents and
staff during nursing care (Baltes, Burgess & Stewart, 1980), residents' dependent behaviors were found to be reinforced by staff.
Independent behaviors, in contrast, were not reinforced and furthermore, tended to be met by dependency-inducing staff behavior. The
authors suggest that their findings reflect the self-reinforcing
nature of dependent behavior on the part of institutionalized elderly
and the lack of reinforcement of autonomous behavior. A later study
(Baltes et al., 1983), involving a more extended observation and a
wider range of social partners, generally confirmed results of the
earlier report regarding the prevalence of dependency-inducing
behavior on the part of social partners of the institutionalized aged.
These studies by Baltes and her associates demonstrated that independence versus dependency-inducing behavior on the part of staff
represents an important context for the study of resident independence
or dependence. They have also demonstrated the feasibility of
observing dependency-inducing behavior of staff in diverse institutional contexts.

Behavioral observations of nursing home staff in response to
dependency inducing behaviors and treating clients as equals were
conducted by Kahana & Kiyak (1984). This research revealed a
considerable range of staff behaviors with frequent instances of
treating residents as equal partners. The fact that observations
were focused on mentally alert patients may explain the greater
prevalence of staff behaviors which do not encourage or reinforce
dependency, than that noted by other researchers who considered staff
behaviors vis-à-vis cognitively impaired elderly.

Some authors focus on the value of nurturant and caretaking
behaviors for quality of patient care. According to Vladek (1980),
high quality of care implies that assistance is readily given with
dressing and bathing. Similarly, "caring" by staff has been cited as
an important predictor of patient satisfaction (Ware & Snyder, 1975),
further suggesting the positive value of caretaking behaviors by

staff. Linn, Gurel & Linn (1977) found that in community nursing homes, the variable most related to patient outcomes (survival, improvement, discharge) was the number of nursing hours devoted per patient.

In a similar vein, Brody (1973) argues that staff behaviors which meet patient dependency needs often facilitate more independent functioning. In other words, when staff behavior enables residents to maintain certain levels of functioning, inappropriate dependency is not likely to arise.

Coping and Lack of Person-Environment Fit

Coping with lack of person-environment fit usually entails a change in the environment or a shift in one's personal beliefs and preferences. Little research has been done to date on the option of obtaining mastery through actually leaving the institutional setting. Nevertheless, it is important to note that the option of leaving the institution is becoming more feasible for some elderly persons. Contrary to the commonly held belief in the permanence of institutional placements, a recent longitudinal study by the authors (Kahana, Kahana & Young, 1985) reveals that twenty-two percent of the newly institutionalized aged returned to community living or voluntarily transferred to other institutions over a two-year follow-up period.

Instrumental control may not be possible or adaptive in those situations where there is a high degree of environmental control or where the older person has insufficient "personal resources" to react to the environment with instrumental coping strategies. Various coping strategies have been delineated, which succeed in controlling such situations (Lazarus & Folkman, 1984). Such strategies include both emotion-focused and problem-focused coping attempts to minimize the importance of the problem or other attempts at cognitive restructuring. These cognitive strategies are similar in nature to secondary control mechanisms (Weisz, Rothbaum & Blackburn, 1984) which may be particularly useful to the frail elderly (White & Janson, 1986). Thus, a potential area of convergence is suggested between the distinct literatures of locus of control and of coping strategies. To the extent that individuals are unable to change their environment and are also unable to come forth with necessary cognitive restructuring, adverse psychological outcomes are very likely. In the case of elderly persons living in a highly controlling institutional setting, continued belief in personal control or attempts to exercise such control may very well contribute to negative outcomes.

Implications for Treatment and Intervention

Efforts to Reduce Learned Helplessness

A final issue to be discussed is the contribution of these theoretical frameworks to the development of intervention strategies. Learned helplessness theory would suggest that if a nursing home resident learns that all attempts to behave in an independent manner, efforts to change the staff's attitudes and behavior, and/or attempts to otherwise gain control over the environment have no impact, then the deficits of learned helplessness would be likely to ensue. In this event, depression, with the accompanying deficits in motivation, affect, and self-esteem, would follow. This prediction would lead us to seek an intervention program that includes modifications of both environment and person characteristics. Specific examples of intervention may include efforts to liberalize institutional policies in order to provide residents with more options and efforts to train staff to be better listeners to the requests and needs of residents. Physical environmental features may also be organized to facilitate resident control (for example lights may be installed to signal resident requests for staff assistance).

A search for relevant intervention strategies in recent litera-ture reveals that there are very few, if any, published studies that have attempted to prevent or reduce the negative outcomes associated with learned helplessness in the institutionalized aged. The intervention studies that have been done to date either relate specifically to the community-dwelling elderly (Priddy et al., 1982; Teitelman & Priddy, 1985), or are based on research which has focused on more general issues of control in nursing home settings with only indirect linkages to helplessness. The work of Priddy and his colleagues (Teitelman & Priddy, 1985) has suggested that the concepts of learned helplessness and depression are useful in developing treatment plans for older individuals in either individual or small group psychotherapy. Some of their recommendations include the promotion of choice, predictability, and positive attributions in the older client. They also recommend the elimination of helplessness-engendering stereotypes, counteracting some of the negative effects of helplessness by providing success experiences, and offering control-enhancing communication skills. By focusing on these issues and encouraging the elderly client to develop realistic goals, the authors suggest that the behavioral deficits of a helplessness depression may be overcome (Teitelman & Priddy, 1985).

Efforts to Increase Control

A number of studies have been conducted involving control-enhancing interventions in nursing homes (Rodin & Langer, 1977; Schulz, 1976). As mentioned earlier, the very process of institutionalization of a frail elderly individual may involve actual or perceived loss of control (Arling, Harkins & Capitman, 1984; Avorn & Langer, 1982). It also has been reported that older nursing home residents perceive themselves as having limited control over their environment (Morganti, Nehrke & Hulicka, 1980). Thus, while some suggest that enhancement of control may lead to positive psychosocial outcomes (Rodin & Langer, 1977), others have warned that efforts to increase the institutionalized adult's independence may have a "boomerang" effect if these interventions are not continued on a long term basis (Schulz & Hanusa, 1978). It may be anticipated (White & Janson, 1986) that efforts to increase the control of frail institutionalized older persons have limited value in an environment where such efforts are likely to be ignored or actively discouraged.

The limitation of these intervention strategies have been well described by White & Janson (1986). They point out that such interventions typically relate to very circumscribed aspects of institutional living. The control developed by such intervention programs cannot be readily implemented in the daily routines of institutional life where restrictions and demand for conformity are prevalent. Thus, therapeutic programs may inadvertently produce greater disappointments and may result in long term adverse sequelae.

This review of literature on interventions indicates that just as the development and manifestations of helplessness are complex processes so too are the factors which impact on therapeutic efforts designed to prevent or ameliorate the mental health problems resulting from loss of control and helplessness.

Efforts to Increase Person-Environment Fit

Interventions in the mental health field have generally focused on effecting changes in individuals in an effort to enhance coping abilities and to diminish adverse psychosocial states. The person-environment fit conceptualization permits a more flexible alternative to intervention which would target intervention to both individuals and environments in order to increase person-environment fit. In institutional settings, environmental manipulations may often be more feasible than will therapeutic efforts to modify behavior of individuals.

A review of interventions using a P-E fit framework has been provided by Kahana & Kahana (1984). It is noteworthy that promising treatment strategies attempt to improve placement and to achieve a better matching of individual residents and staff caregivers or roommates. Proper placements involve development and utilization of assessment strategies for determining personal needs and preferences. In addition, efforts at supporting and enhancing coping strategies of residents to deal with a lack of congruence between their needs and environmental conditions offer useful therapeutic possibilities. Training of staff to be more sensitive to potential areas of P-E incongruence and to display empathetic responses in acknowledging resident discomfort are also important goals. Intervention in a P-E fit framework is generally aimed at setting positive outcome goals rather than simply at ameliorating adverse effects of institution-alization.

Conclusions

Issues of control and dependency represent useful and salient conceptual approaches for understanding post-institutional adaptations of the elderly. Specific formulations regarding learned helplessness have been described here as a rich resource for the understanding of cognitive, behavioral, and emotional deficits among the institutional-ized elderly. If used properly, this framework has great potential for enabling us to have a meaningful impact on the lives of older persons. The very language of learned helplessness implies an iatrogenic disease, thereby providing a basis for remediation. Along with our discussion of this paradigm, we have suggested that there are a number of ways to achieve an understanding of the psychosocial conditions associated with institutional living which focus on understanding and ameliorating environmentally induced deficits such as excess disability and dependency, including issues of control and excess disability.

Our analysis of prevalent conceptualization and research strategies for understanding issues of control and helplessness in institutional settings points to the need for moving beyond relatively static models considering personal outcomes simply as a function of environmental stimuli. Instead, there is a need to specify dynamic components of person-environment transactions which help explain the impact of institutionalization on the elderly.

A congruence model of personal needs for control and environmen-tal presses related to control (P-E congruence) has been proposed and delineated in an effort to specify conditions of both person and environment which may account for adverse post-institutional outcomes such as learned helplessness and excess disability. This model also permits consideration of positive post-institutional outcomes which may be viewed as direct functions of P-E congruence. Such congruence is not simply a *given* environmentally or personally derived condition but is amenable to change through personal coping efforts or environ-mental interventions. The likelihood of increasing P-E fit is related to environmental opportunities for personal coping efforts. Accord-ingly, in a non-contingent environment lack of P-E fit is likely to result in adverse personal outcomes as outlined in the learned helplessness paradigm. In contrast, in contingent environments residents have the opportunity to improve P-E fit through successful coping efforts and achieve positive psychosocial outcomes.

Our conceptualization also attempted to specify mechanisms by which institutional environments exert their influence on elderly residents. Physical environmental features, institutional policies, staff attitudes and staff behaviors have been considered as the specific influences which impinge on institutionalized residents. Specification of environmental features which contribute to institutional control and environmental press for dependency or autonomy is viewed as a critical requisite for operationalizing and empirically testing formulations regarding control and dependency in institutional settings. Similarly, it is necessary to pinpoint salient dimensions and levels of personal needs or preferences for control and to recognize individual differences in these characteristics.

Research is required to examine the utility and heuristic value of the proposed congruence paradigm which integrates elements of several previously proposed conceptual frameworks for considering control and dependency of aged residents in institutional settings. Future research should examine "control" or "dependency" both as personal predispositions and as characteristics of the environment.

The proposed model allows gerontologists to view the institutionalized elderly in a more proactive light than that characterizing previous discussions of control and learned helplessness. It is suggested that issues of control may be profitably studied not only in understanding iatrogenic influences of institutions but also in implementing interventions with institutionalized aged and in assessing survival skills of the frail elderly.

References

Abramson, L., Seligman, M. E. P., Teasdale, J. (1978). Learned helplessness in humans: critique and reformulation. *Journal of Abnormal Psychology, 87*, 49-74.

Arling, G., Harkins, E. B., & Capitman, J. (1984). *Institutionalization and personal control in a panel study of impaired older people*. Paper presented at the Annual Scientific Meeting of the Gerontological Society of America, San Antonio, TX.

Avorn, J., & Langer, E. (1982). Induced disability in nursing home patients: A controlled trial. *Journal of the American Geriatrics Society, 31*, 397-400.

Avorn, J. (1983). Biomedical and social determinants of cognitive impairment in the elderly. *Journal of the American Geriatrics Society, 31*, 137-143.

Baltes, M. M. (1982). Environmental factors in dependency among nursing home residents: A social ecology analysis. In T. W. Wills

(Eds), *Basic processes in helping relationships* (pp. 405-425). New York: Academic Press.

Baltes, M. M., & Baltes, P. B. (1986). *The psychology of control and aging.* Hillsdale, NJ: Lawrence Erlbaum Associates.

Baltes, M. M., Burgess, R., & Stewart, R. (1980). Independence and dependence in self-care behaviors in nursing home residents: An operant-observational study. *International Journal of Behavior Development, 3,* 489-500.

Baltes, M. M., Horn, S., Barton, E. M., Orzech, J. J., & Lago, D. (1983). Social ecology of dependence and independence in elderly nursing home residents. *Journal of Gerontology, 38,* 556-564.

Baltes, M. M., & Reisenzein, R. (1986). The social world in long-term care institutions: Psychosocial control toward dependency? In M. M. Baltes & P. B. Baltes (Eds.), *The psychology of control and aging* (pp. 315-343). Hillsdale, NJ: Lawrence Erlbaum Associates.

Baltes, M. M., & Werner-Wahl, H. (1987). Dependence in aging. In L. L. Carstensen & B. A. Edelstein (Eds.), *Handbook of clinical gerontology* (pp. 204-219). New York: Pergamon Press.

Barton, C. D. (1982). Locus of control and helplessness as reported by residents and staff in four nursing homes. *Dissertation Abstracts International, 43*(4), 1299-B.

Barton, E. M., Baltes, M. M., & Orzech, M. J. (1980). Etiology of dependence in older nursing home residents during morning care: The role of staff behavior. *Journal of Personality and Social Psychology, 38,* 423-431.

Berezin, M. (1963). Some intrapsychic aspects of aging. In N. Zimberg & I. Kaufman (Eds.), *Normal psychology of the aging process* (pp. 93-117). New York: International Universities Press.

Branch, G., & Jette, A. M. (1982). A prospective study of long-term care institutionalization among the aged. *American Journal of Public Health, 12,* 1373-1379.

Brody, S. J. (1973). Comprehensive health care for the elderly: An analysis: The continuum of medical, health and social services for the aged. *The Gerontologist, 13,* 413-418.

Brody, E. M. (1977). Environmental factors in dependency. In A. N. Exton-Smith & J. G. Evans (Eds.), *Care of the elderly: Meeting the challenge of dependency* (pp. 81-95). London: Academic Press.

Byerts, T. (1973). *Housing and environment for the elderly.* Washington, DC: The Gerontology Society.

Clark, M. (1969).   Cultural values and dependency in later life.   In R. Kalish (Ed.), *The dependencies of old people*. Occasional Papers in Gerontology, No. 6, 59-72.   Institute of Gerontology, Michigan: Wayne State University.

Cohler, B. J. (1983).   Autonomy and interdependence in the family of adulthood: A psychological perspective. *The Gerontologist, 23*, 33-39.

Costello, S. E. (1986).   A comparison of depressive symptoms, types of learned helplessness, and perception of stressful life events in the younger and older geriatric population. *Dissertation Abstracts International, 46*(8), 2618-B.

Davis, R. W. (1968).   Psychologic aspects of geriatric nursing. *American Journal of Nursing, 68*, 802-804.

Exton-Smith, A. J., & Evans, J. G. (1977).   *Care of the elderly:; Meeting the challenge of dependency*. New York: Academic Press.

Felton, B., & Kahana, E. (1974).   Adjustment and situationally bound locus of control among institutionalized aged. *Journal of Gerontology, 29*, 295-301.

Fish, M. (1986).   The differential relationship of learned helplessness to dementia, pseudodementia, and depression. *Dissertation Abstracts International, 46*(9), 3055-B.

French, J. P. R., Rodgers, W., & Cobb, S.   (1974).   Adjustment as person-environment fit.   In G. V. Coelho, D. A. Hamburg & J. E. Adams (Eds.), *Coping and adaptation* (pp. 316-333). New York: Basic Books.

Giele, J. Z. (1980).   Adulthood as transcendence of age and sex.   In N. J. Smelser & E. H. Erikson (Eds.), *Themes of work and love in adulthood*. Cambridge, MA: Harvard University Press.

Goffman, E. (1961). *Asylums*. Garden City, NY: Anchor Books.

Goldfarb, A. (1969).   The psychodynamics of dependency and the search for aid.   In R. Kalish (Ed.), *The dependencies of old people*. Occasional Papers in Gerontology, No. 6, 1-15, Institute of Gerontology, Michigan: Wayne State University.

Gottesman, L. E., & Bourestom, N. C. (1974).   Why do nursing homes do what they do? *The Gerontologist, 14*, 501-506.

Gould, R. L. (1972).   The phases of adult life: A study in developmental psychology. *American Journal of Psychiatry, 129*, 521-531.

Gubrium, J. E. (1975). *Living and dying in Murray Manor*. New York: St. Martin's Press.

Harel, Z. (1981). Quality of care, congruence and well-being among institutionalized aged. *The Gerontologist, 21*, 523-531.

Havighurst, R. J. (1973). History of developmental psychology: Socialization and personality development through the life span. In P. B. Baltes & K. W. Schaie (Eds.), *Life span developmental psychology: Personality and socialization* (pp. 209-217). New York: Academic Press.

Henry, W. E. (1968). Personality change in middle and old age. In E. Norbeck, D. Price-Williams & W. W. McCord (Eds.), *The study of personality: An interdisciplinary appraisal*. New York: Holt, Rinehart & Winston.

Hochhauser, M. (1981). Learned helplessness and substance abuse in the elderly. *Journal of Psychoactive Drugs, 13*, 127-133.

Huesmann, L. R. (1978). Special issues: Learned helplessness as a model of depression. *Journal of Psychoactive Drugs, 87*, 1-198.

Hulicka, I. M., Morganti, J., & Cataldo, J. (1975). Perceived latitude of choice of institutionalized and non-institutionalized elderly women. *Experimental Aging Research, 1*, 27-34.

Johnson, C., & Grant, L. (1985). *The nursing home in American society*. Baltimore, MD: Johns Hopkins University Press.

Kahana, E., & Coe, R. M. (1969). Self and staff conceptions of institutionalized aged. *The Gerontologist, 9*, 364-367.

Kahana, B., & Kahana, E. (1984). Stress reactions. In P. Lewinsohn & L. Teri (Eds.), *Clinical geropsychology* (pp. 139-169). New York: Pergamon Press.

Kahana, E., Liang, J., & Felton, B. (1980). Alternative models of person-environment fit: Prediction of morale in three homes for the aged. *Journal of Gerontology, 35*, 584-595.

Kahana, E., Kahana, B., & Young R. (1985). Social factors in institutional living. In I. W. Peterson & J. Quandagno (Eds.), *Social bonds in later life: Aging and interdependence* (pp. 389-419). Beverly Hills, CA: Sage Publications.

Kahana, E. (1975). A congruence model of person-environment interaction. In P. G. Windley, T. Byerts & E.G. Ernst (Eds.), *Theoretical developments in environments for aging* (pp. 181-214). Washington, DC: Gerontological Society of America.

Kahana, E. (1982). A congruence model of person-environment interaction. In M. P. Lawton, B. G. Windley & T. O. Byerts (Eds.), *Aging and the environment: Theoretical approaches* (pp. 97-120). New York: Garland Publishing.

Kahana, E., & Kiyak, H. A. (1984). Attitudes and behavior of staff in facilities for the aged. *Research on Aging, 6,* 395-416.

Kahn, R. L. (1975). The mental health system and the future aged. *The Gerontologist, 15,* 24-31.

Kalish, R. A. (1969). *Dependencies of old people. Ann Arbor: University of Michigan Institute of Gerontology.*

Kasl, S. V. (1972). Physical and mental health effects of involuntary relocation and institutionalization of the elderly -- a review. American Journal of Public Health, 62, 377-384.

Kennelly, K. J., Hayslip, B., & Richardson, S. (1985). Depression and helplessness induced cognitive deficits in the aged. *Experimental Aging Research, 11,* 169-173.

Kuypers, J. A. (1972). Internal-external locus of control, ego functioning and personality characteristics in old age. *The Gerontologist, 12,* 168-173.

Langer, E. J., & Rodin, J. (1976). The effects of choice enhanced personal responsibility for the aged: A field experiment in an institutional setting. *Journal of Personality and Social Psychology, 34,* 191-198.

Lao, I. (1974). The development trend of the locus of control. *Personality and Social Psychology, Bulletin 1,* 348-350.

Lawton, M. P. (1980). *Environment and aging.* Monterey, CA: Brooks/Cole.

Lawton, M. P., & Nahemow, L. (1973). Ecology and the aging process. In C. Eisdorfer & M. P. Lawton (Eds.), *Psychology of adult development and aging* (pp. 619-674). Washington, DC: American Psychological Association.

Lazarus, R. S., & Folkman, S. (1984). *Stress, appraisal, and coping.* New York: Springer.

Lewin, K. (1951). *Field theory in social sciences.* New York: Harper & Row.

Lieberman, M. A., & Tobin, S. S. (1983). *The experience of old age, stress, coping, and survival.* New York: Basic Books.

Lieberman, M. A. (1974). Relocation research and social policy. *The Gerontologist, 14*, 494-501.

Linn, M. W., Gurel, L., & Linn, B. S. (1977). Patient outcome as a measure of quality of nursing home care. *American Journal of Public Health, 67*, 337-342.

Maiden, R. J. (1981). The attribution of learned helplessness and depression in the elderly. *Dissertation Abstracts International, 42*(3), 1181-B.

Marlowe, R. A. (1973). *Effects of environment on elderly state hospital relocatees.* 44th Annual Meeting of the Pacific Sociological Association, Scottsdale, Arizona.

Moos, R. H., & Igra, A. (1980). Determinants of the social environments of sheltered care settings. *Journal of Health and Social Behavior, 21*, 88-98.

Moos, R. H., & Lemke, S. (1984). *The multiphasic environmental assessment procedure.* Palo Alto: Stanford University Veterans Administration Hospital.

Morganti, J. B., Nehrke, M. F., & Hulicka, I. M. (1980). Resident and staff perceptions of latitude of choice in elderly institutionalized men. *Experimental Aging Research, 6*, 367-384.

Murray, H. A. (1938). *Exploration in personality.* New York: Oxford University Press.

Neugarten, B. (1964). A developmental view of adult personality. In J. E. Birren (Eds.), *Relations of development and aging* (pp. 176-208). Springfield, IL: Charles C. Thomas.

Noelker, L. (1975). *Friendship and intimacy in nursing homes.* Unpublished doctoral dissertation, Case Western Reserve University.

Pastalan, L. A. (1983). Environmental displacement: A literature reflecting old-person-environment transactions. In G. D. Rowles & R. J. Ohta (Eds.), *Aging and milieu* (pp. 189-203). New York: Academic Press.

Patrick, L. F. (1985). Life event types and attributional styles as predictors of depression in the elderly. *Dissertation Abstracts International, 45*(12), 3719-A.

Piaget, J. (1950). In translation by M. Piercy and D. E. Berlyne (Eds.), *The psychology of intelligence.* (Original French edition, 1974). London: Routledge & Kegan Paul Ltd.

152   *E. Kahana, B. Kahana and K. Riley*

Pinder, M. M. (1983). The impact of a short-term training program on learned helplessness among staff and residents of nursing homes. *Dissertation Abstracts International, 44*(5), 1298-A.

Priddy, J. M., Teitelman, J., Kivlighan, D. M., & Fubermann, B. S. (1982). Overcoming learned helplessness in elderly clients: Skills training for service providers. *Educational Gerontology, 8,* 507-518.

Raps, C. S., Peterson, C., Jones, M., & Seligman, M. E. P., (1982). Patient behavior in hospitals: Helplessness, resistance, or both? *Journal of Personality and Social Psychology, 42,* 1036-1041.

Reichard, S., Livson, F., & Peterson, P. C. (1962). *Aging personality: A study of eighty-seven older men.* New York: Wiley & Sons.

Riley, M., & Foner, A. (1968). *Aging and society, Vol. 1. An inventory of research findings.* New York: Russell Sage Foundation.

Rodin, J., & Langer, E. J. (1977). Long-term effects of control relevant to intervention with the institutionalized aged. *Journal of Personality and Social Psychology, 35,* 897-902.

Ryckman, B. M., & Malikoski, M. (1975). Relationship between locus of control and chronological aged. *Psychological Reports, 36,* 655-658.

Schulz, R. (1976). The effects of control and predictability on the psychological and physical well-being of the institutionalized aged. *Journal of Personality and Social Psychology, 43,* 563-573.

Schulz, R., & Hanusa, B. (1978). Long-term effects of control and predictability-enhancing interventions: Findings and ethical issues. *Journal of Personality and Social Psychology, 36,* 1194-1201.

Schwartz, A. N. (1974). Staff development and morale building in nursing homes. *The Gerontologist, 14,* 50-54.

Segal, S., & Moyles, E. (1979). Management style and institutional dependency in sheltered care. *Social Psychiatry, 14,* 159-165.

Seligman, M. E. P. (1975). *Helplessness: On depression, development and death.* San Francisco: Freeman.

Shanas, E. (1979). The family as a social support system in old age. *The Gerontologist, 19,* 169-174.

Solomon, K. (1982). Social antecedents of learned helplessness in the health care setting. *The Gerontologist, 22,* 282-287.

Stern, G. (1970). *People in a context.* New York: Wiley & Sons.

Taylor, S. E. (1979). Hospital patient behavior: Reactance, helplessness, or control. *Journal of Social Issues, 35,* 156-184.

Teitelman, L. E., & Priddy, J. M. (1985). *Helplessness, pseudo-helplessness, and psychotherapy.* Paper presented at the annual meetings of the Gerontological Society of America, New Orleans.

Tobin, S. S., & Lieberman, M. A. (1976). *Last home for the aged.* San Francisco: Jossey-Bass.

Tuckman, J., & Lorge, I. (1954). The influence of changed directions on stereotypes about aging: Before and after instruction. *Education and Psychological Measurement, 14,* 128-132.

Vladek, B. (1980). *Unloving care: The nursing home tragedy.* New York: Basic Books.

Ware, J. E., & Snyder, M. K. (1975). Dimensions of patient attitudes regarding doctors and medical care services. *Medical Care, 13,* 669-682.

Weisz, J. R., Rothbaum F., & Blackburn, T. (1984). Standing out and standing in: The psychology of control in America and Japan. *American Psychologist, 39,* 955-969.

White, C. B., & Janson, P. (1986). Helplessness in institutional settings: Adaptation or iatrogenic disease? In M. M. Baltes and P. B. Baltes (Eds), *Aging and the psychology of control* (pp. 297-313). New Jersey: Lawrence Erlbaum Associates.

Wittels, I., & Botwinick, J. (1974). Survival in relocation. *Journal of Gerontology, 29,* 440-443.

*Psychological Perspectives of Helplessness
and Control in the Elderly, P.S. Fry (ed.)*
© *Elsevier Science Publishers B.V. (North-Holland), 1989*

Chapter Six

SITUATIONAL PERCEPTIONS OF CONTROL IN THE AGED

Virginia L. FITCH
The University of Akron

Lee R. SLIVINSKE
Youngstown State University

Abstract

Control is an issue of importance throughout the life span.
Generalized perceptions of having control have been
associated with such positive outcomes as greater life
satisfaction and increased physical and psychological well-
being. A number of studies suggest these generalized
expectancies do not significantly decrease with age.
However, individuals also form perceptions of their degree
of control in specific situations based on their personal
abilities, the resources available to them from the
environment, and the demands of the situation. Situational
perceptions of control are subject to modification as
abilities, resources, and demands fluctuate. The aged are
particularly susceptible to decreases in situational
perceptions of control. Two primary factors are the real
changes associated with aging, so-called status passages,
and the cultural youth bias and dread of aging so pervasive
in this society. Status passages occur throughout life, but
such passages are frequently terminal events for the aged
including deterioration of health, retirement, and loss of
significant others. Cultural biases are based on negative
images of aging as a time of nonproductivity, decreased
social worth and decline. A conceptual framework based on
the theory of person-environment fit is utilized for
examining situational perceptions of control in the aged.
Person-environment fit is defined as a relational concept
derived from the interactions of environmental properties
and individual characteristics. It is argued that the individual is more likely to experience positive consequences
when his/her abilities are consistent with environmental
demands and when his/her needs are consistent with environmental supplies. A high degree of congruence would be
associated with feelings of being in control and well-being,

*and over time, with health, adaptive behavior and growth.
If misfit should occur to a sufficient degree, feelings of
lack of control, helplessness and dissatisfaction may
develop immediately. If the discrepancy persists over time,
dysfunction, maladaptive behavior, or illness may result.
Dimensions of congruence which are particularly salient to
the aged are discussed and approaches to intervention
consistent with the conceptual framework are presented.*

Introduction

Control is an issue of importance throughout the lifespan. Generalized perceptions of having control have been found to be associated
with such positive outcomes as greater life satisfaction and increased
physical and psychological well-being (Schulz, 1976; Tobin & Lieberman, 1976).   Similarly, other studies of both animal and human
subjects have demonstrated the profound impact loss of control has on
cognitive and emotional functioning and on the motivation to react
(Miller & Seligman, 1975; Seligman, 1975), to the extent that it may
result in the development of physical illness, psychiatric symptomatology and death (Suls, 1982).   Several studies suggest these generalized expectancies do not decrease significantly with age (Wong &
Sproule, 1984; O'Brien & Kabanoff, 1981; Lao, 1974).   However,
individuals continuously form perceptions of their degree of control
in specific situations based on their personal abilities, the
resources available to them from the environment, and the demands of
the situation. Situational perceptions of control are more subject to
modification as abilities, resources, and demands fluctuate.

The aged are particularly susceptible to decreases in situational
perceptions of control.   Several factors contribute to their greater
susceptibility including 1) the greater physical vulnerability
associated with aging, 2) the apparent noncontingent nature of many
events experienced by the aged, 3) societally limited opportunities to
exercise control, and 4) the internalization of negative stereotypes
by some of the aged.

The purpose of this chapter is to present a conceptual framework
based on the theory of person-environment fit to explain situational
perceptions of control in the aged. First, a review of the literature
regarding situational control appraisals is presented.   Second, a
theoretical rationale for applying that framework to the aged is
provided.   Finally, approaches to intervention consistent with the
conceptual framework are presented.

A Theoretical Approach for Situational Control Appraisals

Many researchers of locus of control have concluded that understanding
the perceptions and attributions of control made in specific contexts

requires the development of situation-specific measures of locus of control (Phares, 1976; Rotter, 1975). Individuals have been found to alter their interpretations of causality in specific situations while maintaining a somewhat consistent belief about causal expectations (Harper, 1984). Beliefs about causality may be relatively consistent due to self-selection of familiar and similar environments. Generalized expectancies are most applicable where cues from the environment are ambiguous (O'Brien, 1984; Phares, 1976) while situation specific expectancies are most applicable when situational cues are well-defined and the means to attain reinforcers explicit (Carlson, 1979; Ramanaiah & Adams, 1981).

Several efforts have been made to develop a more specific application of control. A brief review of some of these will follow.

Situation-Specific Research

Research regarding situational control appraisals variously have focused on specific goals, activities, contexts or populations. Although labeled situational approaches, several approaches more appropriately might be termed domain specific since they deal with classes of situations. For example, Wallston, Wallston, Kaplan and Maides (1976, p. 580) utilized the locus of control concept to develop and validate the Health Locus of Control Scale (HLC) measuring health beliefs. Their hope was to develop an approach that "would provide more sensitive predictions of the relationship between internality and health behaviors" than that provided by generalized locus of control scales. They originally treated health locus of control as unidimensional with health externals perceiving their health as determined by factors outside of their control and health internals perceiving health as the result of their own behavior. In their later work they reconceptualized health locus of control as a multidimensional concept. Three different dimensions were identified, paralleling those developed by Levenson (1974), based on their hypothesized source of control. These included internality, chance externality and powerful others externality (Wallston & Wallston, 1981).

Lachman, Baltes, Nesselroade and Willis (1982) developed three domain specific scales, also modeled after those developed by Levenson (1974), to assess beliefs and attributions about intellectual functioning. They were developed specifically for use with the elderly. Although related to Levenson's generalized scales, they concluded the measures were not redundant and were useful in understanding attributions of intellectual aging outcomes.

Other attempts have been made to assess domain specific control. Each has proven useful in understanding control perceptions with regard to certain activities. These include research into locus of control and economic outcomes (Gurin & Gurin, 1970), crowding (Schmidt & Keating, 1979), academic achievement of children (Crandall,

Katkovsky, & Crandall, 1965), environmental activism (Huebner & Lipsey, 1981), and daily activities (Ryden, 1984).

Several other approaches though labeled examinations of situational control, seem to be examinations of generalized expectancies since they cut across settings and behaviors. For example, Paulhus and Christie (1981) in their examination of control identified three behavioral spheres. In the first sphere, situations of personal achievement, perceived control is termed personal efficacy. This involves achieving control over objects such as repairing a car. The second sphere involves achievements in social interactions and includes activities such as achieving a position of influence within the family or other significant groups or developing a friendship. This sphere is labeled interpersonal control. The final sphere, called sociopolitical control, takes into consideration the conflicts between individual goals and social and political systems. They suggest that an individual may have different control expectations in each sphere which could serve to generate a control profile of his/her expectancies in dealing with the world.

Based on social learning and attribution theories, Lefcourt, Von Baeyer, Ware and Cox (1979) conceptualized an approach for studying locus of control for a series of specific goals. Their approach has been applied to the study of affiliation and achievement with university undergraduates. They investigated the salience of four sets of attributions for each goal: 1) stable internal attributions where causality is attributed to skill and ability; 2) unstable internal attributions deriving from fluctuations in motivation and effort; 3) stable external attributions based on contextual characteristics; and 4) unstable external attributions due to luck or fate. Although acknowledging some reservations about their model, namely the necessity to consider the possible causes of control attributions specific to each goal, they emphasize the importance of examining goal specific control beliefs in understanding behavioral complexities (Lefcourt, 1981).

In research on the psychological adjustment of the elderly, Reid and Ziegler (1981a) examined their beliefs about the controllability of important reinforcements. Guided by Rotter's theory, they hypothesized that the extent to which an elderly person perceives himself or herself as able to affect desirable outcomes is central to well-being. Although their work focused on a variety of reinforcements based on interviews with elderly, subsequent analysis revealed their approach to be unidimensional. They further concluded it probably explored generalized expectancies rather than situation specific ones.

A primary advantage of both categories of approaches is that they may be useful in achieving greater predictability of behavioral outcomes in specific areas. Where comparisons have been made with more general measures of locus of control, the domain specific measures have demonstrated greater sensitivity in detecting changes in control beliefs particularly when these changes are age related. Lachman (1986) compared the usefulness of the *Levenson Locus of Control Scales*, the *Multidimensional Health Locus of Control Scale* and the *Personality in Intellectual Aging Contexts Control Scales* in a series of three studies. The sample consisted of college students and elderly from sixty to ninety-one years of age. No age differences were found with the generalized measures. However, the health and intellectual scales were better predictors of behavioral outcomes for the elderly subjects than the generalized measures, but were not for the young. In general, the elderly were more external on intelligence and health specific measures. Compared to college students, they more often attributed intellectual aging outcomes to chance and health outcomes to powerful others. Similar results regarding health were obtained in another study comparing the elderly to a middle-aged group (Saltz & Magruder-Habib, 1982). Reid and Ziegler (1981a) in a 5-year study examining intraindividual change in desired control for a sample ranging from 60 to 100 years of age, found that 65% manifested decreased perceived control and 13% showed an increase while 22% demonstrated no change. Although there is considerable disagreement on the direction and extent of age related change in control (for a discussion of this see Skinner & Connell, 1986), changes in certain domains such as intellectual functioning, health, social, and physical domains would seem particularly salient to the elderly (Lachman, 1986; Bradley & Webb, 1976) rendering more specific conceptualizations helpful to researchers working with this population.

The primary question here is whether these more specific approaches actually meet the need, identified by Rotter (1975), for examinations of control in specific situations. Reid and Ziegler (1981a) expressed some doubts. Certainly domain specific research developed out of a recognition that the personality construct locus of control was affected by situational influences (Endler & Edwards, 1978; Reid, 1977). However, each situation or setting involves numerous dimensions on which control appraisals are made (Folkman, 1984). Although there may be some dimensions in common across settings and others unique to a setting, dimensions may vary in importance between individuals and between settings. Therefore, in understanding control related outcomes, both the internal and external determinants of control perceptions in each situation should be examined on the dimensions identified as salient.

An Interactional Approach

Several studies have demonstrated that the behavior and cognitions of individuals may vary from setting to setting (Magnusson & Endler, 1977; Pervin & Lewis, 1978); furthermore, the coping processes employed may depend largely on the particular environmental context presenting demands (Argyris, 1968; Mischel, 1968). These and other studies have culminated in an increasing interest in research on how people fit into their particular setting.

There are two basic approaches to the study of behavior. The tendency has been for research to emphasize either internal or external determinants of behavior, although neither view totally denies the importance of the other. The controversy between the two has to do with whether individual differences or situations are more important in the determination of behavior.

Caplan (1979) suggested that some responses are determined primarily by individual attributes, some by environmental attributes, and still others by the interaction between the two. Therefore, a theoretical orientation such as person-environment fit, which provides for an examination of all these factors, would seem to have many advantages over other approaches which limit the scope of their inquiry to either individual or environmental characteristics. Numerous studies indicate the desirability of a match, fit, or congruence between the individual and various elements in his/her environment (Pepitone, 1969; McMichael, 1978; White, 1974; Rosenberg, 1969; McAdoo, 1985).

The concept of person-environment fit refers to the degree of congruence between the individual's needs and abilities and the demands and resources of his/her environment. Person-environment fit by definition can be said to be simultaneously concerned with control and the importance of control in specific areas to the individual. To the extent that abilities are sufficient to meet environmental demands and expectations in a setting, an individual can be expected to experience feelings of mastery and influence in that setting. The degree to which his/her needs are met by situational supplies, however, will determine its importance to him/her. This seems consistent with Rotter's emphasis on outcome expectancy and reinforcement value.

Person-environment fit is a relational concept derived from the interaction of environmental properties and individual characteristics. The responses exhibited in a given environment and consequences experienced depend on the degree of congruence and the length of time over which it persists.

Support for the Concept of Person-Environment Fit

Historically, the concept of fit between people and their environments has emerged from various disciplines including anthropology (Meade, 1952), sociology (Langner & Michaels, 1963; Levi-Strauss, 1969), and psychology (Lewin, 1951). It has been studied directly in a variety of settings. Murray (1938; 1951) developed a need-press model of behavior with needs inferred from the spontaneous behavior manifested by the person and the environment defined in terms of alpha press (referring to "objective" situational stimuli) and beta press (referring to the individual's subjective interpretation of the stimuli). Using Murray's need-press theory, Stern (1970) measured college environments and students along several dimensions including achievement standards, group life, order lines and constraints. A lack of fit along these dimensions was related to attrition while congruence was related to continued enrollment and satisfaction. In a more recent examination of university students in residence halls, the concept was found to be useful as an indicator of distress and strain (Tracey & Sherry, 1984). In the work environment this approach has been found to be associated with such positive outcomes as less psychological strain (Caplan, Cobb, French, Harrison & Pinneau, 1975; Defares, Brandjes, Nass & Van der Ploeg, 1984), higher performance ratings and feelings of competence (Lorsch & Morse, 1974), and greater job satisfaction (Harrison, 1978; House, 1972).

Kahana, Liang, and Felton (1980) conducted studies with elderly residents of nursing homes excluding those with incapacitating physical or mental impairments. Congruence on some dimensions was strongly related to morale. In similar research with discharged psychiatric patients, it has been found to result in decreased symptomatology (Lehmann, Mitchell, & Cohen, 1978) and greater stability in functioning (Coulton, Holland, & Fitch, 1984). In the latter study, although one-third of the sample were judged to be seriously impaired at the time of discharge, the majority achieved a degree of adjustment sufficient to maintain community tenure for the duration of the study. This suggests that the interaction between person and environment was more critical for outcome than any prior characteristic of the person. Kabanoff and Ashton (1984) found that fit between a person's political values and those of the immediate social milieu was associated with self reports of greater general life satisfaction in a sample of Australian undergraduates.

Application of the Concept of Interaction

The conceptual framework utilized here is presented in Figure 1. The concepts and hypothetical relationships presented are those believed to be important in understanding the situational control appraisals made by the aged. In addition to permitting an examination of both internal and external determinants of situational perceptions, the framework allows for an exploration of the relationship between actual control and perceptions of control. Presumably, perceptions of losing control are based on a corresponding real loss of control. However, one of the most striking factors in the literature on control and aging is the paucity of research on the relationship between actual control and control perceptions. The results of some studies suggest understanding this relationship may be crucial in developing effective control-enhancing interventions with the elderly. The positive increases in the well-being of an institutionalized aged sample, achieved by Schulz (1976), came about by enabling them to

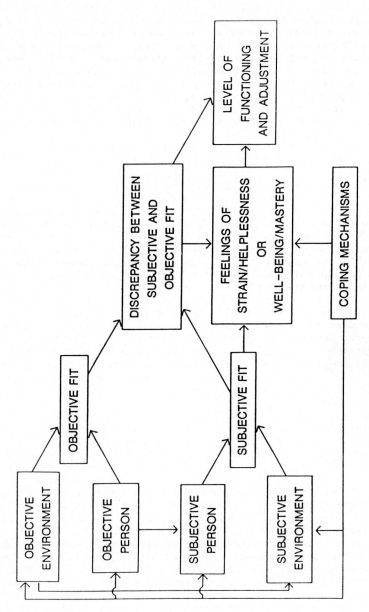

Figure 1.--Representation of Conceptual Approach

either predict or control the timing of visits. This involved giving them actual control. In a follow-up of the aforementioned study, Schulz and Hanusa (1978) found that the participants who had manifested improvements in physical and psychological health status deteriorated after termination of the controllable event. Where perceptions of having control are not supported through continued experience, the benefits of enhancing perceived control appear to be short-lived. Also assessing the long term effects of increased control in nursing home residents (Langer & Rodin, 1976), Rodin and Langer (1977) found the responsibility induced group to exhibit greater improvement in health than the comparison group. The key factor is that in the latter situation the enhanced controllability of events continued.

The model proposed by French, Rodgers and Cobbs (1974) offers a method of assessing actual control and control perceptions in a situation. They distinguish two meanings of environment: the *objective environment* that exists independently of the individual's perception of it and the *subjective environment* as it is perceived by the individual. Correspondingly distinctions are also made between the *objective person* as he/she really is, including the individual's attributes that are relatively lasting, such as needs, values, and abilities; and the *subjective person* or self-concept, referring to the person's perception of these attributes. Harrison (1978) indicates that good adjustment occurs when there is a low discrepancy on each of the four concepts.

The importance of all four concepts in understanding control appraisals of the elderly is supported by several sources. For example, Bandura (1981) views the self-efficacy problems of the aged as derived from reappraisals and faulty appraisals of their abilities. The reappraisals are necessitated by the real physical changes that occur with age although he suggests these may be more than compensated for by their increased knowledge and experience. Misappraisals may result when the abilities of the elderly are compared to those of the young in a society that defines youth as the ideal. Langer (1983) suggests that decreases in self-esteem and activity level in the aged result from attributing problems to the aging process rather than to the environment and from negative labels placed on the elderly by significant portions of the environment.

Several studies indicate the importance of both subjective and objective concepts in understanding control related behavior. For example, both perceived health status and actual health status of cardiac patients have been found to be equally important to morale and adjustment. Subjects who perceived their health to be better were more likely to have resumed prior activities including work and social involvement. They also rated their morale higher than did those who perceived their health as poor (Garritz, 1973).

In a 6-month study of the relationship between perceived control and placement of a portion of the sample in a nursing home, Arling,

Harkins and Capitman (1986) found that institutionalization reduced perceptions of personal control. A decline in perceived control was observed in all but was greater among the less educated and more functionally impaired. This suggests that although institutionaliza- tion brought about a loss of actual control for everyone, the differential abilities of the residents mediated between the ex- perience of loss of control and the perception.

The emphasis on subjective aspects of control seems to have resulted from the greater predictive power of perceptions for behavioral outcomes. In a reformulation of learned helplessness, Abramson, Seligman and Teasdale (1978) concluded that perceiving an aversive environmental event as uncontrollable is more important than whether it is actually controllable or not. Their work has been supported by a number of studies (Brewin, 1985; Peterson & Seligman, 1984; Skinner, 1985). This is well and good if the primary concern is predicting control behavior. However, when the goal is understanding control behavior, its antecedents, including real events, must be examined. Only a few attempts have been made to examine the relation- ship between objective and subjective determinants of behavior although the need for such research has been acknowledged (French, Rodgers & Cobb, 1974; Kahana, 1978; Pervin, 1968; Sells, 1963). A major reason for this is the apparent difficulty of obtaining objective measures. French, Rodgers and Cobb (1974) attempted to measure the objective and subjective fit of a group of high school students along two dimensions, affiliation and intelligence. Only a weak correlation was found between objective and subjective fit. However, it appeared that similar dimensions were not being measured which would account for the weak relationship.

Some research suggests that both measures are useful and explain unique aspects of behavior. A study by Coulton, Holland and Fitch (1982) explored the relationship between objective measures and subjective measures on commensurate dimensions and the community adjustment of discharged psychiatric patients. Subjective fit was found to be predictive of stability in functioning while objective fit was predictive of rehospitalization. These findings are supported by Tracey and Sherry (1984). In their study of college student distress, the effects of actual lack of fit and perceived misfit were indepen- dent.

Aging and Loss of Control

Kuhl (1986) notes that in current research on control and aging, the causal chain views loss of control as occurring first, followed by perceived loss of control, reduction in motivation, reduced perfor- mance and, finally, accelerated aging. He acknowledges that this causal chain may proceed differently for some individuals. It is our contention that situational control perceptions may be reduced due to changes in ability or the environment or the perception of change.

As individuals age significant losses of personal control may result from declines in ability. Two sources of change have to be considered: real declines and perceived declines in ability. The relationship between the two is highly complex and a one-to-one correspondence cannot be assumed.

The real changes associated with aging are well documented and, though numerous, are highly individualized. The senses are vulnerable to deterioration and impairment from disease. Visual deficits, where present, pose severe problems to adjustment and, even when treatable, the treatment itself may be experienced as threatening. The hearing loss associated with aging interferes with communication and integration, may increase isolation, and lead to feelings of suspicion and paranoia. Decreasing ability in taste differentiation (Newman & Newman, 1983) may contribute to a disinterest in food and, when paired with other factors such as illness or dental problems, may lead to problems of malnutrition.

Regarding declines in physical capabilities, Marshall (1973) noted that ability to engage in moderate activity remains about the same at seventy as at forty, but the aged have more difficulty recuperating after prolonged exertion. Respiratory, circulatory and digestive systems function less efficiently. A general decline, referred to as behavioral slowing (Birren, Woods, & Williams, 1980), may be manifested in behavioral response as seen in a slowing of motor responses, reaction time, memory skills, and information processing, particularly on complex rather than routine tasks. Although intellectual competence for the majority of elderly either remains constant or actually improves with age, for some, changes in cognitive abilities do occur. General health declines with age although the elderly as a whole are healthier than the general public assumes. Over 80 percent have at least one chronic illness and multiple conditions are often found. However, the majority report being able to carry on normal activities (National Center for Health Statistics, 1979) with some adjustments.

The experience of such declines is highly variable and even their occurrence does not necessarily result in the perception of loss of control. The meaning accorded the change in ability by the individual is an important factor. This, undoubtedly, involves the degree of decline and the alteration necessitated in preferred activities. One examination of the association between daily activities and self sufficiency for individuals over sixty indicated that a daily structure including productive and leisure activities is critical for self-esteem (Mullins & Hayslip, 1986). Decker and Schulz (1985), in a study of the well-being of middle-aged and elderly spinal cord injured, found they reported somewhat lower well-being than similar aged nondisabled people in previous research. Those who viewed their disability more favorably reported high levels of perceived control, were employed, had higher income and educational levels and reported higher religiosity. These findings suggest that certain factors such as having more options available for exercising control, positive sources of self-validation, and social supports may mediate between the occurrence of functional impairment and the perception of loss of control. This is supported by Phifer and Murrell (1986) who examined factors in the development of depressive symptoms in a probability sample of 1,233 adults over fifty-five. They concluded that health and social support played both additive and interactive roles in depressive onset.

Furthermore, performance in at least some areas may remain high if it is attributed to internal causes. Lachman, Steinberg and Trotter (1987) investigated the relationship of control beliefs and attributions on memory self-assessments to memory performance across two trials. Forty-seven elderly adults participated. Those with stronger internal control beliefs made higher self-assessments and had higher performance at the first trial. Greater decrements in self-assessments and performance across trials were found for those who attributed their initial higher performance to internal, stable, and global causes.

In summary, perceptions of declines in ability may result from actual declines and from misappraisals of ability. The elderly may be more prone to such false attributions than are younger individuals. The findings of Prohaska, Parham and Teitelman (1984) support this. They examined two age cohorts of females, with one group ranging in age from 18 to 28 and the other from 60 to 84, and subjected them first to noncontingent failure and then to response contingent tests. Older participants manifested lower success expectations and poorer performance on the latter than did younger subjects. Their findings suggest that younger individuals attribute failure to effort while older individuals attribute their failure to ability and, therefore, experience more deleterious effects.

Loss of personal control also may come about through participation in environments that are not amenable to the control efforts of the elderly, through events that are beyond the control of any individual but which are more likely to occur to the aged, and through the misperception that events/environments are beyond the capacity of the aged person to control. A comparison of three groups of elderly over 68 years of age based on living accommodations (living in a health care facility, living with or near family, and living in their own homes) found that control perceptions were consistent with the actual control available in their living accommodations. Furthermore, measures of performance and perceptions of control corresponded (Tiffany, Tiffany, Camp & Dey, 1984). Some environments in which the elderly interact more than do other segments of the population may be less controllable. Nursing homes and retirement facilities are environments where research has documented the effects of reduced opportunities for control.

The term learned helplessness has been utilized to explain the generalized perception of uncontrollability which occurs after the experience of repeated uncontrollable aversive events. This concept may be applied to the responses exhibited by the aged who must adapt to multiple losses many of which occur simultaneously. These losses, including retirement, death of spouse and friends, relocation, decreased mobility, financial limitations and the like, are often more debilitating than physical declines. Pitcher and Hong (1986) found some support for this. The result of their analysis of an older male cohort suggest that decreases in individual perceptions of control may come about due to a reduction in opportunities and resources resulting from environmental changes and altered social conditions. Although such changes need not and do not always result in learned helplessness, they can result in debilitation if the aged individual fails to distinguish between events/changes which are controllable and which are not or if he/she attributes failure to control to age. In a study involving the attributions of task performance made by both young and elderly female judges, failure on the part of performers described as old was attributed to age. For young performers, success was attributed to age (Banziger & Drevenstedt, 1982). Solomon (1982) indicates that the elderly are even more likely to accept the negative stereotypic view of the aged than are others with a concomitant reduction in expectations and an increase in passivity. Furthermore, in some environments the elderly may be sanctioned if they display characteristics inconsistent with the stereotype. In one study elderly nursing home patients with a higher locus of desired control were more likely to be identified as "poor" patients by nursing staff than were those with lower locus of desired control (Mullins, 1982). This suggests misperceptions of the controllability of environments by the elderly may be derived, at least in part, from feedback from important elements of the social environment as well as acceptance of negative stereotypes. Studies providing evidence for the presence of ageism in clinical diagnosis (Perlick & Atkins, 1984; Settin, 1982) support this view. In addition to negative messages, changes in social conditions, including role loss and loss of reference groups, deprive the aged of much daily feedback regarding their competencies and create a susceptibility to negative societal labeling (Holahan & Holahan, 1987).

Discrepancies Between Actual Control and Control Perceptions

A number of studies of psychiatric patients indicate the importance of perceptions that are congruent with important elements in the environment. Rogers, Gendlin, Kiesler, and Truax (1967) found therapy to be more successful when clients and their therapists held similar perceptions of their therapeutic relationships. Furthermore, Moos (1972) suggests that effective program operation may be dependent on the agreement between clients and staff as to the nature of the program. Successful adaptation to an environment does not require a totally accurate perception of reality (Mechanic, 1974). However, if the individual's perception of reality is too extreme from that which is acceptable to other inhabitants of the environment, successful adaptation may be hindered.

A reasonable degree of similarity can be expected when the individual maintains good contact with reality. However, as they become more dissimilar, problems may occur. Inaccurate perceptions may result in behavior inappropriate to the situation whereas accurate perceptions should result in more appropriate responses. Although all individuals vary in their perceptions of the same event at any particular moment and over time, perceptions of situational control by the elderly may differ, at times markedly, from the perceptions of individuals who are middle-aged or younger. The comparison of an individual's perception of situational control with the actuality of control may indicate the extent to which control beliefs are rational or dysfunctional. Although illusions of control or lack of control are not necessarily dysfunctional, in some instances they may be. Decisions about the functionality/dysfunctionality of beliefs must necessarily be based on knowledge of the situation, the person, and potential outcomes. Illusions of control may be used to transcend self-imposed limitations (Langer, 1983; Piper & Langer, 1986). However, illusions of competence when too extreme, may lead the elderly to engage in action that invites failure or that places them at risk. The study, previously described, of the positive association between perceived health status and adjustment of cardiac patients (Garritz, 1973) suggests some potential dangers. For example, illusions of competence may be an important factor in recovery from illness for the elderly; however, they may lead to physical exertion that jeopardizes recovery. Thus, it seems important that beliefs of control not differ too greatly from actual controllability.

Illusions of incompetence or lack of control seem to be related to a state of learned helplessness (Seligman, 1975) but are not identical. Learned helplessness is a generalized perception whereas illusions of incompetence are context specific. Where such illusions are held, individuals fail to act in situations that are response contingent. They, in fact, give up.

Responses of the elderly to gaining or losing control can be defined in terms of person-environment fit. An event is stressful to the extent that it makes demands the individual is not able to meet. The negative emotional impact of even an aversive event is ameliorated when an individual perceives that he/she has some degree of influence over the situation. In a sample of nursing home residents, those who experienced enhancement of personal responsibility and choice exhibited marked improvement in alertness, participation in activities, and in well-being when compared to a control group (Langer & Rodin, 1976).

A large discrepancy between actual control and beliefs of control also can be expected to contribute to feelings of distress and strain

on the part of the elderly and ultimately to helplessness. Perceptions of control, when too extreme from actual control, may be
associated with helplessness, giving up, and debilitation in the aged.
For example, the elderly are told they have options, choices they may
exercise, and control they may use. If the environment does not
support their attempts to exercise control, repeated failures may lead
to feelings of incompetence and helplessness. Situational perceptions
of uncontrollability prevent the elderly from responding even when
events are response contingent.

Coping Mechanisms

The experience of strain or distress by the elderly invariably lead to
the employment of coping mechanisms. There is general agreement that
the functions of coping are highly complex (Menaghan, 1983), but the
nature of the process underlying the choice of coping response is less
clear. Furthermore, our understanding of the concept seems to be in
the process of evolving.

Coping has been variously defined in the literature. At times
the concept has been used as coextensive with adaptation; at other
times it has been used to refer to specific adaptive processes that
are somewhat narrow in scope. In the latter vein, Lazarus (1966) in
his earlier work applied the term *coping* to situations of threat,
while Haan (1969) differentiated coping from defense. The scope of
the term has since expanded. Murphy (1974) defined it as any attempt
at mastering a situation that is perceived as potentially threatening,
frustrating, challenging, or gratifying. This expanded the definition
of coping to include more positive concepts although the process
continued to focus on threat and frustration. Lazarus and Launier
(1978) defined coping mechanisms as:

> . . . effort, both action-oriented and intrapsychic, to
> manage (i.e., master, tolerate, reduce, minimize) environ-
> mental and internal demands and conflicts among them, which
> tax or exceed a person's resources. (p. 311)

More recently these have been categorized as problem-focused and
emotion-focused, respectively (Folkman & Lazarus, 1980).

Coping efforts of the elderly can be directed toward the person,
the environment, or both. They can be directed toward altering the
transaction through problem-solving, regulating the emotions,
maintaining of options, managing effective distress, and maintaining
self-esteem (Folkman & Lazarus, 1980; Lazarus & Launier, 1978;
Mechanic, 1974; Murphy, 1974). In general, people use a mixture of
both problem-focused and emotion-focused coping. The context of the
stressor has been found to be influential in the choice (Lazarus,
1984). Their effectiveness is a function of the particular situation
in which they are utilized and the extent to which their use leads to

behavior inconsistent with reality. On the one hand people maintain self-respect and energy for action through perceptions that enhance their self-esteem (Adams & Lindeman, 1974), while on the other, too great a reliance on such methods by the aged may result in self-endangerment and, ultimately, in feelings of helplessness.

A study of the relationship of coping responses to health status among older women found that emotion-focused coping responses (i.e., positive-cognitive coping and passive-cognitive coping) had important direct effects particularly for those with multiple chronic health problems. The former was effective in buffering the effects of physical impairment on life satisfaction and subjective health assessments while the latter prevented negative health assessments from generalizing to decreased life satisfaction. Direct action coping was found to have little effect (Lohr, Essex & Klein, 1988). These findings suggest that where stressors are chronic and less amenable to change emotion-focused responses that modify the meaning of noncontingent events in positive ways enhance control perceptions and self-esteem. In such instances direct action coping may result in perceptions of uncontrollability and helplessness.

A final point should be noted with regard to coping. Perceptions of being in control are not always desirable. If an individual is subjected to repeated failure, such a belief, over time, would result in a lowering of self-esteem. A realization of helplessness may be the most accurate and beneficial to an individual in some circumstances (Averill, 1973).

To summarize, loss of control in a situation, whether real or illusory, will lead to coping responses. These responses may be directed at altering the person, the environment, and/or perceptions of the same. The functionality of the response depends on the situation, the nature of the stressor and whether the response leads to greater vulnerability. Many events experienced by the aged are not amenable to direct action suggesting the importance of understanding the benefits of both forms of coping.

Level of Functioning and Adjustment

Becoming ill has been shown to be one way in which individuals of all ages respond to strain in their social environment (Moos & Insel, 1974). A number of studies show prolonged and recurrent maladaptation to the social environment to be related to various illnesses, including physical and mental disorders (Lloyd, 1980; Wildman & Johnson, 1977). Thus, strain can lead to various responses ranging in severity from increased anxiety, sleeplessness, development of illness, and finally a deterioration in level of adjustment.

The effects of aging on any one individual are not singular but multiplicative and affect numerous aspects of life. Adjustment to the stressful effect of change and loss is a significant challenge for the elderly.   Langer (1983) indicates that the experience of several events involving loss of control may force the recognition that one is old and engender a negative self-concept.   Such self-images often are wrongly attributed to the aging process rather than to situational and social factors which would   have similar effects regardless of age. The development of negative self-concepts will increase the likelihood of self-blame even when situational attributions of uncontrollability are warranted.   Initially, this will result in decreased motivation to deal with the situation and, over time, in loss of ability through disuse.

Level of functioning and adjustment among the elderly is related, to some extent, to very real physical, psychological, and social changes, but to an even greater extent to the individual interpreta- tions placed on those events.   Where the elderly erroneously conclude they are incompetent, helpless, and lack the skills needed, they will behave in a manner consistent with this belief.   Through lack of use, their skills will erode, further affirming their helplessness. Adjustment also is directly related to the degree of similarity between actual control and perceptions of control.   Lack of correspon- dence between the two may result in negative feedback from the environment and experiences of failure, all threatening adjustment.

Person-environment fit is not a static concept.   Individuals grow and develop throughout the lifespan; their needs and their capabili- ties change somewhat.   Similarly, environments change.   Certain need-meeting resources become scarce while others become more plentiful.   Environmental demands on the individual also vary. Therefore, the individual and environment are in constant transaction as the individual tries to maintain or improve fit over time.   When faced with a poor fit denoting loss of control, the aged individual has several options: change the environment or the perception of it; change personal abilities/attributes or self-perceptions; or leave the environment in pursuit of one that provides a better fit. Alternatively, more than one of the above options may be utilized in an effort to improve fit.

Although some circumstances appear to lead, almost universally, to feelings of strain and distress, a great many situations appear benign for most but produce distress in a few.   A situation may be evaluated as threatening by some, challenging by others, and ir- relevant by still others.   The assessment made is a function of the aged individual's vulnerability in a given situation.   Research indicates that the coping behaviors people employ are more important to functioning and to health than factors inherent in the situation (Antonovsky, 1974; Lazarus & Launier, 1978; Mechanic, 1974; Murphy, 1974; White, 1974).   A large body of research provides support for the view that maladjustment results when individuals perceive their capabilities as being taxed to the extreme.   Given the variety of stressful experiences to which the aged are vulnerable why don't more elderly exhibit poor adjustment? A number of factors seem to be involved. First of all, the salience of the stressor, in this instance, perceptions of situational uncontrollability, to the individual is crucial. Loss of control is not a sufficient basis for assuming that maladjustment will occur or even that stress will occur (Grant, Yager, Sweetwood, & Olsen, 1982). The individual's perception of the situation and its importance must be examined (Dohrenwend & Dohrenwend, 1974; Monroe, 1982). Brown (1974) emphasized the unique meanings accorded events by different individuals. The importance of the individual's perception is further highlighted by a study of perceptions of change and their relationship to illness in industrial workers. Thurlow (1971) found a stronger relationship between illness and subjective perceptions than between illness and objective perceptions.

A second factor may be that the internal and external resources necessary for successful coping are differentially available to the aged. These resources are thought to mediate between long term stressful elements and maladaptive behavior (LaRocco, House, & French, 1980; Williams, Ware, & Donald, 1981). For the elderly, dealing with chronically aversive circumstances, including reduced finances, multiple losses, negative labeling and the like, internal and/or external resources may be taxed to the limit.

Given this conceptual frame of reference, it may be assumed that adjustment to aging will be more successful if the elderly interact in environments that match, to a degree, their needs and capabilities and if the differences in subjective perceptions of control and actual control are small.

Issues in the Application of the Framework

In applying the theoretical framework of person-environment fit to situational perceptions of control, two issues require further discussion. The first is the importance of directionality and its meaning on various dimensions. This question has received increased attention from researchers of person-environment fit. Their findings suggest that the directionality of the discrepancies in fit should be examined. For example, the model used by French, Rodgers and Cobb (1974) considered only a deficiency of environmental supplies relative to individual needs to have a negative influence; excess supplies or ability were not considered to have any effect. They did, however, qualify their assumption by noting that the direct relationship between the dependent variable (e.g., functioning, coping, etc.) and fit on a particular supply may be affected by the interrelationships between fit on various supplies. For example, supply on one dimension in the environment may have an inverse relationship to supply on another dimension. An oversupply of support for an individual in a particular environment may also imply that there is an undersupply of autonomy for his/her needs. Furthermore, if an individual has an excess of ability over that required by environmental demands, lack of challenge, and stagnation, deterioration of ability may result. Therefore, assumptions about directionality of incongruence must be made with care because of the probable complexity of the relationships.

Kahana (1978) examined three conceptualizations of congruence. One, the non-directional model, assumes that zero mismatch between abilities and demands and needs and supplies leads to the best outcome and holds that any lack of congruence, whether from over- or under-supply, results in equally negative outcomes. Two, the one-directional model assumes that only undersupply and insufficient ability will result in unfavorable outcomes. This model may be problematic for at least some dimensions. Three, the two-directional model considers that both an undersupply and an oversupply and both insufficient ability and underutilization of ability may have negative results though the effects of both may be different. In her analysis, for some dimensions, undersupply had negative consequences while for others, both undersupply and oversupply resulted in similar negative conditions. Although both the non-directional model and the two-directional model explained almost the same amount of variance, the two-directional model allowed a closer exploration of the connection between fit and outcome. A study by Kiyak, summarized by Kahana (1978) obtained similar results.

Dimensionality

A second issue that needs consideration is the multidimensional nature of situational control and the dimensions of fit which are important both to the elderly and their environments. Both the individual and the environment must be measured along the same dimensions (French et al., 1974; Lewin, 1951; Murray, 1938). Researchers attempting to measure the variability of person-environment interaction have found it to be multidimensional in nature with the dimensions involved varying somewhat from setting to setting. Moos and Tsu (1977) identified several adaptive tasks involving control issues related to physical illness. They appear to reflect situational dimensions that range from those that are illness-related (dealing with pain/discomfort, dealing with treatment procedures) to more general tasks (support and affiliation needs). These could be assumed to vary in importance between settings.

An examination of relevant research suggests that a number of dimensions have relevance across settings while others assume more importance as the setting and characteristics of those occupying the setting change. A comparison of the dimensions found to be important in research in such diverse settings as community psychiatric treatment environments (Moos, 1974), nursing facilities for the elderly (Kahana, 1978), and chronically ill living at home (Coulton, 1979), reveals a number of quite similar dimensions which could prove to be "core" dimensions. These include support, autonomy, and order among others.

Furthermore, the dimensions of fit identified as important by researchers have focused more on the need-resource aspect of congruence rather than the ability-demand aspect. In using this conceptual framework for examining situational perceptions of control, an equal emphasis on both aspects for each dimension is important.

Conclusions and Suggestions For Intervention

The devastating effects of loss of control on the elderly have been well-documented. In general, individuals with an external belief are thought to be more vulnerable to stressful events than those with an internal belief. Lefcourt (1982) suggests that since research has found external beliefs to be an obstacle to successful coping and associated with lower self-esteem and depression, the goal of therapy might naturally focus on shifting external beliefs to more internal ones. However, if generalized expectancies of control are person attributes, they may be resistant to change. Nevertheless, perceptions of situational control are amenable to change. Several studies have demonstrated that perceptions of having control in particular settings may be enhanced through interventions designed to increase choice and predictability (Langer & Rodin, 1976; Mercer & Kane, 1979; Schultz, 1976; Slivinske & Fitch, 1987). The theoretical framework presented here provides some suggestions for intervention with the elderly.

First, interventions that are compatible with the older person's subjective perceptions of control will be more effective than those that are incompatible. This is supported by research on the outcomes of health promotion activities (Brown, Muhlenkamp, Fox, & Osborn, 1983), cardiovascular treatment (Strickland, 1979), and drug administration programs (D'Altroy, Blissenbach, & Lutz, 1978). Where interventions contradict subjective reality, it is unlikely that they will be utilized consistently if at all since control belief is more relevant to behavior than control reality (Langer 1983).

Second, the provision of some change to increase controllability in a setting, appropriate though it may be, is not sufficient to insure the elderly person's adjustment will be improved in that setting. The change must be accurately perceived for the desired consequences to occur. This raises questions about the value of professional assessments in planning effective interventions if the elderly are not intimately involved in the process. These difficulties may be dealt with by asking the person about his/her capabilities and needs and about the environment in order to obtain his/her beliefs. Specific suggestions advanced by the person for skill enhancement or environmental change should be incorporated since this creates shared control over treatment. A study of two groups of elderly, one in an institution and the other in the community, who were given the opportunity to assume partial control over their activities program found that both manifested an increase in satisfaction with their lives and the facilities. They, further, showed an increase in personal control (Byrd, 1983).

Third, a comparison of subjective perceptions with actual control can be used to evaluate responsiveness to and effectiveness of treatment. Both illusions of control and the reality of control should be considered in developing control enhancing interventions for the elderly. Quite clearly, even if opportunities for control are provided, they will not be utilized unless accompanied by a belief that effort can achieve the desired outcome. The reverse also is true. Enhancement of skills will not result in an increase in self-sufficiency if other messages reinforce low self-esteem. This is supported by a study examining the effects of increasing opportunities for personal control in elderly nursing home residents. Although all subjects increased control in areas that were identified as significant to their living situations, no increases were observed in measures of perceived control or self reported happiness (Hutchison, Carstensen, Silberman, et al., 1983). It may be that elements in the environment contradicted and negated their positive experiences.

Illusions of control and actual control are mutually reinforcing Research on the effects of congruence between treatment and control belief illustrate this point. However, actual control may impose limits on enhancement of control beliefs. Furthermore, encouraging control beliefs that are inaccurate may lead to greater debilitation by exposing the individual to more experiences of failure.

References

Abramson, L. Y., Seligman, M. E. P., & Teasdale, J. D. (1978). Learned helplessness in humans: Critique and reformulation. *Journal of Abnormal Psychology, 87,* 49-74.

Adams, J. E., & Lindeman, E. (1974). Coping with long-term disability. In G. Coelho, D. Hamburg & J. Adams (Eds.), *Coping and adaptation* (pp. 127-138). New York: Basic Books.

Antonovsky, A. (1974). Conceptual and methodological problems in the study of resistance resources and stressful life events. In B. S. Dohrenwend & B. P. Dohrenwend (Eds.), *Stressful life events: Their nature and effects* (pp. 245-258). New York: Wiley & Sons.

Argyris, C. (1968). Conditions for competence acquisition and therapy. *Journal of Applied Behavioral Science, 4,* 147-177.

Arling, G., Harkins, E. B., & Capitman, J. A. (1986). Institutionalization and personal control: A panel study of impaired older people. *Research on Aging, 8,* 38-56.

Averill, J. R. (1973).   Personal control over aversive stimuli and its relationship to stress. *Psychological Bulletin, 80,* 286-303.

Bandura, A. (1981).   Self-referent thought: A developmental analysis of self-efficacy.   In J. H. Flavell & L. Ross (Eds.), *Social cognitive development* (pp. 200-239).   Cambridge: Cambridge University Press.

Banziger, G., & Drevenstedt, J. (1982).   Achievement attributions by young and old judges as a function of perceived age of stimulus person. *Journal of Gerontology, 37,* 468-474.

Birren, J. E., Woods, A. M., & Williams, M. V. (1980).   Behavioral slowing with age: Causes, organization and consequences.   In L. W. Poon (Ed.), *Aging in the 1980's* (pp. 293-308).   Washington, DC: American Psychological Association.

Bradley, R. H., & Webb, R. (1976).   Age-related differences in locus of control orientation in three behavior domains. *Human Development, 19,* 49-55.

Brewin, C. R. (1985).   Depression and causal attributions: What is their relation? *Psychological Bulletin, 98,* 297-309.

Brown, G. W. (1974).   Meaning, measurement and stressful life events. In B. S. Dohrenwend & B. P. Dohrenwend (Eds.), *Stressful life events: Their nature and effects* (pp. 217-243). New York: Wiley & Sons.

Brown, N., Muhlenkamp, A., Fox, L., & Osborn, M. (1983).   The relationship among health beliefs, health values, and health promotion activity. *Western Journal of Nursing Research, 5,* 155-163.

Byrd, M. (1983).   Letting the inmates run the asylum: The effects of control and choice on the institutional lives of older adults. *Activities, Adaptation and Aging, 3,* 3-11.

Caplan, R. D. (1979).   Social support, person-environment fit and coping.   In L. O. Ferman & J. P. Gardua (Eds.), *Mental health and the economy* (pp. 89-137). Kalamazoo, MI: Upjohn Institute.

Caplan, R. D., Cobb, S., French, J. R. P., Harrison, V., & Pinneau, S. (1975).   *Job demands and worker health: Main effects and occupational differences* (pp. 75-160).   Cincinnati: National Institute for Occupational Safety and Health, (HEW Publication No. NIOSH).

Carlson, J. G. (1979). Locus of control and frontal muscle action potential. In N. Birbaumer & H. Kimmel (Eds.), *Biofeedback and self-regulation* (pp. 242-259). Hillsdale, NJ: Lawrence Erlbaum Associates.

Coulton, C. (1979). Developing an instrument to measure person environment fit. *Journal of Social Service Research, 3,* 421-435.

Coulton, C., Holland, T., & Fitch, V. (1982). *Matching patients with community environments.* Unpublished manuscript. Cleveland: Case Western Reserve University.

Coulton, C., Holland, T., & Fitch, V. (1984). Person-environment congruence and psychiatric patient outcome in community care homes. *Administration in Mental Health, 12,* 71-88.

Crandall, V. C., Katkovsky, W., & Crandall, V. J. (1965). Children's beliefs in their control of reinforcement in intellectual academic achievement. *Child Development, 36,* 91-109.

D'Altroy, L., Blissenbach, H., & Lutz, D. (1978). Patient drug self-administration improves regimen compliance. *Hospitals, 52,* 131-132.

Decker, S. D., & Schulz, R. (1985). Correlates of life satisfaction and depression middle-aged and elderly spinal cord injured persons. *American Journal of Occupational Therapy, 39,* 740-745.

Defares, P. B., Brandjes, M., Nass, C. H., & Van der Ploeg, J. D. (1984). Coping styles and vulnerability of women at work in residential settings. *Ergonomics, 27,* 527-545.

Dohrenwend, B. S., & Dohrenwend, B. P. (1974). *Stressful life events: Their nature and effects.* New York: Wiley & Sons.

Endler, N. S., & Edwards, J. (1978). Person by treatment interactions in personality research. In L. A. Pervin & M. Lewis (Eds.), *Perspectives in interactional psychology* (pp. 141-170). New York: Plenum Press.

Folkman, S. (1984). Personal control and stress and coping processes: A theoretical analysis. *Journal of Personality and Social Psychology, 46,* 839-852.

Folkman, S., & Lazarus, R. S. (1980). An analysis of coping in a middle-aged community sample. *Journal of Personality and Social Psychology, 21,* 219-239.

French, J. R. P., Rodgers, W., & Cobb, S. (1974). Adjustment as person environment fit. In G. V. Coelho, D. A. Hamburg & J. E. Adams (Eds.), *Coping and adaptation* (pp. 316-333). New York: Basic Books.

Garritz, T. F. (1973).   Social involvement and activeness as predictors of morale six months after myocardial infarction.   *Social
Science and Medicine, 7,* 199-207.

Grant, I., Yager, J., Sweetwood, H., & Olsen, R. (1982).   Life events
and symptoms.   *Archives of General Psychiatry, 39,* 598-605.

Gurin, G., & Gurin, P. (1970).   Expectancy theory in the study of
poverty.   *Journal of Social Issues, 26,* 83-104.

Haan, N. (1969).   A tripartite model of ego functioning values and
clinical and research applications.   *Journal of Nervous and Mental
Disease, 148,* 14-30.

Harper, D. C. (1984).   Application of Orem's theoretical constructs to
self-care medication behaviors in the elderly.   *Advances in Nursing
Science, 6,* 29-46.

Harrison, R. V. (1978).   Person-environment fit and job stress.   In C.
L. Cooper & R. E. Payne (Eds.), *Stress at work* (pp. 175-205).   New
York: Wiley & Sons.

Holahan, C. K., & Holahan, C. J. (1987).   Life stress, hassles and
self efficacy in aging: A replication and extension.   *Journal of
Applied Social Psychology, 17,* 574-592.

House, J. S. (1972).   *The relationship of intrinsic and extrinsic
motivations to occupational stress and coronary heart disease risk.*
Unpublished dissertation.   Ann Arbor: University of Michigan.

Huebner, R. B., & Lipsey, M. W. (1981).   The relationship of three
measures of locus of control to environmental activism.   *Basic and
Applied Social Psychology, 2,* 45-58.

Hutchison, W., Carstensen, L., Silberman, D., et al. (1983).
Generalized effects of increasing personal control of residents in a
nursing facility.   *International Journal of Behavioral Geriatrics,
1,* 21-32.

Kabanoff, B., & Ashton, R. (1984).   Conservatism, locus of control and
life satisfaction: A person/environment fit analysis.   *Australian
Psychologist, 19,* 19-23.

Kahana, E. (1978).   *A congruence model of person-environment interaction.*   Unpublished manuscript.   Detroit: Wayne State University.

Kahana, E., Liang, J., & Felton, B. (1980).   Alternative models of
person-environment fit: Prediction of morale in three homes for the
aged.   *Journal of Gerontology, 35,* 584-595.

Kuhl, J. (1986). Aging and models of control: The hidden costs of wisdom. In M. M. Baltes & P. B. Baltes (Eds.), *The psychology of control and aging* (pp. 1-33). Hillsdale, NJ: Lawrence Erlbaum Associates.

Lachman, M. E. (1986). Locus of control in aging research: A case for multidimensional and domain specific assessment. *Psychology and Aging, 1,* 34-40.

Lachman, M. E., Baltes, P. B., Nesselroade, J. R., & Willis, S. L. (1982). Examination of personality-ability relationships in the elderly: The role of the contextual assessment made. *Journal of Research in Personality, 16,* 485-501.

Lachman, M. E., Steinberg, E. S., & Trotter, S. D. (1987). Effects of control beliefs and attributions on memory self-assessments and performance. *Psychology and Aging, 2,* 266-271.

Langer, E. J. (1983). *The psychology of control.* Beverly Hills, CA: Sage.

Langer, E. J., & Rodin, J. (1976). The effects of choice and enhanced personal responsibility for the aged: A field experiment in an institutional setting. *Journal of Personality and Social Psychology, 34,* 191-198.

Langner, T., & Michaels, S. (1963). *Life stress and mental health.* Glencoe, IL: Free Press.

LaRocco, J., House, J., & French, J. R. P. (1980). Social support occupational stress, and health. *Journal of Health and Social Behavior, 21,* 202-218.

Lao, R. C. (September, 1974). *The developmental trend of the locus of control.* Paper presented at the American Psychological Association, New Orleans, LA.

Lazarus, R. S. (1966). *Psychological stress and the coping process.* New York: McGraw-Hill.

Lazarus, R. S. (1984). The costs and benefits of denial. In B. S. Dohrenwend & B. P. Dohrenwend (Eds.), *Stressful life events and their contexts* (pp. 131-156). New Brunswick, NJ: Rutgers University Press.

Lazarus, R. S., & Launier, R. (1978). Stress-related transactions between person and environment. In L. A. Pervin & M. Lewis (Eds.), *Perspectives in interactional psychology* (pp. 287-326). New York: Plenum Press.

Lefcourt, H. M. (1981).   The construction and development of the multidimensional-multiattributional causality scales.   In H. M. Lefcourt (Ed.), *Research with the locus of control construct, Volume 1* (pp. 245-277). New York: Academic Press.

Lefcourt, H. M. (1982).   *Locus of control: Current trends in theory and research.*   Hillsdale, NJ: Lawrence Erlbaum Associates.

Lefcourt, H. M., Von Baeyer, E. L., Ware, E. E., & Cox, D. J. (1979). The multidimensional multiattributional causality scale: The development of a goal specific locus of control scale.   *Canadian Journal of Behavioral Science, 11*, 286-304.

Lehmann, S., Mitchell, S., & Cohen, B. (1978).   Environmental adaptation of the mental patient.   *American Journal of Community Psychology, 6*, 115-124.

Levenson, H. (1974).   Activism and powerful others: Distinctions within the concept of internal-external control.   *Journal of Personality Assessment, 38*, 377-383.

Levi-Strauss, C. (1969).   *The elementary structures of kinship.* Boston: Beacon Press.

Lewin, K. (1951).   *Field theory in social science.*   New York: Harper & Row.

Lloyd, C. (1980).   Life events and depressive disorder reviewed. *Archives of General Psychiatry, 37*, 541-548.

Lohr, M. J., Essex, M. J., & Klein, M. H. (1988).   The relationships of coping responses to physical health status and life satisfaction among older women. *Journal of Gerontology, 43*, 54-60.

Lorsch, J. W., & Morse, J. J. (1974).   *Organizations and their members: A contingency approach.* New York: Harper & Row.

Magnusson, D., & Endler, N. (1977).   *Personality at the crossroads: Current issues in interactional psychology.*   Hillsdale, NJ: Lawrence Erlbaum Associates.

Marshall, W. A. (1973).   The body.   In R. R. Sears & S. Feldman (Eds.), *The seven ages of man.* Los Altos, CA: William Kaufman.

McAdoo, H. P. (1985).   Racial attitude and self-concept of young black children over time.   In H. P. McAdoo & J. L. McAdoo (Eds.), *Black children: Social, educational, and parental environments* (pp. 213-242). Beverly Hills, CA: Sage.

McMichael, A. (1978).   Personality, behavioral and situational modifiers of work stressors. In C. Cooper & R. Payne (Eds.), *Stress at work* (pp. 275-297). New York: Wiley & Sons.

Meade, M. (1952). Some relationships between social anthropology and psychiatry. In F. Alexander & H. Ross (Eds.), *Dynamic psychiatry* (pp. 401-448). Chicago: University of Chicago Press.

Mechanic, D. (1974). Social structure and personal adaptation: Some neglected dimensions. In G. Coelho, D. Hamburg & J. Adams (Eds.), *Coping and adaptation* (pp. 32-44). New York: Basic Books.

Menaghan, E. G. (1983). Individual coping efforts: Moderators of the relationship between life stress and mental health outcomes. In H. B. Kaplan (Ed.), *Psychosocial stress: Trends in theory and research* (pp. 123-144). New York: Academic Press.

Mercer, S., & Kane, R. A. (1979). Helplessness and hopelessness among the institutionalized aged: An experiment. *Health and Social Work, 4*, 91-116.

Miller, W. R., & Seligman, M. E. P. (1975). Depression and learned helplessness in man. *Journal of Abnormal Psychology, 80*, 206-210.

Mischel, W. (1968). *Personality and assessment.* New York: Wiley & Sons.

Monroe, S. (1982). Assessment of life events. *Archives of General Psychiatry, 39*, 606-610.

Moos, R. H. (1972). The community oriented programs environment scale. *Community Mental Health Journal, 8*, 28-37.

Moos, R. H. (1974). *Evaluating treatment environments.* New York: Wiley & Sons.

Moos, R. H., & Insel, P. (1974). *Issues in social ecology: Human ecology.* Palo Alto: National Press.

Moos, R. H., & Tsu, V. (1977). The crisis of physical illness: An overview. In R. Moos (Ed.), *Coping with physical illness* (pp. 1-19). New York: Plenum Press.

Mullins, D., & Hayslip, B. (1986). Structure of daily activities and self-efficacy. *Clinical Gerontologist, 4*, 48-51.

Mullins, L. C. (1982). Locus of desired control and patient role among the institutionalized elderly. *Journal of Social Psychology, 116*, 269-276.

Murphy, L. (1974). Coping, vulnerability and resilience in childhood.

In G. Coelho, D. Hamburg, & J. Adams (Eds.), *Coping and adaptation* (pp. 69-100). New York: Basic Books.

Murray, H. A. (1938). *Exploration in personality*. New York: Oxford University Press.

Murray, H. A. (1951). Toward a classification of interaction. In T. Parsons & E. Shils (Eds.), *General theory of action* (pp. 434-464). Cambridge: Harvard University Press.

National Center for Health Statistics. U. S. Department of Health, Education, and Welfare (1979). *The national nursing home survey-- 1977 survey for the United States*. Washington, DC: DHHS Publication.

Newman, B. M., & Newman, P. R. (1983). *Understanding adulthood*. New York: Holt, Rinehart & Winston.

O'Brien, G. E., & Kabanoff, B. (1981). Australian norms and factor analysis of Rotter's internal-external control scale. *Australian Psychologist, 16*, 184-202.

O'Brien, G. E. (1984). Locus of control, work, and retirement. In H. M. Lefcourt (Ed.), *Research with the locus of control construct, Volume 3* (pp. 7-72). New York: Academic Press.

Paulhus, D., & Christie, R. (1981). Spheres of control: An interactionist approach to assessment of perceived control. In H. M. Lefcourt (Ed.), *Research with the locus of control construct, Volume 1* (pp. 161-188). New York: Academic Press.

Pepitone, A. (1969). *Attraction and hostility*. New York: Prentice Hall.

Perlick, D., & Atkins, A. (1984). Variations in the reported age of a patient: A source of bias in the diagnosis of depression and dementia. *Journal of Consulting and Clinical Psychology, 52*, 812-820.

Pervin, L. A. (1968). Performance and satisfaction as a function of individual environment fit. Psychological Bulletin, 69, 56-68.

Pervin, L. A., & Lewis, M. (1978). *Perspectives in interactional psychology*. New York: Plenum Press.

Peterson, C., & Seligman, M. E. P. (1984). Causal explanations as a risk factor for depression: Theory and evidence. *Psychological Review, 91*, 347-374.

Phares, E. J. (1976). *Locus of control in personality*. Morristown, NJ: General Learning Press.

Phifer, J. F., & Murrell, S. A. (1986). Etiologic factors in the onset of depressive symptoms in older adults. *Journal of Abnormal Psychology, 95,* 282-291.

Piper, A. I., & Langer, E. (1986). Aging and mindful control. In M. M. Baltes & P. B. Baltes (Eds.), *The psychology of control and aging* (pp. 71-89). Hillsdale, NJ: Lawrence Erlbaum Associates.

Pitcher, B. L., & Hong, S. Y. (1986). Older men's perceptions of personal control: The effect of health status. *Sociological Perspectives, 29,* 397-419.

Prohaska, T., Parham, I., & Teitelman, J. (1984). Age differences in attributions to causality: Implications for intellectual assessment. *Experimental Aging Research, 10,* 111-117.

Ramanaiah, N. V., & Adams, M. L. (1981). Locus of control and attribution of responsibility for academic performance. *Journal of Personality Assessment, 45,* 309-313.

Reid, D. W. (1977). Locus of control as an important concept for an interactionist approach to behavior. In D. Magnusson & N. Endler (Eds.), *Personality at the crossroads* (pp. 185-192). Hillsdale, NJ: Lawrence Erlbaum Associates.

Reid, D. W., & Ziegler, M. (1981a). The desired control measure and adjustment among the elderly. In H. M. Lefcourt (Ed.), *Research with the locus of control construct, Volume 1* (pp. 127-159). New York: Academic Press.

Reid, D. W., & Ziegler, M. (November, 1981b). *Longitudinal studies of desired control and adjustment.* Paper presented at the joint meetings of the Gerontological Society of America and the Canadian Association of Gerontology, Toronto, Canada.

Rodin, J., & Langer, E. J. (1977). Long term effects of a control relevant intervention with the institutionalized aged. *Journal of Personality and Social Psychology, 35,* 897-902.

Rogers, C., Gendlin, E., Kiesler, D., & Truax, C. (1967). *The therapeutic relationship and its impact.* Madison: University of Wisconsin Press.

Rosenberg, M. (1969). *Conceiving the self.* New York: Basic Books.

Rotter, J. B. (1975). Some problems and misconceptions related to the construct of internal versus external control of reinforcement. *Journal of Consulting and Clinical Psychology, 43,* 56-67.

Ryden, M. B. (1984). Morale and perceived control in institutionalized elderly. *Nursing Research, 33,* 130-136.

Saltz, C., & Magruder-Habib, K. (November, 1982). *Age as an indicator
of depression and locus of control among non-psychiatric inpatients.*
Paper presented at the meeting of the Gerontological Society of
America, Boston, MA.

Schmidt, D. E., & Keating, J. P. (1979). Human crowding and personal
control: An integration of the research. *Psychological Bulletin,
86,* 680-700.

Schulz, R. (1976). Effects of control and predictability on the
psychological well being of the institutionalized aged. *Journal of
Personality and Social Psychology, 32,* 563-763.

Schulz, R., & Hanusa, B. (1978). Long term effects of control and
predictability enhancing interventions: Findings and ethical
issues. *Journal of Personality and Social Psychology, 36,* 1194-
1201.

Sells, J. B. (1963). *Stimulus determinants of behavior.* New York:
Ronald Press.

Settin, J. M. (1982). Clinical judgement in geropsychology practice.
Psychotherapy: Theory, research and practice, 19, 397-404.

Seligman, M. E. P. (1975). *Helplessness.* San Francisco: Freeman.

Skinner, E. A. (1985). Action, control judgements, and the structure
of control experience. *Psychological Review, 92,* 39-58.

Skinner, E. A., & Connell, J. P. (1986).   Control understanding:
Suggestions for developmental framework. In M. M. Baltes & P. B.
Baltes (Eds.), *The psychology of control and aging* (pp. 35-69).
Hillsdale, NJ: Lawrence Erlbaum Associates.

Slivinske, L. R., & Fitch, V. L. (1987).   The effect of control
enhancing interventions on the well-being of elderly individuals
living in retirement communities. *The Gerontologist, 27,* 176-181.

Solomon, K. (1982). Social antecedents of learned helplessness in the
health care setting. *The Gerontologist, 22,* 282-287.

Stern, G. (1970). *People in context.* New York: Wiley & Sons.

Strickland, B. R. (1979).   Internal-external expectancies and
cardiovascular functioning.   In L. C. Perlmuter & R. A. Monty
(Eds.), *Choice and perceived control* (pp. 183-205). Hillsdale, NJ:
Lawrence Erlbaum Associates.

Suls, J. (1982).   Social support, interpersonal relations and health: Benefits and liabilities.   In G. Sanders & J. Suls (Eds.), *The social psychology of health and illness* (pp. 57-71).   Hillsdale, NJ: Lawrence Erlbaum Associates.

Thurlow, H. (1971).   Illness in relation to life situation and sick role tendency. *Journal of Psychosomatic Research, 15,* 73-88.

Tiffany, P. G., Tiffany, D. W., Camp, C. J., & Dey, K. A. (1984). Relationship between experienced control and domiciles of elderly persons. *Psychological Reports, 54,* 731-736.

Tobin, S., & Lieberman, M. (1976).   *Last home for the aged.*   San Francisco: Jossey-Bass.

Tracey, T. J., & Sherry, P. (1984).   College student distress as a function of person environment fit.   *Journal of College Student Personnel, 25,* 436-442.

Wallston, B. S., Wallston, K. A., Kaplan, G. D., & Maides, S. A. (1976).   Development and validation of the health locus of control (HLC) scale.   *Journal of Consulting and Clinical Psychology, 44,* 580-585.

Wallston, K. A., & Wallston, B. S. (1981).   Health locus of control scale.   In H. M. Lefcourt (Ed.), *Research with the locus of control construct, Volume 1* (pp. 189-243).   New York: Academic Press.

White, R. W. (1974).   Strategies of adaptation: An attempt at systemic description.   In G. Coelho, D. Hamburg & J. Adams (Eds.), *Coping and adaptation* (pp. 47-68).   New York: Basic Books.

Wildman, R., & Johnson, D. (1977).   Life change and Langer's 22-item mental health index.   *Journal of Health and Social Behavior, 18,* 179-188.

Williams, A., Ware, J., & Donald, C. (1981).   A model of mental health, life events and social supports applicable to general populations. *Journal of Health and Social Behavior, 22,* 324-336.

Wong, P., & Sproule, C. (1984).   Attributional analyses of locus of control.   In H. M. Lefcourt (Ed.), *Research with the locus of control construct, Volume 3* (pp. 309-360).   New York: Academic Press.

Psychological Perspectives of Helplessness
and Control in the Elderly, P.S. Fry (ed.)
© Elsevier Science Publishers B.V. (North-Holland), 1989

Chapter Seven

CONTROL AND DEPENDENCY IN RESIDENTIAL CARE SETTINGS FOR THE ELDERLY: PERSPECTIVES ON INTERVENTION

Paul A. MUNSON

Health and Welfare Canada, Ottawa, Ontario, Canada

Abstract

Residency for the elderly in a long-term care institution has been described as fostering a diminished sense of personal control and increased dependency behavior and helplessness. The development of dependency and the decline of personal control has also been associated with poorer psychological adjustment and physical health. This chapter examines the relationships among social cognition and operant learning approaches to dependency behavior and personal control in the context of long-term residential care settings. Principal behavior domains of residents which are at risk for diminished personal control are described with special attention to the regulation of social interaction, privacy, and self-care activities. A review of the existing research on planned interventions to enhance personal control and independent behavior of elderly residents in residential care is presented with a critical examination of the validity of the findings and their implications for the management of residential care settings. The characteristics of elderly residents and the properties of care settings which influence personal control and dependency behavior of residents are discussed to identify potential entry points for intervention activities. Particular emphasis is given to caregiver/recipient interaction as a potential therapeutic modality. The chapter concludes with considerations for developing control enhancing interventions and more effective experimental evaluation of approaches to intervention.

Introduction

The first reports of studies carried out to examine the effects of
enhanced personal control on the psychological well-being and health
of elderly persons in residential care settings appeared more than ten
years ago (Langer & Rodin, 1976; Schulz, 1976). Since that time the
belief that enhancing control will result in positive benefits for
elderly residents in residential care settings has gained general
acceptance. More recent research has left behind the question of
whether a positive relationship between control enhancing interventions and well-being can be demonstrated and attention has been
directed to other issues such as variants of control constructs
(Reid, 1984; White & Janson, 1986), control related concepts such as
mindfulness (Chanowitz & Langer, 1980) and the nature of helping
relationships (Karuza, Rabinowitz & Zevon, 1986). The studies which
have been conducted to directly test the effectiveness of a control
enhancing intervention for promoting psychological adjustment or
improved health are few in number and have as yet not been critically
reviewed. One of the purposes of this chapter is to examine the
information provided by these studies in order to assess the strength
of the evidence supporting the idea that control enhancing interventions have beneficial effects for the elderly in residential care.
The principal studies which form the foundation of control intervention research are ones by Schulz (1976) and Langer and Rodin (1976)
along with their follow-up studies (Rodin & Langer, 1978; Schulz &
Hanusa, 1978) which were conducted to evaluate possible long-term
effects of the control interventions. These studies are reviewed
first and are followed by a discussion of subsequent research. The
reader should be advised that this is not an attempt to disparage
either the individual researchers or their work. Rather, the purpose
of this critique is to clarify the level of certainty which may be
accorded the results that have been reported.

    The review of intervention research is followed by a discussion
of factors in institutional care settings that serve to restrict
personal control. A milieu based approach to control intervention is
described and the chapter concludes with proposed recommendations for
research designed to assess control enhancing interventions.

Foundations of Control Enhancing Intervention Research

Schulz (1976) hypothesized that among the elderly feelings of
helplessness and depression as well as accelerated physical decline
were, at least in part, attributable to loss of control. Schulz's
study was designed to separately evaluate the effects of control and
predictability on psychological adjustment and physical well-being of
residents in a retirement home. The intervention was based on social
visits by college students with control and predictability manipulated
through the scheduling and the duration of the visits. Residents in
the control condition were given decision control over both the

scheduling and the duration of the visits. Residents in the predict condition were informed by the visitor when the visit would take place and how long the visit would be. A third group of residents was visited on a random schedule. Visitations in the predict and random conditions were yoked to visitations in the control condition to equate for the frequency and duration of visits. Manipulation checks on the residents' perceptions regarding who controlled the scheduling and the duration of visits demonstrated that the source of control was accurately perceived with the control group differing from the other two visitation groups. The effects of the intervention on the dependent measures of psychological well-being, activity level and health status were evaluated by three orthogonal comparisons: (a) no-treatment versus random; (b) predict versus control; and (c) no-treatment plus random versus predict plus control. Schulz (1976) reported positive outcomes on health status, psychological status and activity level for the combined control and predict group of residents when compared to the combined no treatment and random group. There were no differences between the predict and control and hence no demonstrated benefit to control over that of predictability.

While this approach to evaluating the data makes clear the lack of difference between the predict and the control groups it does not fully explore the differences among the three intervention groups. The question of whether the predict and control manipulations produce any benefit to the residents beyond the effect of the visitation alone is not directly answered. If this issue is set aside and it is assumed that the predict and control visitation conditions did differ from the random visitation condition in their effects on the residents, the reason for such an outcome would be unclear. The study does not demonstrate in any way that a greater generalized expectancy for control or predictability in one's daily life was produced for the residents in the predict or control conditions. The simple fact that they correctly perceived the nature of the control relationships governing the visitations does not provide direct support for the idea that they experienced a generalized sense of greater control or predictability in their day-to-day life. The beneficial effects produced for subjects in the predict and control conditions may have been caused in part by the development of a personal relationship with the visitor which enhanced self-esteem and perceived importance to others. Certainly more courteous and deferential treatment was accorded the residents in the predict and control conditions and greater openness was exhibited by the visitor in the control condition through the invitation to the resident to call at anytime. It is possible that these differences may have engendered differences in the quality of the social relationships in the three visitation conditions. Although Schulz (1976) administered measures to assess how much the residents liked the visitors and how much they enjoyed the visits the mean scores and the statistical evaluation of these measures were not reported with the results.

It would seem that the results of this study do not provide strong evidence that a greater sense of control was either produced or that it was associated with the enhanced well-being of the residents. Although predictability may be conceptualized as an important aspect of control, why then should the predictability provided by the experimental procedure stand apart from the already existing predictability, which is typical of residential setting for the elderly, in producing an enhanced level of functioning of the residents? Previous research which has demonstrated beneficial effects of enhanced predictability has been in the context of coping with aversive events (Averill, 1973). It is not clear why increasing predictability in a benign and highly predictable environment should result in increased zest for life or improved health. Schulz's (1976) own comment that the residents in the predict and control groups may have benefitted from the opportunity to look forward to a positive event provides an interpretation of the results which is equally plausible as one based on increased predictability.

Schulz's (1976) study has been frequently cited as demonstrating the beneficial effect of greater pedictability and control on the physical health of the residents. This conclusion rests primarily on the analysis of pre- to post intervention change scores of subjects' self-reports of the quantity of medication taken. Schulz (1976) does not provide any information on the response format of this measure. Were the residents expected to recall accurately both the number of pills and dosage in milligrams of their daily medication? Does the +2.40 change score for the Random visit group represent a mean increase in the number of pills or the combined daily dosage of all types of medication in milligrams? If this measure assesses change in daily dosage in some standardized unit, does it represent a change in health status or habituation to the effects of medication? Interpretation of the relative differences between groups on this measure as demonstrating that the intervention inhibited physical decline does not seem warranted. The only other measure that demonstrated a significant difference between Schulz's combined pairs of experimental groups was the single-item Likert scale of health status completed by the activities director. This was taken as a post-intervention measure only. Since no independently assessed health status measure was administered before the intervention procedure and the relative physical health of the residents in each of the four groups is unknown it would seem reasonable that interpretations of a positive impact on health status should be accepted with caution.

In a follow-up study Schulz and Hanusa (1978) attempted to evaluate the potential long-term impact of the predictability and control intervention on health and psychological well-being. Direct access to participants in the original study was not permitted but ratings of health status and "zest for life" by the activities director were obtained for each resident at periods of 24, 30 and 42 months after the intervention procedure. Significant differences between the predict and control groups and the random and no-treatment groups were not found at any of the three follow-up periods. The failure of the predict and control groups to demonstrate superior health status or zest for life during the follow-up period has been interpreted as a possible result of a change in control expectancies following the termination of the intervention (Schulz & Hanusa, 1978). Interpretations of this type are purely speculative given that nothing is known about the subjects' control expectancies. The fact that four randomly selected groups of individuals in the same residential setting are rated as having essentially the same level of functioning after a two-year interval with no known differential treatment should not require explanations based on shifts in subjective appraisal of personal control.

The idea that enhancing the personal control of the elderly in residential care would have a broad ranging beneficial impact on the quality of life of the residents received further impetus from the study conducted by Langer and Rodin (1976). The intervention procedure employed in this study attempted to manipulate control through enhanced responsibility and choice. The enhanced responsibility and choice intervention consisted of three components: (1) subjects attended a talk given by the administrator of the nursing home in which they were encouraged to take responsibility for events in their day-to-day life and which also emphasized options for choice and personal influence, (2) a few days later residents were visited on an individual basis by the administrator to emphasize the expectancies expressed in the preceding talk, (3) residents were given the opportunity to choose a plant and to take responsibility for its care. In the second experimental condition subjects also attended a talk by the administrator but received a message which described existing services in the home and the staff's willingness to meet the needs of the residents. This message may be considered to be one which communicates an expectation for dependency (Rodin, 1980). Langer and Rodin (1976) reported improvement for the experimental group over the comparison group on measures of happiness, activity and well-being, using both self-report measures and ratings by nurses. This study is frequently cited as a demonstration of beneficial effects of enhanced control on psychological adjustment and physical health (Beck, 1982; Gatz, Popkin, Pino & VandenBos, 1985; Kuhl, 1986; White & Janson, 1986). A follow-up study by Rodin and Langer (1977) even suggests that the responsibility induction manipulation in the original study may have affected mortality rates of the two groups of subjects.

While the Langer and Rodin (1976) study has become one of the two landmark studies of research in control interventions the effects reported by Langer and Rodin (1976) appear to have been accepted in an uncritical manner. To begin with the critical assumption that the intervention was effective in modifying control beliefs is unsupported by the data reported by Langer and Rodin (1976). There were no significant differences between the responsibility induced group and the comparison group on a self-report measure of control. Despite this fact, the study has often been described as demonstrating the effects of enhanced control. To describe the source of influence on the behavior of the residents as one of induced responsibility, or as induced responsibility and enhanced choice, is also unwarranted given that no measures were taken to determine whether perceived choice and responsibility were greater following the experimental manipulation. Regardless of whether the Langer and Rodin (1976) study is cast in an induced responsibility framework (Beck, 1982; Langer & Rodin, 1976) or in a control framework (Krantz & Schulz, 1980) there is no evidence that such changes took place in the subjects. In fact, since control was measured and no difference was found it is perhaps more reasonable to conclude that the manipulation had no effect on control.

If there is no evidence for group differences on the intervening constructs of control, induced responsibility or enhanced choice, what may account for the reported differences between the two groups of residents on self-report measures of happiness and activity and on the nurses ratings of well-being and activity? It may simply have been the case that the two groups of residents were not comparable to begin with. There was no true random assignment of subjects to the two experimental groups but rather the groups were composed of residents from two different floors of the facility. Even if residents were assigned to a particular room on the basis of availability as Langer and Rodin (1976) report this does not insure that the procedure was random nor does it preclude the possibility that differences in characteristics of the two groups did not emerge over time due to different social environments on the two living units. One simple check on the comparability of the two groups of residents, and to an extent on the assumption of random assignment, would have been a comparison of the mean age of the two groups of residents but this information was not provided by Langer and Rodin (1976).

The data presented by Langer and Rodin (1976) even suggest that differences in activity patterns of the two groups of residents may have existed prior to the intervention. Subjects in the comparison group spent only sixty percent as much time as subjects in the experimental treatment group visiting with other "patients" at the pretest evaluation. One additional point with respect to the comparability of the two groups is that the self-report measures for the experimental group were based on forty-five subjects while those of the comparison group were based on twenty subjects. In terms of the percentage of subjects in the original experimental groups these numbers represent 96 percent of the treatment and 45 percent of the comparison group. The obvious questions which present themselves are what events accounted for the disproportionate loss of subjects in the comparison group and were the participating subjects different from their group cohorts? Were there then differences between the two experimental groups in age, proportion of males and females, or functional ability? Other reviews have pointed out that the proced- ures of the study failed to adequately control for experimenter bias and treatment contamination due to awareness by the nursing staff (Mosher-Ashley, 1987). If one accepts the Langer and Rodin (1976) study at face value it is not only a demonstration of a successful control intervention but also one of the most remarkable illustrations of the effects of a persuasive communication on behavior.

Rodin and Langer (1978) conducted a follow-up study to examine the long term effects of the enhanced responsibility manipulation on elderly people in residential care. Despite the fact that there was no evidence that an increased sense of responsibility, self-determination or control had been successfully induced in the residents in the treatment group, self-report and nurses' rating of resident behavior were carried out on a residual sample of residents from the first study. As with the original Langer and Rodin (1976) study there is a question whether the two groups of subjects included in the analyses were comparable at the time the experimental manipulation was administered. Again the mean ages of the two samples were not reported nor the proportion of males and females. A further problem with this follow-up study is that the scales used as dependent measures were different from those used in the original work. Although these measures may have some utility in comparison of the two groups at the time of the follow-up, the use of such measures in the calculation of change scores from the measures used in the original study is essentially unsound from a methodological standpoint.

Rodin and Langer (1978) also reported differences between the responsibility induced group and the comparison group on mortality rates, a remarkable effect for a brief intervention that had no clearly demonstrable effect on the mediating variable of control at the time it was administered. However the reported difference in mortality rates was in fact not significant (Rodin & Langer, 1978), yet reference to the effect of induced responsibility on mortality is still frequently reported (Banziger & Roush, 1983; Kuhl, 1986; Moos & Lemke, 1985; Slivinske & Fitch, 1987). In one case the "significantly lower death rate" has come back to life (Piper & Langer, 1986) and the note of erratum has apparently vanished like a spirit.

In a subsequent study by Rodin and White (described in Rodin, 1980) in which the responsibility-induced intervention manipulation of Langer & Rodin (1976) was replicated, there was again no effect on nursing home residents' perceptions of control. More important is the fact that subjects in the responsibility-induced intervention group also failed to demonstrate any gains on measures of activity or well-being. These results clearly render suspect the reliability of the induced-responsibility manipulation as a technique for affecting the beliefs and behaviors of geriatric residents in care settings.

Mercer and Kane (1979) investigated the effects of an induced-responsibility intervention similar to that employed by Rodin and Langer (1978) on residents' activity, hopelessness and psychosocial adjustment. Their study was carried out in two nursing homes with one home assigned to the treatment intervention condition and the other serving as the no-treatment control. The two subject groups did not differ at the time of pretest on any of the experimental measures but did so on the proportion of males and females in each setting (treatment 3% male, no-treatment 40% male) as well as mean number of years in residence (longer in no-treatment), educational level (lower in no-treatment) and perceived choice over admission into nursing home (less choice in the no-treatment group). Residents were given a talk by the administrator which encouraged them to take responsibility for events in their lives and identified decision-making opportunities that were available to the residents. The message was reinforced by the administrator who spoke to each resident individually and at this time they were given the opportunity to care for a plant. Subjects were tested before the intervention and at the end of the intervention period of five weeks. Subjects in the intervention group showed an increase on a thirteen-item self-report measure of activity relative to residents in the no-treatment group. Subjects in the intervention condition showed an increase on activity and a decreased score on the *Beck Hopelessness Scale*. Decrease in hopelessness was strongly correlated with increase in activity (r = .62). Over the five-week period of the study residents in the no-treatment group declined on staff ratings of behaviors related to psychosocial adjustment while subjects in the treatment group did not. Staff ratings were composed of independent ratings by the day nurse, night nurse and social worker.

Mercer and Kane (1979) did not employ any measure of perceived control so the effect of the intervention procedure on control beliefs is unknown. The possibility that the measure of hopelessness could in some sense be regarded as an indirect measure of control is a small one. The scale has been shown to be only weakly correlated with direct measures of control (Quinless & McDermott Nelson, 1988) and the items reflect pessimism and negative outcome expectancies rather than control related concepts (Beck, Weissman, Lester & Trexler, 1974).

The inferential limitations of this study which arise from the methodological weaknesses, ones which are the same as those of the Langer and Rodin (1976) study, are acknowledged by Mercer and Kane (1979) when they state that "one cannot know whether the behavioral changes that were reported resulted from changes in choice and control, from the resident being treated with greater respect and concern, or from a general Hawthorne effect secondary to the study" (p. 108). The possibility is also present that initial differences between the groups or other uncontrolled factors in the two settings contributed to differences found between the groups at the post intervention evaluation.

Banziger and Roush (1983) again replicated the Langer and Rodin (1976) procedure for induced responsibility but substituted giving residents a bird feeder rather than a plant to care for. In addition to the control intervention group the study utilized two comparison groups; a dependency group similar to the comparison group in Langer and Rodin (1976) and a no-treatment control group which received only the pretest and posttest measures. Subjects were reportedly assigned to each condition by random assignment. Although there was a constraint on assigning subjects to the control intervention group such that both residents of a room were assigned to the same condition, the experimental groups were not evaluated for comparability in age or scores on pretest measures. The results suggest that nursing home residents in the induced-responsibility group increased in self-reported control, happiness, and activity while such gains were not present for subjects in the dependency or the no-treatment groups.

The more serious problem with this study is that the experimenters helped deliver the enhanced responsibility manipulation and also served as interviewers for the administration of pretest and posttest measures. Furthermore, subjects in the control intervention condition would have bird feeders hanging outside their window at the time the experimenters were administering the posttest measures. Consequently the study is open to sources of experimenter bias particularly through demand characteristics arising from the experimenters visiting subjects individually to emphasize the control-relevant and dependency-relevant communications. In addition no statistical evaluation of between groups comparisons were made with analysis of variance or, more appropriately, analysis of covariance. Instead t-tests were used to evaluate change within each group.

In all there have been four studies which have employed essentially the same procedure as an intervention for enhanced control as originally described by Langer and Rodin (1976). Only the study by Banziger and Roush (1983) provides evidence that the induced-responsibility manipulation may have affected control beliefs and the validity of this outcome is uncertain given the sources of experimenter bias which existed in the procedure. Three of the studies reported beneficial outcomes for the residents in terms of self-reported activity and well-being while one found no beneficial effects. The fact that Rodin and White (described in Rodin, 1980) found no beneficial consequences of this intervention should call into question the findings originally reported by Langer and Rodin (1976) as well as the likelihood that the intervention produced any long-term effects as suggested by Rodin and Langer (1976). If it is to be accepted that such brief interventions have both powerful and long-term effects then it should be possible to better articulate and measure the process that is responsible for the changes in behavior.

The next study to be considered was not conceived as an intervention based on enhanced control, however the results provide some information on the relationship of control to psychological adjustment. The purpose of the study by Moran and Gatz (1987) was to evaluate the effectiveness of two types of group therapy for adults in nursing homes. The study was carried out in two proprietary nursing homes with the design replicated in each. Subjects were randomly assigned to one of three experimental groups, insight-oriented group therapy, task-oriented group therapy, or waiting-list control. No differences existed among the subjects in the three conditions in distribution of age, sex, race, or length of residence. The groups met once a week for twelve weeks with each session lasting 75 minutes. In the task-group, residents worked to develop a welcoming project to help new residents upon entering the home, a focus that could be described as problem solving and other-directed. In contrast many of the planned topics for the insight-oriented group touched on control related behavior, e.g., problem-solving behavior and self-efficacy. Issues which emerged in the insight group included lack of control over personal space, diet, possessions, finances, visitors, status, noise, and roommates. Participants in both the therapy groups demonstrated significant increases in expression of internal locus of control while participants in the waiting list group became slightly more external in their control beliefs. The proportion of subjects increasing in internality were comparable for the two groups, eighty percent in the task-group and seventy percent in the insight-group. Although both intervention groups showed increases in internal control only the task-group demonstrated improvement in life satisfaction as measured by the *Life Satisfaction Index-A*. This would suggest that change in life satisfaction was independent of change in control. Furthermore, inspite of their enhanced sense of control, the participants in the two treatment groups did not show enhanced performance on a measure of active coping relative to participants in the waiting-list group. It would appear that an increase in perceived control may not be sufficient to lead to increased life satisfaction or more active coping in day-to-day life. The results of this study stand in contrast to the suggestion by Schulz and Hanusa (1980) that increase in control is more important than the absolute level of control.

A study by Slivinske and Fitch (1987) was conducted to determine whether a control enhancing intervention would promote positive health and psychological effects of non-institutionalized elderly living in a retirement community. Participants were drawn from three retirement communities and randomly assigned to one of two experimental groups, control intervention and no-treatment. The control enhancing intervention spanned a period of twenty weeks and consisted of bi-weekly educational classes for ten weeks and tri-weekly physical fitness classes for the full twenty-week period.

The educational classes provided knowledge and skill development relevant to environmental mastery and control. Participants in the no-treatment condition were engaged in a variety of group activities and recreational events that did not emphasize information or skill development related to more effective daily living. Perceived control was measured by a thirty-five item scale with demonstrated reliability and concurrent validity. Participants also were assessed on a self-administered *Wellness Index* which was also demonstrated to have good reliability and discriminant and concurrent validity. Participants in the control intervention group showed significant gains in perceived control relative to their counterparts in the no-treatment group.

Analyses of the three subscales of the control measure showed that the treatment group enhanced perceptions of predictability, interpersonal power, and choice relative to participants in the no-treatment group. The treatment group showed positive and significant change relative to the no-treatment group on self-report measures of physical health, social resources, economic resources and spirituality. There were no differences between the two groups on the measures of morale or activities of daily living. Although the self-report measure of physical health suggests that the intervention was beneficial no significant differences were found between the two groups on muscular strength and flexibility, the number of times medical care was sought, number of days ill, or number of days hospitalized. One would have to suspect that if any true health benefits did result from the intervention that they would largely be attributable to the exercise program. The lack of any effect on the measure of activities of daily living may be attributable to the generally high level of functioning of participants of both groups. What is of interest here is that a well demonstrated increase in control was not associated with a positive impact on morale. Here again the possibility may exist that level of functioning of the subjects in this study was already sufficiently high such that relatively little change could be effected. In any case the intervention employed by Slivinske and Fitch (1987) goes well beyond a simple control enhancement intervention.

The body of evidence provided by these studies does not give strong support to the idea that enhancing the level of personal control of elderly people living in residential care settings will promote psychological and physical well-being. Not a single study demonstrates both a change in control beliefs and gains in measures of psychological or physical well-being while adequately controlling for confounding variables and sources of experimenter bias. The studies by Moran and Gatz (1987) and Slivinske and Fitch (1987) indicate that even when control is enhanced, improved morale does not necessarily follow.

All of the preceding studies have been characterized by one common feature. The target of the intervention has been the resident of the care setting. In the majority of these studies the intervention attempted to enhance the level of residents' control beliefs through brief exposure to control experiences with the expectation that the sense of enhanced control would affect other domains of daily activity and persist over time. There must however be some level of concordance between the residents' perception of control and the actual control options available to the residents. In order for short-term interventions which are directed at influencing control beliefs to have sustained effects, the subsequent experiences of the individual must confirm and support the appraisal of personal control.

Care Delivery and Resident Control

When the control beliefs of the elderly in residential care settings
are examined it is apparently the case that control for the residents
is greatly reduced relative to their community based cohorts or to
their previous patterns of daily living (Arling, Harkins & Capitman,
1986). There are many attributes of residential care settings which
may be considered to restrict the degree of control available to
residents. These restrictive elements can be arbitrarily partitioned
into two domains. One is the care delivery service composed of all
the staff members and volunteers associated with a facility and the
organizational structures, both explicit and implicit, that regulate
the standing patterns of behavior that take place in the setting. The
other is the physical setting itself which may either limit the range
of activity available to a resident or coerce the resident to
participate in undesired behavior (Howell, 1980; Moos & Lemke, 1985).
The control restricting factors associated with the physical setting,
such as multiple resident rooms and large communal dining areas, will
not be discussed in this chapter but are simply noted as a potential
area for control intervention research.

For geriatric residents in institutional settings the reduction
in control and personal efficacy has been shown to be a product of the
care-giving system as well as that of the individual's reduced
physical capabilities (Barton, Baltes & Orzech, 1980). Although the
routines of care settings are established to provide a high standard
of care, delivery of care tends to be more efficient if there is less
variation in the needs of the recipient. Consequently, there are
forces operating in institutional settings which act to limit personal
choice and behavioral autonomy. Mikulic (1971) has documented that
independent behavior of geriatric residents during morning care
activities was reinforced less frequently by care staff than was
dependent behavior. Mikulic's findings have been supported by more
recent work by Barton et al. (1980). In sequential analyses of
resident-staff interaction, it was established that independent
behavior in self-care activities by residents was followed more
frequently by staff behaviors that reinforce dependent behavior
rather than independent behavior. When residents engaged in dependent
behavior it was followed by dependence-supportive behavior from the
staff. The absence of reinforcement by staff of independent behavior
communicates to the resident a lower level of expectation for
self-control of behavior and for the initiation of self-care activity.

The tendency of nursing staff to selectively support dependent
behavior may stem from staff attitudes regarding the recipient's
apparent needs or from values associated with caregiver role. In a
large sample study of personnel from seven nursing homes Bagshaw and
Adams (1986) found a positive coorelation between negative attitudes
toward the elderly and a custodial ideological orientation toward
resident care. The dependency supporting behaviors that stem from
such an orientation plus the presence of negative attitudes should act

to diminish the sense of control in the recipients of care. Staff at the nurse aide level were less empathic and more custodial in orientation than staff at the registered nurse or licensed practical nurse level. The differences between these groups may be due to any one of the other variables that distinguish them, such as level of education. However, the possibility that the the attitudes of nursing staff at the aide level are shaped by the demands of the job role should also be considered.

A second source of staff influence on the behavior of elderly residents may be through the communication of attitudes to the residents which reflect diminished respect and the expectancy for dependent behavior (Rodin & Langer, 1980). Negative expectancy for behavioral competency can be communicated through expressive manner and style as well, for example talking down to residents (Caporeal, 1981; Caporeal, Lukaszewski & Culbertson, 1983). As a consequence, residents' awareness of negative appraisal from others and stereotyped attitudes regarding ability can lead to a diminished expectancy for effective functioning and increased dependency (cf. Langer & Benevento, 1978). The absence of strong demands for personal responsibility and staff acceptance of dependency behavior on the part of residents in extended care settings may support the development of helplessness and dependency (Avorn & Langer, 1982). Self-care activities may be lost to dependency even though the capability for self-care is present (Kennedy & Kennedy, 1982).

Caregiver Based Intervention

The previous studies indicate that one avenue for influencing both dependency behaviors and the perception of control of residents in long-term care settings is through their interactions with care staff. By training nursing and care staff to be aware of their potency as sources of social reinforcement and providing them with guidelines for supporting the behavioral independence of the residents the benefits associated with enhanced independence and control should be promoted. The objective is to create a control enhancing intervention that actually restores some of the behavior and decision control to the resident on a continuing basis.

The practice of structuring a psychosocial intervention program which employs caregiver/recipient interaction as a treatment modality has been applied in special care nursing (Baltes & Lascomb, 1975; Gardner, 1979), psychiatric nursing (Miller, 1978), and geriatric care (Weiss, 1969). Common features of programs of this type include instruction of care staff based on a simple heuristic model to guide interaction with the recipient, and the provision of some skill training in observing behaviors and executing appropriate responses. Program maintenance is variously supported by supervision, self-monitoring aids, or task group discussion (Hussian, 1981).

There are several reasons why a milieu based program of this type should be effective.   First is the fact that an individual's behavior patterns are integrated with and supported by the behavior of other people, particularly in institutional settings (Baltes & Reisenzein, 1986).   Second, direct care staff have more frequent contact and spend a greater amount of time with the resident than do professional staff.   If consistency of behavior is maintained by staff in interactions with the resident, the potential for modifying designated behaviors and providing therapeutic benefit is substantial (cf. Baltes & Zerbe, 1976).   In addition, programs of this type typically do not interfere with or affect the quality of the primary care activities of the staff since the therapeutic interaction co-occurs with care activity (Burg, 1979).

Munson and Seyfort (1987) developed a staff training program for health care workers which was designed to employ caregiver/recipient interaction as a therapeutic modality for geriatric residents in long-term care facilities.   The general purpose of the short-term training program was to provide the health care worker with information and skills that would facilitate the execution of care activities and at the same time promote personal control and expand the range of behavioral competencies of geriatric residents.   In conjunction with the training program a controlled evaluation was incorporated into the first delivery of the program.   The purpose of the evaluation was to determine whether the training program would, indirectly through the health care workers, promote greater personal control and positive psychological adjustment of the residents.

The content of the inservice training was structured to provide health care workers with an understanding of changes in physical and mental functioning that can influence emotion and behavior of elderly residents.   Emphasis was given to losses in personal control and increased dependency.   The first four sessions were devoted specifically to changes in control, dependency and depression, as well as care approaches for supporting independent functioning of residents. Sessions five through eight addressed basic behavior management skills, communication skills, working with the organically impaired and confused residents, and family issues.   It was predicted that residents receiving care from health care workers who participated in the training program would demonstrate a greater level of perceived control, and show improved functioning on measures of psychological adjustment.

Program Delivery

The training program was conducted with one instructional unit presented on each of eight consecutive weeks.   Each unit of material was repeated in four sessions to cover all sets of health-care workers on both day and evening shifts and a video tape of each instructional unit was made available to workers on night shift to provide program coverage to all three shifts. Brief on-floor visits with health-care workers were carried out during the training program and the three-month follow-up period. The purpose of these visits was to support health-care workers' understanding and application of concepts presented during training through discussion of specific resident care and behavior management problems.

The evaluation of the training program was based on comparison of a treatment group with a no-treatment group. Assessments of residents in both groups were made at three times: 1. before training program delivery; 2. immediately after program delivery; and 3. three months after program delivery.

The treatment group was made up of residents on a single living unit who received daily care primarily from health care workers participating in the training program. The control group was made up of residents from a different living unit who received daily care from health care workers who had not participated in the training sessions.

The nursing supervisors from the two units each identified an initial group of thirty residents who were alert and whose health was expected to remain stable over the next several months. These residents were then asked to participate in three personal interviews, each to be held several months apart. A total of thirty-eight residents agreed to participate, nineteen in both the treatment group and the no-treatment group. The groups were comparable in the proportion of male and female participants with fourteen female participants in each group. The mean age of the participants in the treatment group and no-treatment groups were 80.2 and 83.6 years respectively. The two groups were also comparable in terms of physical capability based on nursing records of activities of daily living. Three participants in each group were lost over the course of the study due to transfers to other care settings. Interviews were conducted by five research assistants who had experience working with the elderly but who were unfamiliar with the nature or purpose of the project. Each assistant was assigned an equal number of interviews from both experimental groups.

Health Care Worker Assessment

The program objectives were to encourage health care workers to view residents in a way which would promote physical and emotional independence and foster a positive sense of personal control in the residents. The attitudes of health-care workers toward the residents were assessed at the beginning and at the end of the training program on a fifteen-item semantic differential scale (Osgood, Suci, & Tannenbaum, 1957). The verbal anchors were selected to include terms that are common descriptors of geriatric residents, e.g., dependent-independent, cooperative-uncooperative, and spirited-dispirited.

The individual semantic differential scale items are convention-
ally grouped together to represent three dimensions of evaluation:
affect (e.g., like-dislike), potency (e.g., strong-weak), and activity
(e.g., active-passive). A related measures t-test comparison of the
pretraining and posttraining measures found attitudes of staff toward
the residents to be more positive on both the affective and potency
dimensions at levels that were statistically significant, t (10) =
2.32, p < .05 and t (10) = 2.96, p < .01 respectively. No significant
change occurred for staff's perception of resident activity. These
findings support the idea that following training, staff viewed the
residents they worked with as being both more pleasant and more
capable than they had at the beginning of the training.

The systematic observation of resident care activities of staff
who participated in the training program was not carried out because
the necessary organizational support for this type of activity could
not be developed within the scope of this project. In addition the
union representing the careworkers was preparing for negotiations of
contract renewal. Without the proper support, the monitoring of staff
care activities could have engendered program resistance and problems
between the staff, the employee's union and management. Since the
behavior of health-care workers on the care unit was not monitored,
the ways in which caregiver/recipient interactions may have changed as
a result of the training remains an area for further study.

Assessment of Resident Adjustment

The primary purpose of the training program was to enhance residents'
quality of life. The specific objective was to foster an increased
sense of personal control for residents and to facilitate positive
adjustment to life within the long-term care facility. Resident
perception of control was assessed by a control questionnaire
developed specifically for work with the elderly (Reid, Haas &
Hawkings, 1977). Resident adjustment was assessed in two ways. The
first was by the revised *Philadelphia Geriatric Center Morale Scale*
(Lawton,1975) which was presented to residents in individual interviews along with the control scale. The second measure was information on activities of daily living and adjustment from the nursing
unit records which was taken at the same periods as the resident
interviews. The nursing records contained information on residents'
level of functioning on twenty-four items in four domains of daily
activity: mobility, eating, personal hygiene and dressing. Ability
to perform each activity was rated at one of three levels: independent, needs some assistance, or needs total help. Nursing staff
evaluation of an individual resident's level of orientation was
rated on four levels: 1 = alert, 2 = slightly forgetful, 3 = moderately confused, and 4 = completely confused. Resident adjustment to the
environment was evaluated by a simple dichotomous judgment.

Residents in the treatment group increased in their perception of control over the period of the project relative to their counterparts in the no-treatment group. A repeated measures analysis of variance of the expectancy for control scores over the three Time periods yielded a significant Group x Time interaction, F (2, 52) = 6.24, p < .01. This indicates that the relative differences in perception of control between the two groups changed over time. There were no differences between the two groups on the measures of desire for control.

At the time of initial testing the two groups of residents were substantially different from one another with respect to their expectancies for control in daily life. Based on the the sum of the control expectancy items the treatment group had lower expectations for control (M = 17.8) than did the no-treatment group (M = 21.4), F (1, 34) = 10.69, p < .01. The treatment group had lower scores than the control group on every one of the seven items which measured expectancy for control.

Immediately following the inservice training program participants in the treatment groups had shown increases in their expectancy for control making them comparable to the residents in the no-treatment group. Residents in the two group did not differ based on the sum of the control expectancy items. After a period of three months, residents in the treatment group scored slightly higher than residents in the no-treatment group on the summed measure of expectancy for control. An analysis of the control expectancy scores using the pretraining control scores as the covariate yielded a significant difference between treatment and the no-treatment group, F (1, 20) = 4.29, p < .05. The results support the interpretation that the staff training intervention promoted an increased sense of control for residents in the treatment group.

Psychological Adjustment

Scores for the two groups on the interview measure of morale were essentially the same at each time period and showed no change over the duration of the project. The repeated measures analysis of total scores on the *Philadelphia Geriatric Center Morale Scale* yielded no significant effects for Group or Time main effects nor for the Group x Time interaction. Similarly, there were no significant effects for any of the the three factor components of the scale. The low correlation of the *Philadelphia Geriatric Center Morale Scale* with expectancy for control at the pretreatment interview (r = .13) indicates a lack of relationship between adjustment and perception of control as measured by these two instruments, at least for this group of subjects. Although the factor structure of the *Philadelphia Geriatric Center Morale Scale* has been validated on samples of the elderly (Lawton, 1975; Morris & Sherwood, 1975), its sensitivity and reliability for measuring change in a program evaluation context have not been previously demonstrated.

The absence of change on the *Philadelphia Geriatric Center Morale Scale* and the low correlation of this scale with the measure of control raises a number of issues concerning the relationship between personal control and psychological well-being of the elderly in residential care, and the adequacy of self-report measures for both variables. One explanation for the absence of change in the treatment group on the *Philadelphia Geriatric Center Morale Scale* is, of course, that the magnitude of change in control was not sufficient to influence the self-report measure of adjustment. Alternatively, it may be the case that the *Philadelphia Geriatric Center Morale Scale* functions more as a measure of trait adjustment rather than one of state adjustment and is relatively insensitive to short term change in residents' life satisfaction. This may be due to both the yes/no format of the items which limits gradations in evaluation, and the nature of the items, which focus on attitudes toward life in general rather than present day evaluations.

Nursing Staff Assessment of Adjustment and ADL Functioning

In contrast to the self-report measure of morale the ratings of resident adjustment by the supervisory nursing staff indicate that the intervention may have beneficially affected adjustment. At the preprogram measurement, residents on the treatment unit were assessed as slightly but not significantly less well-adjusted to the environment than their counterparts on the control unit, the proportions of adjusted residents on each unit being 33% and 40% respectively. Immediately following the completion of the training program differences between the two groups on adjustment to the environment were essentially unchanged. After the three-month posttraining interval the treatment group showed greater adjustment than the control group, a reversal in the order of ratings of the two groups from that found in the pretraining and the posttraining ratings. The percentage of adjusted residents in the treatment group was eighty-seven while that of the no-treatment group remained at the forty percent level of the the previous two periods. The difference in proportions between the two groups at the third measurement period was significant, $X^2_1 = 7.01$, $p < .01$.

If one accepts the ratings of resident adjustment by the supervisory nursing staff as a valid indicator of resident adjustment, then it appears that in addition to enhancing control the intervention also enhanced the well-being of the residents. It is important to note that improved functioning of the treatment group was developed even though the cognitive capacity of this group was lower than that of the no-treatment group, as demonstrated by their rated level of orientation. The repeated measures analysis of residents level of orientation yielded a significant Group main effect, $F (1, 27) = 8.54$, p < .01. The treatment group was evaluated by nursing staff as having a lower level of orientation ($M = 1.64$) than the no-treatment group ($M = 1.19$) over the three periods of assessment.

The treatment and no-treatment groups did not differ over the course of the study on any of the measures of activities of daily living. With functional status remaining unchanged over the course of the study the increase in perception of control and the gains in adjustment cannot be attributed to positive gains in functional ability. On the other hand it is equally clear that the intervention did not promote any change in functional status for the residents. The limitations that the functional capabilities of the resident may impose on interventions for enhancing personal control is one area which merits consideration in future research.

The study by Munson and Seyfort (1987) has demonstrated that staff training based intervention is a viable approach for control enhancement. However, the intervention procedure of this study is a relatively weak one as far as producing major changes in the way that care staff interact with the residents. Eight hours of training which covers a diverse range of topics is not very intensive. A program of this type could be structured to put more emphasis on social reinforcement of independent behavior and incorporate methods of behavior monitoring. This would provide care staff with information about their own behavior and would also make staff aware of the product of their efforts in terms of the functional capability of the residents.

Control Relationships for Caregivers and Residents

There may be some value in considering the care workers and the residents in long-term care settings to be linked in an hierarchical control network. If control is conceptualized as the relative degree of influence in determining the activity one engages in, the timing of activity, and the range of settings in which activity takes place, the degree of personal control available to the care worker is seen to be very limited. When the health-care worker is expected to assist in the morning care of twenty residents and see that they are all dressed and in the dining area at the prescribed time, the opportunities to encourage the resident to engage in choice behaviors in the selection of clothes to be worn, or to patiently give encouragement while the resident attempts to independently carry out part of dressing and grooming are severely limited. If a health-care worker takes extra time with one resident they are often painfully aware of two facts; their own job performance may be criticized by their nursing supervisor and some other resident is not getting the attention they need. Certainly staffing ratios are one factor that affect these problems. But other policy features of residential settings also contribute to the constraints on the health-care worker and the resident. It may be the food service workers who determine the time and the number of seatings for meal services with these issues negotiated in their contracts. An intervention based on shifting from a single breakfast service to two would reduce the time demands of morning care for care workers and allow them to be more supportive of the residents' independent behavior. In addition it would give the residents increased choice and control over their daily routine.

The training intervention conducted by Munson and Seyfort (1987) appeared to have a positive impact on the health-care workers' sense of control. Although this was not considered at the initiation of the project and no measures were taken, the health-care workers expressed a greater sense of control over their work. This may be the result of a better understanding and appreciation for some of the factors which influence the behavior of the residents or because of actual gains in behavior management skills. One issue for future investigations of control intervention is that control perceptions of care staff as well as those of the resident could be considered. An intervention that promotes the degree of control of the direct care staff as well as that of the residents will more likely be self-sustaining. Alternatively, an intervention which attempts to enhance control of residents by imposing further demands and constraints on health-care workers may not have long-term effectiveness.

Another aspect of caregiver/resident interaction that may have a bearing on residents' sense of control is the degree of familiarity that the resident has with the caregiver. In large residential facilities staffing of care workers is often not based on resident living groups. Careworkers may receive weekly or daily assignments to different floors and may choose to rotate shifts. Part-time staff are used to fill in for staff during vacation or sick leave. Consequently residents in long-term care settings may not have the consistency of contact with a worker which is needed for feelings of familiarity and trust to develop. The issues of social familiarity and trust should become more important as a resident's functional capability declines. One would expect that receiving bathing or toileting assistance from a few health-care workers that were well-known would provide the resident with a greater sense of control than being required to receive assistance from a greater number of relative strangers. When the most private activities of daily life become exposed to strangers the integrity and value of the person become diminished. A preliminary examination of instances of aggressive behavior by residents directed against careworkers by the participants in the Munson and Seyfort (1987) study suggests they are linked to situations involving toileting assistance or assisting the resident in changing undergarments. These activities require the violation of personal space and clearly convey to the resident their loss of control over basic self-care activities. The frustration and arousal that is likely produced in these situations plus the physical proximity of the careworker as a target of aggression may contribute to the instigation of aggressive action.

One additional consideration for a staff-based intervention is the consistency of staff treatment which the residents receive. The way in which health-care workers interact with the residents is very diverse. A common example is attention-seeking behavior. A resident who makes frequent and unnecessary requests for assistance or attention may be treated in a firm but fair manner by one aide who chooses not to meet unnecessary requests. The next day a different aide will find it easier to give in to the resident because it is personally less troublesome than it is to continue to listen to the resident's requests.

Considerations for Future Research

Several factors affecting the relationship of control to measures of adjustment need to be considered in future control intervention research. The level of constraint in the care setting appears to have a direct effect on the control beliefs of the residents and to affect the relationship between control and measures of life satisfaction and adjustment. Wolk (1976) reported that in a low constraint setting residents had a stronger sense of internal control which was positively associated with adjustment. In a setting with greater environmental constraint, the relationship betweeen control and adjustment was not present. Fawcett, Stonner and Zepelin (1980) found that the majority of the variance in life satisfaction for a group of nursing home residents was accounted for by perceived institutional constraint. Since environmental constraint is a factor which potentially affects both control beliefs and adjustment, considering the relationship of control to well-being without information characterizing the level of constraint in the situational context will make clear and meaningful interpretation of research results less likely. The absence of environmental constraint measures in research also limits the comparison of findings across settings and studies.

Functional dependency of residents is another factor which appears to affect morale and control beliefs directly (Ryden, 1984). It is also associated with environmental context at least to the extent that different facilities serve clients requiring different levels of care. The likelihood that the care setting directly influences the level of functional dependency has been considered by a number of researchers. The equating of experimental groups on age, length of stay and health status does not ensure that groups are also equivalent on level of dependency. A direct measure of functional status more adequately assesses the effects of this variable and may be a particularly important consideration when behaviors such as resident activity are used as outcome measures to assess the effectiveness of an intervention.

Ryden (1984) has examined the relationships between functional dependency, control and morale in intermediate care and skilled nursing care settings. For residents in intermediate care facilities

level of control over eight areas of daily activity was moderately
correlated with morale as was functional dependency. For residents in
skilled nursing care, who had lower levels of functional ability,
control over daily activities was much more strongly associated with
morale whereas functional dependency was not associated with morale.
For the resident in skilled nursing care who has already experienced
significant decline in functional ability, control over self-care
activites may take on greater significance for morale. This may be due
in part to the fact that these activities constitute a greater
proportion of the total behavioral repertoire. Also as actual control
diminishes the relative psychological value placed on the behaviors
which do remain may take on greater significance. A resident in
skilled care may not place as great a value on being able to visit
with friends as on being able to put on their own socks. Ryden has
suggested that in a skilled nursing facility residents who are more
self-determining would represent an elite group and may consequently
have more satisfying interactions with staff. In contrast residents
in intermediate care may be having their initial encounter with
functional dependency and have not yet come to terms with their
change in functional ability. In addition they may feel relatively
more disadvantaged than their peers.

An outline of an hypothesized relationship between functional
dependency, domains of personal control and the continuum of residential settings for the elderly is presented in Figure 1. While there
would certainly be a fair degree of heterogeneity of functional
ability and overlap in the domains of control relevant behavior within
setting type, the sphere of behavior over which the resident can exert
control should contract as functional ability declines. This does
not imply that control takes on less importance with decline in
functional status. It may well be the case that experiences of
control take on greater psychological importance as functional
dependency declines. This model is presented here primarily as an
heuristic for considering how control may best be manipulated and
measured in intervention research. As an example, a control intervention based on visits from college students such as the one employed by
Schulz (1976) may have little benefit for residents low in functional
ability because the intervention does not affect control in the sphere
of activity that holds the greatest importance for the resident on a
day-to-day basis. In contrast an intervention that restores some
degree of control over grooming and eating would be expected to have a
more beneficial impact on the residents' sense of well-being. With
respect to intervention assessment, if there is a gradient of control
relevant behaviors associated with functional dependency then using
the same measure of control in all settings may not be effective.

Overall the research on control interventions has demonstrated a
neglect for the use of measures with established reliability and
validity. This is most clearly the case for the reported dramatic
findings of control interventions on the health of elderly residents.

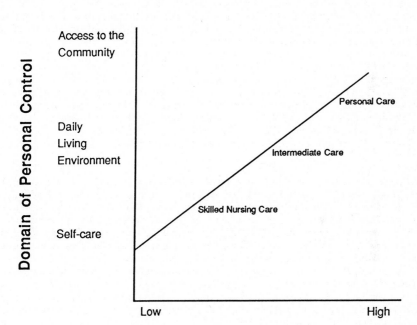

Figure 1

Hypothesized Relationship Between Functional Dependency
and Principal Domain of Personal Control

If health status is to be considered as one of the outcome measures
in control intervention research then the concept of health status
needs to be more clearly defined and measures with demonstrated
reliability and validity must be employed. Judgments by higher level
institutional staff such as nurses and activities directors are
inherently weak as valid indicators of health status because these
individuals often have infrequent contact with residents, particularly
in large settings. Consequently their judgments are susceptible to
the carry over effects of previous information and the influence of
comments by others about the residents. The necessary assumption that
they have uniform frequency of contact and information about all
residents in a setting is probably unfounded.

Conclusions

It should be clear from this review that as of yet the beneficial
effects of control enhancing interventions on psychological well-
being or the health of elderly residents in long-term care settings
has not been demonstrated. This conclusion unfortunately is contrary
to the apparently common belief that such effects have been demonstrated. The misfortune here is that researchers will turn their
attention to other issues and the questions relevant to control
interventions will not be investigated. Apart from the generally
poor methodology which has characterized the majoriy of the control
intervention studies one of the more serious limitations is that the
interventions have not been designed to make any direct changes in the
control contingencies available to the resident. No broadly based
control intervention has as yet been specifically directed at the
factors within the residential care environment that have been
documented as contributing to dependency. The interventions have been
short-term activities superimposed on the existing organizational and
behavioral routines of the setting which leave the existing structure
of dependency reinforcing contingencies intact. One distinction for
future research is whether a control intervention is an integrated
component of the care delivery setting and process or whether it is
an extraneous program that coexists with care delivery. The care
delivery staff should be considered as one of the more potent
avenues for introducing control interventions. By providing care
staff with behavioral alternatives which help to promote choice and
independence for the resident, the social contingencies which reduce
control and support dependency can be altered. The potential power in
staff based intervention approaches is that gains in control and
reduced dependency can be supported on a continuing basis.

References

Arling, G., Harkins, E. B., & Capitman, J. A. (1986). Institutiona-
    lization and personal control: A panel study of impaired older
    people. *Research on Aging, 8,* 38-56.

Averill, J. R. (1973). Personal control over aversive stimuli and its relationship to stress. *Psychological Bulletin, 80,* 286-303.

Avorn, J., & Langer, E. J. (1982). Induced disability in nursing home patients: A controlled trial. *Journal of the American Geriatric Society, 30,* 397-400.

Bagshaw, M., & Adams, M. (1986). Nursing home nurses' attitudes, empathy, and ideologic orientation. *International Journal of Aging and Human Development, 22,* 235-247.

Baltes, M. M., & Lascomb, S. L. (1975). Creating a healthy institutional environment: The nurse as a change agent. *International Journal of Nursing Studies, 12,* 5-12.

Baltes, M. M., & Reisenzein, R. (1986). The social world in long-term care institutions: Psychosocial control toward dependency? In M. M. Baltes & P. B. Baltes (Eds.), *The psychology of control and aging* (pp. 315-343). Hillsdale, NJ: Lawrence Erlbaum Associates.

Baltes, M. M., & Zerbe, M. B. (1976). Independence training in nursing-home residents. *The Gerontologist, 16,* 428-432.

Banziger, G., & Roush, S. (1983). Nursing homes for the birds: A contol-relevant intervention with bird feeders. *The Gerontologist, 23,* 527-531.

Barton, E. M., Baltes, M. M., & Orzech, M. J. (1980). Etiology of dependence in older nursing home residents during morning care: The role of staff behavior. *Journal of Personality and Social Psychology, 38,* 423-431.

Beck, A. T., Weissman, A., Lester, D., & Trexler, L. (1974). The measurement of pessimism: The hopelessness scale. *Journal of Consulting and Clinical Psychology, 42,* 861-865.

Beck, P. (1982). Two successful interventions in nursing homes: The therapeutic effects of cognitive activity. *The Gerontologist, 22,* 378-383.

Burg, M. M. (1979). Use of a self-recording and supervision program to change institutional staff behavior. *Journal of Applied Behavior Analysis, 12,* 363-375.

Caporeal, L. R. (1981). The paralanguage of caregiving: Baby talk to the institutionalized aged. *Journal of Personality and Social Psychology, 40*(5), 876-884.

Caporeal, L. R., Lukaszewski, M. P., & Culbertson, G. H. (1983). Secondary babytalk: Judgments by institutionalized elderly and their caregivers.   *Journal of Personality and Social Psychology*, 44, 746-754.

Chanowitz, B., & Langer, E. J. (1980).   Knowing more (or less) than you can show: Understanding control through the mindlessness-mindfulness distinction.   In J. Garber & M. E. P. Seligman (Eds.), *Human helplessness* (pp. 97-129).   New York: Academic Press.

Fawcet, G., Stonner, D., & Zepelin, H. (1980).   Locus of control, perceived constraint and morale among institutionalized aged. *International Journal of Aging and Human Development*, 11, 13-23.

Gardner, K. G. (1979).   Supportive nursing: A critical review of the literature.   *Journal of Psychiatric Nursing*, 17, 6-18.

Gatz, M., Popkin, S. J., Pino, C., & VandenBos, G. R. (1985). Psychological interventions with older adults.   In J. E. Birren & K. W. Schaie (Eds.), *Handbook of the psychology of aging* (2nd Ed.) (pp. 755-785).   New York: Van Nostrand Reinhold.

Howell, S. C. (1980).   Environments and aging.   In C. Eisdorfer (Ed.), *Annual review of gerontology and geriatrics* (pp. 237-260). New York: Springer.

Hussian, R. A. (1981).   *Geriatric psychology: A behavioral perspective*.   New York: Van Nostrand Reinhold.

Karuza, J., Jr., & Rabinowitz, V. C., & Zevon, M. A. (1986). Implications of control and responsibility on helping the aged.   In M. M. Baltes & P. B. Baltes (Eds.), *The psychology of control and aging* (pp. 373-396).   Hillsdale, NJ: Lawrence Erlbaum Associates.

Kennedy, R. W., & Kennedy, A. B. (1982).   Absence of purposeful behavior: Issues in training the profoundly impaired elderly.   In A. M. Horton (Ed.), *Mental health interventions for the aging* (pp. 69-83).   New York: Praeger.

Krantz, D. S., & Schulz, R. (1980).   A model of life crisis, control, and health outcomes: Cardiac rehabilitation and relocation of the elderly.   In A. Baum & J. E. Singer (Eds.), *Advances in environmental psychology: Applications of personal control* (Vol. 2, pp. 23-59).   Hillsdale, NJ: Lawrence Erlbaum Associates.

Kuhl, J. (1986).   Aging and models of control: The hidden costs of wisdom.   In M. M. Baltes & P. B. Baltes (Eds.), *The psychology of control and aging* (pp. 1-33).   Hillsdale, NJ: Lawrence Erlbaum Associates.

Langer, E. J., & Benevento, A. (1978).   Self-induced dependence. *Journal of Personality and Social Psychology*, 36, 886.

Langer, E. J., & Rodin, J. (1976). The effects of choice and enhanced personal responsibility for the aged: A field experiment in an institutional setting. *Journal of Personality and Social Psychology, 34,* 191-198.

Lawton, M. P. (1975). The Philadelphia Geriatric Center Morale Scale: A revision. *Journal of Gerontology, 30,* 85-89.

Mercer, S., & Kane, R. A. (1979). Helplessness and hopelessness among the institutionalized aged: An experiment. *Health and Social Work, 4,* 91-116.

Mikulic, M. (1971). Reinforcement of independent and dependent behavior by nursing personnel: An exploratory study. *Nursing Research, 20,* 162-163.

Miller, T. W. (1978). A model for training nursing staff as primary counsellors for psychiatric service. *Journal of Psychiatric Nursing, 16,* 28-33.

Moos, R. H., & Lemke, S. (1985). Specialized living environments for older people. In J. E. Birren & K. W. Schaie (Eds.), *Handbook of psychology of aging* (2nd Ed.) (pp. 864-889). New York: Van Nostrand Reinhold.

Moran, J. A., & Gatz, M. (1987). Group therapies for nursing home adults: An evaluation of two treatment approaches. *The Gerontologist, 27,* 588-591.

Morris, J. N., & Sherwood, S. (1975). A retesting and modification of the Philadelphia Geriatric Center Morale Scale. *Journal of Gerontology, 30,* 77-84.

Mosher-Ashley, P. M. (1987). Procedural and methodological parameters in behavioral-gerontological research: A review. *International Journal of Aging and Human Development, 24,* 189-228.

Munson, P., & Seyfort, B. (1987). *The effect of a short-term inservice training for care workers on perceived control and psychological adjustment of geriatric residents.* Unpublished manuscript.

Osgood, C. E., Suci, G. J., & Tannenbaum, P. H. (1957). *The measurement of meaning.* Urbana, IL: University of Illinois Press.

Piper, A. I., & Langer, E. J. (1986). Aging and mindful control. In M. M. Baltes & P. B. Baltes (Eds.), *The psychology of control and aging* (pp. 71-89). Hillsdale, NJ: Lawrence Erlbaum Associates.

Quinless, F. W., & McDermott Nelson, M. A. (1988). Development of a measure of learned helplessness. *Nursing Research, 37,* 11-15.

Reid, D. W. (1984). Participatory control and the chronic-illness adjustment process. In H. M. Lefcourt (Ed.), *Research with the locus of control construct: Extensions and limitations* (Vol. 3, pp. 361-389). New York: Academic Press.

Reid, D. W., Haas, G., & Hawkings, D. (1977). Locus of desired control and positive self-concept of the elderly. *Journal of Gerontology, 32,* 441-450.

Rodin, J. (1980). Managing the stress of aging: The role of control and coping. In S. Levine & H. Ursin (Eds.), *Coping and health* (pp. 171-202). New York: Plenum Press.

Rodin, J., & Langer, E. J. (1977). Long term effects of a control-relevant intervention with the institutionalized aged. *Journal of Personality and Social Psychology, 35,* 897-902.

Rodin, J., & Langer, E. J. (1978). Erratum. *Journal of Personality and Social Psychology, 36,* 462.

Rodin, J., & Langer, E. J. (1980). Aging labels: The decline of control and the fall of self-esteem. *Journal of Social Issues, 36,* 12-29.

Ryden, M. B. (1984). Morale and perceived control in institutional-ized elderly. *Nursing Research, 33,* 130-136.

Schulz, R. (1976). Effects of control and predictability on the physical and psychological well-being of the institutionalized aged. *Journal of Personality and Social Psychology, 33,* 563-573.

Schulz, R., & Hanusa, B. H. (1978). Long term effects of control and predictability enhancing interventions: Findings and ethical issues. *Journal of Personality and Social Psychology, 36,* 1194-1201.

Schulz, R., & Hanusa, B. H. (1980). Experimental social gerontology: A social psychological perspective. *Journal of Social Issues, 36,* 30-46.

Slivinske, L. R., & Fitch, V. L. (1987). The effects of control enhancing interventions on the well-being of elderly individuals living in retirement communities. *The Gerontologist, 27,* 176-181.

Weiss, J. (Ed.) (1969). *Nurses, patients, and social systems.* Columbia, MO: University of Missouri Press.

White, C. B., & Janson, P. (1986). Helplessness in institutional settings: Adaptation or iatrogenic disease? In M. M. Baltes & P.

B. Baltes (Eds.), *The psychology of control and aging* (pp. 297-313). Hillsdale, NJ: Lawrence Erlbaum Associates.

Wolk, S. (1976). Situational constraint as a moderator of the locus of control-adjustment relationship. *Journal of Consulting and Clinical Psychology, 44,* 420-427.

*Psychological Perspectives of Helplessness
and Control in the Elderly, P.S. Fry (ed.)*
© *Elsevier Science Publishers B.V. (North-Holland), 1989*

Chapter Eight

COGNITIVE SOCIAL LEARNING THEORY OF CONTROL AND AGING, PARTICIPATORY CONTROL AND THE WELL-BEING OF ELDERLY PERSONS

David W. REID and Gloria STIRLING

York University

Abstract

Despite the growing literature on control and aging there are few studies where both theory and practical intervention techniques have been specifically developed to facilitate seniors having more control. Impeding this development have been: (1) ethical dilemmas in implementing such research, (2) the complexity of accommodating the multiple variables determining outcome measures within natural settings, and (3) reliance on overly simple interpretations of psychological control. This chapter critically reviews the studies which attempted to demonstrate that giving seniors a greater sense of control, benefits the seniors. The ethical, practical and conceptual limitations of these studies are discussed in light of recent theoretical advances made by a number of authors. To assist the theoretical advances a reconceptualization of psychological control is presented and described in the form of a new theory. In order to illustrate the theoretical advances from these theoretical improvements and applied research, the results of two recently completed field studies are discussed. One of these studies utilized an experimental design that was integrated within a nursing service to show how control can be facilitated among hospitalized seniors. In the second study the ways in which physicians interacted with patients was systematically varied to demonstrate that patients responded more favorably to physicians who behaved in ways that would give seniors more control. The design of both studies was guided by the concept of Participatory Control, which emphasizes that the experience of control is interactive. The experience of control is constantly in terms of a perceived balance between internal and external forces that are seen to determine one's condition. It is this balanced interplay that affects the control the senior has, and can explain how even disabled and dependent seniors can maintain control.

Introduction

The Inadequacy of Control Concepts for Studying Aging

The limitations of our understanding of control and aging become clear when we try to apply psychological control concepts in field settings. Much of the past psychological control research has remained at the preliminary stage of providing data that demonstrate theoretical ideas. It is time we tested the utility of these theories in applied settings, for it is in the application where problems and subsequent improvements can occur. Despite considerable correlation research demonstrating that seniors receiving better adjustment scores on a variety of measures also report having a greater sense of control, there are relatively few studies demonstrating that one can increase the senior's control and in doing so contribute to the well-being of the elderly citizen (Slivinske & Fitch, 1987). The few studies which have been done are either limited methodologically (e.g. Langer & Rodin, 1976; Rodin & Langer, 1977) or else are not practical and have ethical problems (e.g. Schulz, 1976; Schulz & Hanusa, 1978). We feel the problem with applying control concepts reflects not only the considerable methodological and ethical difficulties, it also reflects the inadequacies of control concepts for understanding aging phenomena.

Past conceptualizations of psychological control have not explained why control is relevant to the process of aging. If we cannot conceive of why or how psychological constructs such as predictability, choice and behavioral control apply to the process of becoming old, then what utility have these constructs for understanding aging? On the one hand, we have a growing gerontology literature outlining the multitude of physiological, psychological and sociological changes with aging. The literature on lifespan developmental phenomena emphasizes aging as a dynamic process of change. Obviously a 70 year old is, feels and behaves very differently from either a teenager or a 30 year old. On the other hand, we have an extensive literature of psychological control that has not focused on the process of change. For example, much of the research on control indicates that in most instances having control is more desirable than not having control no matter what the age. There also a few studies that compare locus of control scores across age groups and cohorts. But there is a lack of research on whether psychological control naturally changes as part of the aging process. For example, if one has had a relatively strong sense of control throughout one's life, surely that sense of control at 70 years of age differs from when one was 30 years and a teenager, respectively. In grade school behavior control may have been critical to one's sense of control (e.g. in order to be able to play games and sports). However, at 70 years of age behavioral ability may not be as central as knowledge and analytical ability for decision making and advising others on what to do. What we lack are theoretical concepts to direct the necessary research into the aging process.

There is a trend towards the development of psychological control concepts that are more applicable to studying aging. The purpose of this chapter is to add impetus to this trend. We begin this in the first sec|ion by encouraging a reconsideration of the use of control constructs for applied research into aging. We next summarize the seminal research of Langer and Rodin (1976) and Schulz (1976) in order to explain how their work provided a beginning to the application of control concepts to understand aspects of aging. These semilal studies provide a backdrop for the third section, where we discuss recent theoretical developments that have applied significance and contribute to the trend we are emphasizing. The fourth section complements the earlier sections by presenting a reconceptualization of psychological control that is more dynamic and accommodating to the multitude of variables affecting the aging process. The fifth section explains this re-interpretation of control within the Cognitive Social Learning Theory of Control (Reid & Ziegler, 1981; Reid, 1984) which was developed to guide research into social-psychological aspects of aging. It is from this theory that we developed the concept of Participatory Control discussed in section six. Participatory Control explains how interpersonal transactions between patients and their health care professionals can maintain the experience of being in control in situations where changes in health and institutional pressure would otherwise erode the patient's control. Two recent studies guided by this concept are summarized. One of these studies illustrates the application of a control concept to facilitate the adjustment of hospitalized geriatric patients.

A Reconsideration of the Use of Control Constructs
for Research on Aging

Past formulations of psychological control have been deterministic, mechanistic, rigid and inadequate for addressing the complexity of both the social systems context and the persons to whom they are applied. Despite some consideration of a more interactional applica-tion (Reid, 1977) control concepts have mainly been used as stable, unidimensional phenomena not influenced by the context within which they are studied or applied. By deterministic we refer to the implicit assumption that by changing one phenomena (e.g., either by teaching a senior patient how to be more assertive, or advising the staff to give patients more choice in what they might do during the day) one is going to change, in a unidirectional way, the situation or person. By mechanistic we refer to the implication that behaviors and environments are made up of distinct entities (e.g., personal control beliefs, personal efficacy, predictable environment, value of desired outcomes, restricting rather than nonrestricting environments) and that somehow, like parts to a machine, we can add them together to gain a desired outcome. Indeed, the notion that one can teach another to have more control is itself a questionable, deterministic view. In education, we do not teach students to be more intelligent; at best we work with them to facilitate their applying their intelligence. Similarly, if scientists/practitioners can understand what the so-called personal control means to the senior within his/her situation, then perhaps they can facilitate the expression/experience of that control. As part of our reconsideration, therefore, we recommend that a more interactional interpretation of psychological control, addressing the ongoing assimilation/accommodation of the individual to his/her environment, is the more reasonable and as such, more applicable approach to understanding behavior.

There are a number of questions that we advance to guide the reconsideration of the use of psychological control concepts for studying aging. We begin with the question: what is the study of psychological control? Baltes and Baltes (1986) point out that psychological control is a field of study and not a singular theoreti-cal construct. What is it about this field of study that may assist our understanding of aging phenomena? There are many constructs within this field and no definitive theory to unite them. Indeed, as Karuza, Rabinowitz and Zevon (1986) have commented, there has been a myriad of "... control like constructs defined and studied" (Karuza, et al., 1986 p. 376). The notion that they all reflect the same underlying construct is rather untenable. On the contrary, the question should not be whether these constructs *represent* the same underlying construct (which is a pseudo question) but whether they *apply* to the same behaviors?

Why do behavioral scientists continue to discuss constructs pertaining to psychological control? Presumably, the value to the scientists is the adequacy of these conceptualizations for discussing the complex behaviors of people as they interact and/or transact with their environment. Of importance is whether these conceptualizations can be used efficiently in discourse among scientists *and* prac-titioners to explain phenomena associated with aging. We believe these concepts are not used efficiently, and thus we feel there is a need to reconsider their value. Indeed, the proliferation of "control-like constructs" is seen as reflecting the scientists' appreciation of the limitations of past conceptualizations and their wish to advance additional refinements about psychological control. The result is the growing list of terms including: Internal-external locus of control, decisional control, behavioral control, predic-tability, controllability, cognitive control, learned helplessness, personal efficacy, secondary control, primary control, personal causation, proxy control, illusory control, mindlessness-mindfulness, powerlessness, and empowerment. The novice reader of this literature may ask either naively or pejoratively: "Would the real control please stand up?"

If the theorists believe these constructs apply to supposedly different behaviors, can the differences among these behaviors be upheld empirically in natural settings? If they cannot, then what is the utility of having such a diffuse set of constructs? Are the theoretical distinctions only in the minds of the theorists, or can they be both verified empirically and shown to be of differential use in natural settings? If these concepts refer to the same behavior, is it possible there are common themes among these conceptualizations which, if we can identify them, are useful to apply in studies of aging?

While scientists have developed the control constructs as unique attempts to advance our understanding of some forms of behavior, it is their joint advancement that needs to be discerned. The viability of each construct has been supported by (1) the presentation of data to which they apply and (2) the author's reasoning for advancing the use of the construct. But what is it about them all that is advancing this field of research? It is not clear to what extent these terms or conceptualizations are mutually complementary or redundant. Are these multiple constructs just a growing mosaic or menu of terms from which the applied scientist merely chooses the term that makes the best sense to him or her for explaining the behavior studied? We need to know if, how, and why certain constructs are more applicable than others. Answers to questions of application such as these will improve discourse among scientists and practitioners regarding psychological control. Without adequate discourse, the terms will be either ignored or superseded with more constructs. But with each additional control construct within the field, we risk further diffusion and increased confusion. As a group, the constructions of psychological control will lack utility and value if we cannot share an understanding of how they fit with the complexities of daily life.

Simply proposing yet another hypothetical construct that is defined by either a single measurement scale (eg. Rotter's I-E scale) or a specific paradigm (eg. Seligman's Learned Helplessness paradigm) is not the answer. A broader conceptualization is required that meets the needs of both the researcher and the practitioner. It must be broad enough to allow insight into the complex interplay between individuals and their environments. It must also be sufficiently flexible to allow for the development of interventions and for the identification of the complex processes influencing the "control" people feel and respond to within a particular context.

Our appreciation of the need for more applicable conceptualizations of control was spurred by our attempts to understand how seniors suffering from illnesses and having to receive long-term care in a hospital setting are able to adjust to these major changes in their lives. From our data, we inferred that the patient's ability to maintain a sense of control is a key component of this complex adjustment. But how does a patient do this and how might we facilitate this process? As part of our search for a better conceptualization, we critically reviewed previous considerations of psychological control and adjustment (Reid, 1984).

We were particularly alarmed that readers of certain well cited articles such as those by Langer and Rodin (1976) and Schulz (1976) might conclude that merely giving a senior patient a modicum of predictability (e.g., of when a visitor would come) or an activity, such as raising plants, would be a reasonable and practical approach to facilitating control, and thus, encouraging psychological adjust-ment. From a systems theory perspective or an applied psychologist's perspective, any possible benefit from such interventions would be temporary and soon eroded by other aspects of the environmental press on the individual. Too much emphasis has been placed on the findings that even such temporary facilitation of control experiences might be beneficial. The scientific value of these studies lies not in their findings, but rather in their methodological and conceptual limita-tions that spurred further developments in this field of research. To underscore the latter contributions, these studies are summarized in the following section.

Lessons From the Early Applied Research on Control and Aging

The seminal studies of Langer and Rodin (1976) and Schulz (1976) are worth reexamining as they reflect how simplistic our interpretations of psychological control were in the mid 1970's. They also provide a background against which to examine more current interpretations.

In the Langer and Rodin study, one group of nursing home residents were encouraged to have more responsibility for day-to-day events. This encouragement took the form of a talk given by the hospital administrator that emphasized the responsibility the patients had for taking care of themselves. This communication was bolstered by giving each patient in the assembly a plant which s/he was to take care of, as well as the administrator later circulating among the patients to further encourage their taking charge. The patients in an alternate group were given a separate talk by the same administrator that stressed the staff's responsibility for taking care of them. They, too, were each given a plant but told that the staff would take care of the plant. Results from the questionnaire and behavioral rating data indicated that patients in the responsibility group were more active and happier than those in the comparison group.

It is not clear, however, that these outcome differences were due to the experimental manipulations; they may have been due to other differences between the two groups. The study did not have many experimental controls, and there is reason to question whether the independent variable of responsibility induction applied differently between groups. For example, it is likely that patients and staff intermingle and talk of daily activities. It is possible that either patients and/or staff learned of the apparent contradictory messages from the administrator. Knowledge of the contradictory message may have led to the patients not believing the administrator's message or else may have generated a suspicion of differential treatment of patients. We do not know whether either the patients or the staff wanted the plants, or if they already had many plants. The question-naire that the authors used as a manipulation check of whether there were differences between the groups in perceived control found no differences. One might also be skeptical that this intervention, which does not seem very forceful or substantive within the everyday life of a nursing home, should have much impact on activity and happiness. The intervention did not directly alter the relationships between staff and patients.

The patients were not randomly assigned to conditions. Rather, within the 4-floor building patients on one floor were compared with patients on a second floor. At issue, therefore, is the comparability of the patients on the two respective floors. It is possible that the differences between floors on the outcome measures occurred "natural-ly" as a result of factors not taken into consideration in this study. For example, it is possible the patients in the intervention group were either healthier or naturally became more healthy and this accounted for the group differences. An 18 month follow-up (Rodin & Langer, 1977) provides evidence that the two groups did differ in health status and that a greater number (p < .10 trend) of those in the comparison group subsequently died. It is hard to believe that this intervention should have an impact on mortality and morbidity. It is more parsimonious to infer, in light of the follow-up findings, that differences in health contributed to the differences found between the two groups. In any event, the results are far from conclusive.

Rodin and Langer (1977) noted the problem of determining cause in their study and it is in their discussion that we see the growth of inquiry into why a causal link might have occurred. While they admitted that they ". . . had no real way of knowing without direct on-line observation exactly what the process was that generated the obtained improvements" (p. 901) they preferred to interpret their intervention as causal and clinically important. They guardedly stated: "We would like to interpret these effects as suggesting that decline can be slowed or, with a stronger intervention, perhaps can even be reversed by manipulations that provide an increased sense of efficacy in the institutionalized elderly" (p. 901). They inferred that somehow their intervention may have helped to set in motion unknown "processes" that effected the differential outcomes in their data. They stated: "One clear area for further study is the patient-nurse interaction to assess if and how this factor is related to patient health" (Rodin & Langer, 1977, p. 901). The worth of their study was that it was less a demonstration of a particular kind of control and more an attempt to ". . . determine whether the decline in health, alertness, and activity that generally occurs in the aged in nursing home settings could be slowed or reversed by choice and control manipulations..." (Rodin & Langer, 1977, p. 897).

The Schulz (1976) study contained more experimental controls than did the Langer and Rodin (1976) study, in so far as the subjects were randomly assigned to experimental conditions and there were manipulation checks taken to confirm the integrity of the interventions. Patients were assigned to one of four experimental conditions, systematically manipulating the way visitations over 2 months (M = 1.3 times/week for about 50 minutes/visit) took place. In one condition, the subject could determine the frequency, length and time of the visit. In a second condition, the subject was only told of when and how long the visit would be. In a third condition, subjects received the same number and length of visits, but on a unpredictable schedule. In the fourth condition, there were no visitations during the 2-month period.

Schulz (1976) found that the control and predictability conditions combined were associated with a slower pre-post intervention general decline in physical health status and a greater increase in psychological status and activity level indicators than occurred in the unpredictable and no visit conditions combined. It is important to note that, in this well controlled study, there was no difference between predictability and control groups.

Unlike the Langer and Rodin (1976) study, the Schulz (1976) study was more like imposing laboratory conditions in a field setting. In essence, the intervention was not part of the normal undertakings of a nursing home. The study involved the temporary introduction of student visitors to demonstrate that there is a substantive difference in patient response to how the visits were scheduled. But careful reading of the Schulz study shows that the measures used had considerable face validity for the setting, and the study was designed not just to compare differing interpretations of control but also to directly examine factors contributing to the well-being of institutionalized seniors. Schulz (1976) stated: "Finally, we know little about the process through which control and predictability come to have their effects on the individual" (p. 22). He then indicated the need to construct a model to enable a better understanding of the impact of predictability and control on seniors well-being.

Schulz and Hanusa (1978) published follow-up data collected 24, 30 and 42 months after the 1976 study was terminated. The general and alarming finding was that those subjects, who had seemingly benefitted by being in the predictability and control conditions, exhibited significant declines after the study was terminated. Schulz and Hanusa (1978) used these results to underscore the considerable ethical dilemma of undertaking studies that inadvertently first effect improvements and then take them away. If we treat their follow-up data collection as if it were part of an A-B-A repeated measures study of the effect of an intervention, then their follow-up results combined with the initial effects indicate the rather potent impact of the intervention. Such findings sensitizes us to the importance of undertaking investigations in such a way that the experimental interventions can remain beneficial after the study is completed.

Both the well-cited studies of Langer and Rodin (1976) and Schulz (1976) were attempting to use existing conceptualizations of control as a means to understand aspects of aging. Rather than demonstrating the value of illustrating a particular form of control, their findings generated the still unanswered questions of: Why is gaining control beneficial? and, What does "having control" mean in such settings? In other words, they contributed to the development of knowledge by showing us what we *did not know*. From these seminal studies, we now turn to some of the more promising interpretations of psychological control to identify trends towards developing more applicable concepts for studying aging.

Developing Trends Towards a More Interactional Interpretation of Psychological Control

Control Awareness: An Interactional View of Control

Hoff and Hohner (1986) make a point of saying they do not want to contribute yet another construct of control but rather to contribute to a more comprehensive and integrated understanding of psychological control. Their wish to do so follows a critical review of locus of control studies and a detailed analysis of case studies where they attempted to use locus of control concepts to understand behaviors in employment settings. They were particularly interested in the effects of variations in both occupational restrictiveness (e.g., one's occupational status within an organization or blue collar versus white collar workers) and occupationally oriented evaluations (e.g., job satisfaction and career success). Their findings indicated that working conditions that facilitated self-determination and positive job evaluations by employees were positively correlated with internal locus of control beliefs. Restrictive working conditions were associated with external beliefs. Their consideration of the findings and the research methods employed lead them to conclude that "... the relationship between working conditions and locus of control can be described as reciprocal" (p. 351). However, rather than endorse the interpretation that behavior is a product of the interaction of person and environment (cf. Magnusson & Endler, 1977) they view that behavior is itself an interactive process. Their reasoning led them to conclude that the important research questions are (1) how do locus of control and working conditions mutually influence each other? and (2) how can these conditions be applied to understanding occupational careers?

To Hoff and Hohner (1986), the emphasis on either an external determination of behavior (such as a constrictive environment or beliefs in fatalism) or an internal emphasis (such as personal determination through personal effort) imply "a monocausal determination which in reality need not exist" (p. 357). In contrast to this emphasis, they argue that an interactional view is a more realistic interpretation of what happens. They feel people see their behaviors as a consequence of the interplay of personal and external factors with the dominance of each changing from situation to situation. This viewpoint they coin as an *interactional* view of control. They argue that the conceptual advantage of interactional control is that it emphasizes the "quality" of control as more important than the "locus" of control. The interactional view presupposes a differentiation of the person from the environment. The focus is on the "process of control" or awareness, whereby one is both influencing and being influenced (Hoff & Hohner, 1986, p. 360).

The Use Of "Control" In Discourse To Explain Events

Gergen and Gergen (1986) emphasize that personal control should be understood not as a tangible entity that can be directly measured. Rather, personal control is merely a term which people use to explain or communicate. In other words, to study personal control is to study people's use of the term to account for their experiences. From this perspective, people's accounts of personal control are social constructions used for discourse and interactions with others. The validity of personal control lies in the consensus and utility this term brings to people's communication and understanding of events.

Gergen and Gergen (1986) argue that human behavior is best understood as the result of *reasons* people have of events (e.g., expected outcomes) rather than specific *causes*, such as forces of gravity, genetics, etc. From this perspective, therefore, the study of control and aging would benefit from more attention being placed on how people use the personal control construct to account for their experience. For example, if a senior living alone in the community expressed a loss of control, Gergen and Gergen would have us examine, in depth, what this expression means or signifies to the senior. The explanations that the Gergens suggest, would be the substantive aspects of "control" that contribute to the well-being of the elderly person.

Gergen and Gergen explain that personal control is a social construction necessitating interpersonal consensus. In turn, social constructions are influenced by the cultural context within which they are developed. This particular perspective of perceived control may allow a reasonable interpretation for cross cultural differences in aging experience and behaviors. From this we can expect that there may be differences in the way individuals define the meaning of "control" (vis-à-vis aging) across cultures. This emphasis on social context is an added advantage of the Gergens' work. With the exception of the research of Weisz, Rothbaum, and Blackburn (1984) on primary and secondary control, it is not clear that current psychological control constructs address cultural differences in aging phenomena.

Mindfulness versus Mindlessness and Control

Langer and colleagues have conducted a series of studies applying control-related concepts to understanding complex behaviors that have led to the conceptualization of mindfulness versus mindlessness behaviors and the conditions that can create them. This conceptualization permits yet another approach to understanding how the process or interaction of the person with the situation influences the experience of being in control. Piper and Langer (1986) feel that the distinction between mindfulness and mindlessness is necessary in order to implement changes in situations such as nursing homes, so that the deleterious effects of aging and institutionalization can be mitigated.

Piper and Langer (1986) criticized the use of many popular control constructs, such as predictability and illusory control, as reflecting only the perception of the observer rather than the subject. This perceptual approach is seen as flawed, for the lack of control is only defined in terms of outcome. For example, a patient who fails to respond actively to an opportunity is judged as not having control over events. But the patient may herself feel in control. They feel the more reasonable approach is to focus on the subject's experience of control and the process involved in gaining that experience.

Mindfulness is described as a process whereby the subject is aware of making meaning and making distinctions, of knowing he/she is responding, deciding, working and reacting. In other words, the subject is attending to what s/he is doing. Mindlessness, in contrast, is doing things reflexively or automatically and without thought or attention. Even when doing something which is relatively trivial and of little major consequence, the process of being mindful of what one is doing is important. Alternatively, when involved in relatively important tasks or undertakings, one can do so in an inattentive or automatic way, which is experienced as being mindless.

Mindlessness is seen as a state of cognitive inactivity. The consequence of this automatic activity is that individuals do not attend to the events that lead to an outcome. This is not usually a problem when the outcome is predictable (e.g., finding your keys where you usually leave them). However, it can be, when the outcome is unexpected (e.g., not finding your keys where you usually leave them). The latter experience may lead you to feel perplexed, since your lack of attentiveness while disposing of your keys now creates difficulty as you try to recount the events that led up to this outcome. Again, it is such daily routines that lead to mindlessness. While many things are going on in one's life, it is usually good that some tasks can be routinely done while attention is focused on novel and/or important undertakings. But according to Langer and colleagues, what is important is that an individual is always mindful of doing something.

Mindlessness is seen as leading to a reduction of the experience of control. Responding mindlessly reduces the ability of the person to adapt and to learn and to respond in the most effective manner in a changing situation. Mindfulness, on the other hand, can lead to a perception of control, but it is different from merely having behavioral control. According to Piper and Langer (1986) mindfulness leads to the interpretation of control existing ". . . in a mutually defining relationship between the individual and the environment that is anchored in the person, and as such, less likely to be limited by external events or other persons" (p. 74). From this perspective, it is possible for the mindful person to examine the contingencies of exercising behavioral control within a specific environment and to decide to relinquish exercising control. To the observer, such a decision may be interpreted as losing control or being externally controlled. But from our view, it is the person's taking action by deciding whether to respond, in light of their circumstances, which is the key component in adaptive responding. Rothbaum, Weisz, and Snyder (1982) make a similar point in their discussion of a two-process model of control.

From this vantage point, we see mindfulness as contributing to an interactive process rooted in the phenomenology of the individual. It gives a sense of control that is internally validated rather than externally validated in terms of outcomes.

Perceived Control versus Actual Control and Action Control

In recent years, Kuhl has been writing extensively on an information processing model of behavior called Action Control. His model differentiates between a person's perceptions or beliefs about control and this person's experience of having active control. While they can be related they are not mutually exclusive. He stresses that it is the experience of active control over the environment that is important. These experiences, he portends, can be so subtle that a senior citizen can continue to perceive s/he has control when, in fact, s/he does not have actual control. If anything, the perception of lost control may be a result of the loss of actual control. It is less likely that the perception of control will lead to the experience of active control. For example, his reasoning would support the idea that it is the experiences rather than the perception of lack of control that can lead to depression. The perception of lack of control would more likely arrive subsequent to the depressive mood. Thus perception is, at best, secondary to the experience.

For these reasons Kuhl sees his action control model as providing a more indepth, extensive, heuristic and elaborate account of control than existing conceptualizations. He contrasts this model with what he refers to as (1) fragmented and (2) overly simple models currently employed in psychological control research. When addressing fragmentation he points out that each model generally pertains to particular kinds of behavior, and therefore, lacks generalizability to a variety of behaviors. There is need, he feels, to supplement these existing simple models with a more comprehensive theoretical framework.

Current models are described as simplistic in that they provide little explanation for the phenomena they study. Referring to current models as "perceived control models" he points out that the explanations they provide are more typically descriptions of the findings. For example, the finding that self-report of lack of control is correlated with self-report of depression would be "explained" as lack of perceived control contributing to feelings of depression. These perceived control models generally only tell us that detrimental effects, such as apathy, will occur when people perceive that they have little control over an event. These models do not explain how this effect happens.

Kuhl's (1986) model is possibly the most intricate one published and too detailed to fully summarize here. He uses a schematic drawing of a flow-chart path to outline the sequential steps in developing the experience and perception of control. The flow-chart begins with self-perceptions which then lead to subsequent behaviors after going through various steps and junctures in the flow-chart path. Often such schematic drawings are good devices for authors to communicate how they construe complex events. Flow-charts can contribute to improving discourse among scientists and can be useful as heuristic devices. But they can be misread as formulas or overly mechanistic models.

To use Kuhl's own terms, his particular model may be so "fine grained" (Kuhl, 1986, p. 18) and molecular that its application may be problematic. As he notes, applied approaches tend to be at a more molar level of analysis, and we would add that they are so for good reason. Fine-grained distinctions are hard to make and maintain within field settings. However, for the purposes of this chapter there are certain insightful contributions he makes that we feel contribute to the trend towards more interactional and applicable conceptualizations of control.

Kuhl (1986) borrows, in part, from Bandura (1977, 1982, 1986) in underscoring the distinction of action-outcome expectancy from outcome-consequence expectancy. Action-outcome refers to the expectancy that one can perform a behavior to attain an outcome. Outcome-consequence is the expectancy that the outcome would make any difference. An example of the action-outcome expectancy is a geriatric patient who feels she does not have the ability or efficacy to communicate her wants to her physician. An example of outcome-consequence expectancy would be the same patient who feels that while she can communicate her wants, it will have no effect on her physician. A patient who reports having little control may be basing her beliefs on either or both expectancies. However, an intervention to change action-outcome expectancies would be different from an intervention to change outcome-consequence expectations.

Kuhl goes on to differentiate action-outcome expectancy into personal ability and *self-regulatory functions*. In this case, the patient may feel she has the ability to perform the task but not to maintain (self-regulate) the performance repeatedly. What we glean from this is the following extrapolation. For the geriatric patient, deficits in the self-regulation of one's abilities as the result of either physical disabilities (e.g., tremors or slurred speech of Parkinson disease) or disuse of abilities (such as thinking through problems or expressing one's ideas for others to hear) may be central to the experience of reduced control with aging. Thus the lack of perceived control *may not be due to the lack of ability but rather it is due to the difficulty with the exercise of that ability*.

What is notable in this concept is that problems with self-regulatory behaviors can be exacerbated or reduced by environmental and social determinants. Without a challenging environment, one's performance of abilities, such as remembering details or being succinct in the expression of one's ideas, deteriorates (Skinner, 1983). This concept of self-regulation can address the interaction of both the situational context and personal ability to effect the senior's feelings of control. To facilitate a greater sense of control, it is not just the abilities or the belief about control that are the objective, but the self-regulation of the abilities to act upon one's environment, to do what one has the ability to do.

Autonomy versus Control of Behavior

After more than a decade of research into motivation, Deci and Ryan (1987) have further enhanced the use of psychological control to understand complex and often subtle behaviors. Their research has repeatedly shown that when subjects are rewarded for undertaking tasks they enjoy doing, their interest in the tasks is diminished. They called this result the "undermining effect" (Deci & Ryan, 1987). Typical of this research is the following. Children in two randomly assigned groups were each given time to play with a fun toy. Each child in one group was told that s/he would be given a present if s/he played with the toy. Children in the other group were not told about any present. Subsequent to playing with the toy for a few minutes each child was thanked and then asked to remain alone in the room for a few more minutes to play with the toys. The room contained the target toy along with other toys. The behavior of each child was recorded by observers watching each child through a one-way mirror.

The finding was that the children who knew they would receive a present were less inclined to play with (or later report interest in) the targeted toy than were children who did not know they would receive a present. Such effects have been found with subjects in different age groups (Deci & Ryan, 1987).

Deci and Ryan (1987) suggest that most behavior can be interpreted as being more or less self-determined along a continuum ranging from being autonomous to being controlled. Self-determined behaviors refer to those intentional behaviors that are ". . . initiated and regulated through personal choice as an expression of oneself. . . "(Deci & Ryan, 1987, p. 1024). Controlled behaviors are those that are initiated and regulated (i.e., pressured, coerced) by either environmental or intrapsychic forces. As an example, consider the addictive drinking behavior of an alcoholic. She may see herself as initiating the behavior of going to the liquor cabinet and of having the ability and self-efficacy of doing what she wants to do. But her behavior is one of compulsion, and as defined by Deci, it is controlled rather than autonomous. To the observer she had control of her behavior. However, she would report that she did the behaviors but that she did not have control. This example is consistent with previous locus of control research demonstrating that traditional beliefs of internal-external control on a Rotter type scale is independent of beliefs in one's self-control of impulses (Reid & Ware, 1973; 1974).

Deci and Ryan (1987) explain that to influence a person's experience of being autonomous or controlled, one has to consider the "functional significance" of both the behavior and its context to the individual. In a rather simplified way of putting this, Deci (1975) once suggested that every reinforcer can have two meanings. It can reflect how well one is doing, or it can reflect a controlling influence over one's behavior. More recently Deci and Ryan (1987) have chosen to describe the distinction between autonomy supportive versus controlling contexts. The subtlety of the distinction can be determined by so-called contextual factors. These contextual factors include task contingent rewards, such as: being given a prize for completing a task; positive feedback for behavior; imposed deadlines on tasks; and subject's personal orientation towards interpreting his/her behaviors as an expression of his/her autonomy. Deci and Ryan (1987) summarize a series of studies demonstrating that subjects behaving within autonomy supportive rather than controlling environments are more likely to be: (1) creative, (2) better learner, (3) be cognitively more flexible, (4) persistent in their behaviors and (5) happier at what they were doing. Although their work is mainly with children and young adults, their conceptualization of control seems very applicable to our understanding of adjustment to aging.

An example of how the autonomy supportive versus controlling contexts might exist in a nursing home is as follows. Consider the existence of an administratively well-run nursing home having staff who develop a series of programmes for the seniors. These programmes keep the seniors busy in activities such as listening to recitals, taking part in arts and crafts, going on bus tours, and having breakfast together, etc. To an outsider, such a home would appear stimulating and therapeutic to the residents, which it could be. However, if the programmes are imposed and the patients coerced to be involved, then the programmes may inadvertently be quite controlling of the residents and undermine their intrinsic motivation. Similarly, it may be that any well-intentioned procedure to try and cause the seniors to have more control may contribute to the *experience of being controlled*. An example of where giving control may undermine the experience of control is found in the Schulz & Hanusa (1978) study discussed earlier. In this study, the giving of control to the patients and then taking it away may have lead the patients to experience a loss of control. The study itself had inadvertently undermined the patients' autonomy--it had amplified the external control.

The research of Deci and his colleagues provides an important refinement of our conceptualization of psychological control for two reasons. Firstly, they see the traditional formulations of psychological control (e.g., Rotter, 1966; Bandura, 1977) as suggesting that personal control occurs when either one sees a connection between one's action and outcomes or one has the self-perceived ability to undertake an action. But these formulations do not explain that *it is not just being able to be instrumental that is critical*. The distinction of whether the instrumental acts are indeed self-determined or controlled may be critical as well. Secondly, they point out that previous formulations placed emphasis on control of external outcomes (e.g., reinforcements) while not placing emphasis on the possibility that some behaviors are intrinsically motivated. The latter are behaviors that require neither reinforcement nor external feedback from others.

A Reconceptualization of Control

The Trend to Phenomenology: Its Relevance to Aging Phenomena

It is evident from the independent research of Hoff & Hohner, Langer, Kuhl and Deci, respectively, that there is an emphasis on the phenomenology of the control experience and that this experience is a product of the interaction of the person with his/her environment. *The experience of control* is primary whereas the *beliefs of control* are more secondary to the experience. This distinction is consistent with the findings in attitude research. It is commonly found that attitudes and opinions are not always perfectly correlated with behavior and/or feelings. For example, the geriatric patient can express *beliefs* about how nurses, doctors, hospital policy or changes in his/her disease symptoms influence how he/she behaves. But at the same time, the patient may still *feel* in control in this setting.

Alternatively, the experience of not having control can lead the patient to realize that he/she does not have much control. In short, external beliefs can either follow from experiencing a lack of control or represent a perspective of the environment independent of personal experience. Beliefs are not necessarily in one-to-one correspondence with the experience of control. It is the experience that is more central.

A reconceptualization of control, which utilizes a phenomenological perspective, requires a clarification of terms so that confusion with previous conceptualizations can be avoided. The locus of control literature, for example, refers to internal versus external control as beliefs that outside forces such as fate, luck, powerful others versus one's own abilities govern access to outcomes or reinforcements (Rotter, 1966). Similarly, the attribution literature refers to the attribution of causation to phenomena that can be categorized as internal stable, external unstable, etc., (Weiner, 1982). Presumably the attribution of causation to external as distinct from internal events has a differential effect on how people will respond to conditions. The use of external locus of control or causality suggests a unidirectional "cause" of one's outcome or condition. However, in this re-interpretation of control we do not refer to such external events as the *locus* of control. Instead they are factors or forces external to oneself which can govern or influence one's condition. Similarly, the internal factors of ability, energy level and stamina are not the *locus* of control. These are additional factors that, in conjunction with external factors, can influence one's condition or outcome. Rather than refer to external and internal control we prefer to refer to external and internal factors influencing a person's condition or outcomes. This clarification in the use of terms is neither radical nor contrary to recent discussions of psychological control and aging (e.g., Lazarus & DeLongis, 1983). But this change does allow for an interpretation of control that is more applicable to studying adjustment to change and social-psychological aspects of aging.

From the phenomenological perspective it is not the person's beliefs about the external factors that lead to feelings of lack of perceived control, but rather the inability to respond to those external sources. The salience of external sources of influence can undermine one's self-determination. In addition to these external sources, there are also internal factors, such as one's impulses, emotions, physiological limitations and ability to concentrate which also contribute to the person's condition. *To have control is to act upon or in light of the variety of forces both within and without the person that would otherwise determine the person's condition.* This re-interpretation of psychological control facilitates our understanding of how age-associated changes within the individual (e.g., physiological changes) together with changes in the social and physical environment influence the individual. This reconceptualization is also a more interactional interpretation of psychological control than has been typical of prior interpretations, although prior interpretations of control have had some interactional emphasis (Reid, 1977).

People are aware of the physiological, social, and physical changes that accompany their aging. When prompted they can describe how they have changed over time in a variety of ways. These changes range from changes in physical stamina to changes in employment, changes in wealth, changes in understanding, changes in roles, etc. But it is not their acknowledgement of these changes that is impor- tant. Rather, it is the meaning or impact of these changes on them that is important (Lazarus & DeLongis, 1983). And this impact can be measured in terms of the ease and success they have accommodating to these changes. In short, it is the personal capacity to respond to or to act upon these changes that provides the experience of psychologi- cal control. Conversely, the loss of control occurs with the experience of changes to which one is not accommodating or assimilat- ing.

To illustrate this perspective, consider the case where a grandmother, after several years of going to her daughters' homes for Christmas, attempts to host and make a meal for a large family gathering. When she undertakes this task she finds that she has lost some of the speed, dexterity and organizational skills she once had. Despite the final success of the meal, the impact is one of personal stress, and she feels a considerable loss of control. Accompanying this experience will be beliefs that she has lost some of the "control" she previously had. Another grandmother undertakes a similar task and also realizes that she is not as fast or coordinated as she was years earlier. She, too, will report beliefs of having lost her effectiveness in hosting and preparing a large meal for a family gathering. But for this latter grandmother, she may have realized the changes and got on with doing the best she could do under the circumstances. In her case, the sense of control will be there, for she was able to respond to the "changes" she experienced. In short, it is the recognition of the age-related changes *and* being able to respond to the impact of those changes that gives the sense of control. The second grandmother accepted the changes and incorporated them into her purposeful, self-determined activities. She acted upon the factors which otherwise would have reduced her control.

There are two expressions that capture some of the psychological experience of aging. One is that "youth is too valuable to waste on the young." The other, originally an expression in German, is translated as "too soon old; too late smart." The substance of these expressions can be seen in the following case description of a senior professor. As a graduate student this professor had a great sense of his ability, his developing skills and enjoyment of learning. Employment opportunities were available, and his sense of professional growth and instrumentality were strong. He also had considerable energy and time to work long hours to succeed. Decades later, this professor looks back and smiles at how naive he was as a graduate student. Over the years, the professor had learned how deans, anonymous reviewers, bureaucratic policies, committees, government cut-backs and a myriad of other factors influenced his activities and outcomes. Having spent years studying the scholarship of others, he may even realize his own effectiveness as a scholar is not as substantive as he once thought. The professor no longer has the level of energy he had in his youth. As a result of his experiences, the professor's *beliefs* and causal attributions have become much more external. However, the professor realizes that if he only knew as a graduate student what he knows now, he would have been even more successful and happier. Despite these substantive changes with aging, the professor's sense of personal control need not have diminished. Indeed, by being more knowledgeable about the myriad of factors controlling his activities he may have an even greater experience of control, because with experience he knows what forces he has to act upon. Over time, the professor has learned how to respond to change and that the more aware he is of the change the better he can respond to it.

To illustrate the developmental cycle of changes with aging, consider that this professor tries to impart his wisdom by advising his graduate student. But the student reacts to this imposition over her creativity and, exercising her self-determination, does her research her way--even if it is the less effective way. And the professor, realizing she is like he was, thinks: "Alas, too soon old; too late smart."

Cognitive Social Learning Theory Of Control: Why It Was Developed

A theory of control that was more suitable to understanding the phenomena of aging has been proposed (Reid & Ziegler, 1981; Reid, 1984). It is a theory that integrates a phenomenological emphasis with attributional models and previous social learning formulations of control. This theory is the start of a reconceptualization of psychological control that is more appropriate for studying social psychological aspects of aging.

Based on Kurt Lewin's observation that there is nothing so practical as a good theory, this theory was developed to guide research on the psychology of aging. The Cognitive Social Learning Theory Of Control is built upon a catechism of psychology, including the writings of Piaget, Heider, Rotter, Decharms, Riegel, White, Adler, Sullivan and Bowers. The explanatory power of social learning theory concepts, theories of cognitive development, the interactional models of behavior and the findings that people do not necessarily consciously mediate many of the determinants of their experiences and behavior are all relevant to applied research on aging. We, therefore, have drawn from the literature on these aspects of behavior as part of our reconceptualization of control.

This theory was developed in response to several discoveries arising from our attempts to apply control concepts to understand aging phenomena.   From our own research (Reid, Haas, & Hawkings, 1977; Ziegler & Reid, 1979) on the relationship between desired control beliefs and psychological adjustment among the elderly, we realized that our studies were not dealing directly with an important question.   The question was: how does a senior citizen retain the experience of being in control, while aware of substantial losses of previous agility, freedom, etc.?   In some of our studies, we found that seniors living in the community had a greater belief in internal control than did those living in an extended care hospital (Ziegler & Reid, 1979).   We also found that within both the community setting and in the hospital, those who reported more internal control beliefs also received more positive scores on psychological adjustment measures. Looking across our studies of geriatric patients, we realized that as these patients experienced deterioration in health and in the loss of autonomy that comes with hospitalization and dependency on others, they had good reason to have more external beliefs (Reid & Ziegler, 1981).   There was also good reason to believe that these patients were very aware of the loss of their instrumentality, freedom of movement, etc.   Yet despite these changes, somehow seniors could retain the *experience* of control, and to do so seemed beneficial.   Current conceptualizations of control did not answer how seniors can be aware of real changes in their instrumentality or effectiveness and yet retain a sense of control.

Our research had taken a very applied focus.   For example, in one pilot study, we taught patients social skills (e.g., assertiveness) which were specially tailored for their being effective patients.   The patients were being taught, for example, how to make requests effectively without being perceived as a complaining patient who should be ignored.   (The latter is an example of the lack of efficacy the patients had reported in interviews.)   We were successful in obtaining significant improvements in social skills, measured with the use of blind rated pre-post study video tapes of the patients' demonstration of the skills.   But such training had no impact on responses to the *Desired Control Belief Measure*, which is a questionnaire specially designed to assess seniors' expectations of realizing desired outcomes (Reid & Ziegler, 1981).   Furthermore, the patients did not apply their new skills in regular nursing unit activities even though we had used interactions with a nurse as part of the training.

In a following pilot study, we applied cognitive behavior therapy strategies after we surmised that besides changing behavior (i.e., to increase self-efficacy to perform the social skills) we also needed to change expectations about the consequences of undertaking the new skills.   But this did not work as expected either.   Instead, the patients became increasingly more articulate in explaining how the application of their newly learned social skills would not work.   The supervisor (DWR) of the graduate clinical student doing the training realized that the patients were changing the student's expectations and not the other way around as planned. The supervisor then discussed openly with the patients his view of the lack of therapeutic progress with the patients and learned that they had found the sessions to be therapeutic and insightful. The clinical impression was that the patients had become quite instrumental in countering the therapeutic attempts of the graduate student. By doing so, they had developed a consensus among themselves about just how difficult it was to change the hospital staff and how they could respond in light of that knowledge.

This pilot study serves as an illustration of not only the problems encountered in applying conceptualizations of control but also the need for the re-interpretation of psychological control for studies of social psychological aspects of aging. The therapeutic session had facilitated the patients in gaining a control experience, because the sessions had been deliberately designed to encourage the patients to discuss their realities regarding the staff, their impact on themselves and what they could do in response. The result was that the patients gained a better insight into the internal and external factors influencing their condition and, in light of this insight or awareness, made a decision of how they would respond.

What we learned from our applied research was just how mechanistic we were in trying to *change* their control rather than trying to *facilitate* their "control" experience in a way that was concordant with their circumstances. We realized that if psychological control was going to be useful for understanding psychological adjustment of the elderly then our conceptualization of psychological control needed a major overhaul. It was simplistic to assume that increasing control was just a matter of increasing predictability, teaching instrumental behaviors and imposing choice. The existing theories of control did not address the psychological impact of aging. For example, Bandura's and Kuhl's distinctions of personal efficacy (action-outcome expectancy) versus control beliefs (outcome-consequence expectancy) are thoughtful ideas which were operationalized by our use of both behavioral therapy and cognitive therapy. But these distinctions were not enough to explain our pilot study discoveries. As with the Langer & Rodin and Schulz studies, our gain from doing applied research was a better appreciation of how complex the application of control concepts is to aging.

Cognitive Social Learning Theory Of Control: A Distillation

A postulate of this theory is that one of the primary motivations of individuals is to have influence over their environment. Such a motivation is necessary for the adaptive evolution of the species. Among the earliest experiences of the child is the need to alter his/her environment in order to assimilate the environment to him/herself (deCharms, 1968). White (1959) has referred to the intrinsic aspect of this experience as effectance motivation, which he suggests has a neurogenic basis. In order to be nurtured and gratified, the child has to be instrumental in gaining satisfaction from his/her environment. Often the child will be ineffective, leading to the fundamental experience of inadequacy that the child will then attempt to overcome. Adler suggests this experience of inadequacy pervades human existence and guides humans throughout their lives. Humans learn to compensate for these experiences of inadequacy by being instrumental in response to their environments.

Being instrumental is itself rewarding, if Adler, White and deCharms are correct, but being instrumental is also a means to obtaining outcomes (e.g., food, attention) that are rewarding if Rotter and others are also correct. But this distinction of in- strumental action as an end rather than a means to an end is likely a pseudo distinction. For the study of aging, it is better to assume that both operate since both are about having an influence upon the environment. Rather than discern whether there is a difference, as some of the control research has done, it is worthwhile assuming that both are useful considerations. From a phenomenological point of view, the experience of acting upon one's environment (i.e., an end in itself) and the feedback of gaining an outcome as a result of acting on one's environment (i.e., a means to an end) are likely difficult to differentiate. These ends versus means distinctions are more complementary and alike than mutually exclusive. Which aspect of instrumental action is emphasized in applied research will depend on what behaviors are being studied. It is also assumed that the instrumental response to environmental pressures often goes on so reflexively that we are not conscious of their happening.

The process of acting upon the environment is exceedingly complex. As the human develops neurologically and experientially, the process of acting upon the environment takes many interrelated forms and increases in complexity. The psychological control the person has is the experience of personal feedback of his/her acting upon his/her environment. This experience will be quite different between childhood and adulthood because of the changing complexity. In the earliest years, the process can be interpreted as the fundamental experience of physical causation accompanying action and feedback of response. Initially, the experience of causation does not necessitate the conceptual dissociation of "self" from one's "external world." But gradually as the person grows older and develops further mental operations, to use Piaget's term, s/he can increasingly differentiate the "self" from his/her "external world." As the person grows older not only do mental operations become more complex but learning also takes place. This culminates in a greater comprehension of the complexity of the world. The result is that people learn that they have more influence on some aspects of their world than on other aspects. People also learn to recognize situations where they cannot have an influence. This latter recognition is very critical, for then the individual can know when not to respond, which is itself an action. In other words, when recognizing the dominance of external over internal forces, they now can act upon this reality and doing so gives them considerable control. For example, we described our pilot research where patients became more articulate in describing the relatively little input they had in changing the hospital situation. By deciding to not act overtly they were exercising control.

As people age, they realize, with increasing clarity, that their behavior is determined to some extent by themselves and to some extent by variables outside of their control. People will admit they do not understand some of these so-called external variables such as God, Mother Nature, and chemical toxins, *but they believe they are there!* And why do they? These variables are all common "constructions" that help people to respond to life.[1] Their realization of multiple self versus external sources of influence not only reflects experience, it is also a realization necessary for effective adaptation to everyday events. What is necessary is to have an accurate grasp of not only the degree to which one has instrumental input, but also know to what extent there are external factors determining one's behavior and outcomes. This awareness of both internal and external determinants is necessary in order to be able to respond effectively. Psychological control, therefore, incorporates the realization of both internal and external determinants; it is the one acting on the other. From this theory, to believe one has complete instrumental input or no instrumental input is non adaptive.[2]

Cognitive Social Learning Theory Of Control not only conceptualizes control as the experience of acting upon one's environment, having control is also considered as optimized when the results of one's acting upon one's environment coincides with the person's expectations (or appraisal) of the relative dominance of internal and external determinants of his/her situation. We refer to this coinciding as a balance. For example, consider a geriatric patient who, based on past experience, (but misreading his current strength and stamina) expects to be able to undertake heading a patients' committee. But once doing the task he experiences a lack of control because he does not have the degree of stamina he thought he had for the role. His regaining the experience of control necessitates changes in his expectations of the balance of internal to external determinants. It is important to emphasize that such changes are a result of interactions with the environment. Once he has reappraised the situation, the patient may resort to renegotiating the demands or responsibilities of the role, choosing to resign, changing meeting times to the morning hours when he is stronger, saving his energy for the meetings, etc. But before such actions were possible, he needed to reappraise the relative contributions of internal and external factors and then to act upon those. *The experience of control, therefore, is constantly in terms of a perceived balance between his appraisal of internal and external forces that coincides with his reactions to these forces.*

To the extent that we see what we do (and what happens as a result) as not reflecting this balance, we experience a loss of control. This balance is critical for without it we cannot respond effectively. Thus when we experience events as not in our control, we automatically search for external and internal sources as an explanation. It is when our experience of internal versus external sources of influence do not account for events adequately that adaptation to our world becomes difficult. In our earlier example, the grandmother who set upon feeding a large family gathering had trouble adapting because she misread how much she had changed in relation to the task at hand. The other grandmother had not misread her abilities vis-à-vis the external determinants, and thus could adapt.

In daily living, we generally keep a good balance in our perceptions of internal to external forces, and thus we feel in control. We are usually very vigilant and sensitive to variations in the balance. This vigilance is often at a tacit level of interaction with the environment. When not sure of the balance, we will test situations or gather information to see what influence we have; and in cases where we realize the dominance of the external powers, we exert our control by abiding by the external power. We have previously referred to this balance, which fits with experience, as a synchronization (Reid, 1984). However, there are times when people experience an asynchronism in the balance of internal-external forces and this asynchronism is almost always a time of potential crisis. An unexpected loss of a job or a loved one, or a major illness are examples. These are, of course, painful and distressful experiences. We suggest that one factor contributing to the distress is the asynchronism that undermines one's control. These events do not fit the determining balances of internal and external forces as the victim has known them. As a result, when such events occur, we demand to know why. We are driven to find an explanation or a cause. The answers to these questions are necessary in order that the victims can act upon the situation-- *to have control*. It is typical for victims of tragedies, such as spinal trauma and terminal cancer, to search for reasons of their victimization (Bulman & Wortman, 1977; Shanfield, 1980).

An important point is that many of the changes with aging can lead a person to either question or reflect upon the changes that do not generate a great deal of questioning unless they are more of a personal crisis. The reason is that aging changes are often gradual, and we shift our balance among the internal and external forces accordingly. It is when these changes are experienced as sudden that they are referred to as crises, as in the so-called mid-life crises. Thus the 70 year old male knows he cannot play squash with the vigour he could as a 20 year old; and while he may wish otherwise, his not having the vigour is not a problem and does not lead to any experience of loss of control. But had the 20 year old been suddenly impaired so that his performance at playing squash was like that of the 70 year old, then surely the impact would be dramatic and the experience would be, in part, one of a loss of control. Why? The answer is because the 20 year old's experiences do not fit with his existing point of balance between internal-external determinants of behavior. His regaining psychological control will be his realigning the balance of internal-external determinants and then acting upon these.

From this theory, we predict that senior citizens can report beliefs about the dominance of external forces in determining their outcomes of themselves and still either report or be rated as being well-adjusted and satisfied. Previous interpretations of psychological control would suggest that these beliefs, as measured on I-E scales, reflect "external control" beliefs. However, this theory would guide the researcher to look closely at the meaning those external beliefs hold for the respondent (Averill, 1973). They may directly reflect an appraisal of the situation but only indirectly reflect their experiences of responding in light of those beliefs. As we stated earlier, there is not a one-to-one relationship between beliefs and experience.

A prediction from this theory is that persons will not be completely content with being externally controlled. Rather, what is necessary is their being able to respond to these external sources in order to validate or corroborate his/her sense of control. In order to adapt, the individual needs to respond in reaction to or in opposition to his/her perception of events being externally determined (Reid, 1984). When their actions are effective in light of their expectations, then the external forces are not likely to be seen as formidable as they would if the actions did not corroborate expectations. For this reason, those persons who tend to score more internally (or less externally) on an I-E belief measure are generally those who report greater well-being and satisfaction because they experienced more control.

Because control is an interactionist concept (Reid, 1977) it is most difficult to compare peoples' experience of control in differing age groups. Cross-sectional comparisons of age groups on responses to belief inventories are fraught with difficulties conceptually. Longitudinal group comparisons are also limited if environmental determinants of psychological control beliefs do not change uniformly for all members of the group (Lumpkin, 1986). The reason is that control will be interpreted differently by persons in different age groups because their situations differ in multiple ways. The experience of control we have as youngsters has to be different from the control we have as adults. Lachman (1986), for example, reviewed the literature on age differences on generalized I-E control beliefs and found the results to be inconclusive. However, in a series of three cross-sectional studies she found that "elderly adults, in contrast to young adults, acknowledged the salience of external forces and, yet, maintained strong beliefs in their internal control" (p. 39). In addition she found the elderly adults more likely to differentiate among sources of external control, a finding consistent with our earlier point of greater differentiation with aging.

Compensation With Aging: Standing Back and Differentiating In Order To Be Instrumental

A possible criticism of the reconceptualization of psychological control outlined earlier is the implication that one can experience control even in extreme cases where there are very dominant forces influencing a person's condition. One would think that a state of apathy or helplessness would be the more likely outcome than having the experience of control. But this is an incorrect interpretation. As stated earlier, a postulate of this theory is that people need to be instrumental or to influence their environment. *In order to be effectively instrumental, one has to be in control;* and in doing so, one acts in light of the internal and external forces contributing to one's condition. Thus being in control is a necessary condition to being instrumental.   It is when one cannot act upon internal and external forces, because they are not understood or cannot be appraised, that the lack of control is apparent. This interpretation is similar to Seligman's early formulation of learned helplessness to explain the so-called apathetic behavior in his dogs (Seligman, Maier, & Geer, 1968).   The learned helplessness was hypothesized to occur when the dog "learned" that neither responding nor not responding was associated with either shock onset or offset. These conditions are also consistent with the extreme laboratory conditions Weiss (1972) used to effect norepinephrine depletions in the nervous systems of white rats. In this case, the administration of electrical shocks was randomly varied in a way that responding (or not responding) was not contingent to shock.   This research has been used as laboratory analogues of what happens in clinical depression (Weiss, Glazer, Pohorecky, Bailey, & Schneider, 1979). Furthermore, while a person can experience control under conditions where there are very dominant external forces, this does not mean they either prefer or enjoy the situation. But being able to respond under undesirable circumstances is important in order to adapt.

It was earlier stressed that as persons age, both the form by which persons can act upon their environment and their comprehension of the external and internal forces acting upon them become more intricate and complex. The latter can be represented as the person's ability to differentiate various sources of external determinants as well as their differentiation of internal factors that would influence their being instrumental.   The ability to be able to make these differentiations is very important.[3]   Thus a geriatric patient may realize that the relative balance of forces between herself and her primary nurse is such that she has considerable input into determining events.   However, relative to her lawyer she may feel she has little input into determining pending legal settlements with an employer. A patient who feels that, in relation to hospital staff, he has little input, may in contrast find he can have a lot of input in helping other patients who are currently distressed. In both examples, the appraisal of internal and external forces are synchronous with the patient's experience. However, the dominance of the hospital staff in determining outcomes undermines the patient's need to be instrumental. To compensate for his need to be instrumental, he may then accept the "reality" that staff have considerable influence on his living and invest himself in helping other patients. It is not the latter that gives him control, rather it is his ability to make the distinction and respond accordingly.

This ability to make distinctions of when and how to be instrumental allows the person to compensate for when he/she is not instrumental. As people age, there are physiological changes, sensory-motor changes, role changes, etc., which may substantially reduce their ability to be instrumental. However, because of the overall need to be able to respond, what happens is that persons will find other ways by which they can be instrumental. When people become disabled they will compensate by developing other abilities.

The making of distinctions of when and how to be instrumental will be easier for persons who either have a natural inclination to stand back from their situation and to reflect upon it or else are in a setting that encourages such psychological distancing. For example, this standing back can be seen in some forms of humour whereby the person can make fun of themselves and the situation. This standing apart can also occur when one has a confidant with whom to discuss one's situation, choices, contingencies, etc. Thus some forms of humour, social supports (Krause, 1987) and other factors can be important for facilitating the experiencing of control. By doing so, they may buffer the stress of major events or daily hassles. The maxims of "not taking oneself too seriously" and "to know thy limitations" cautions one to stand back and be realistic about one's condition. The practices of planning, organizing and problem solving all have this characteristic of (often momentarily) standing apart and taking into consideration the internal and external factors one has to act upon or in light of.

When seniors are institutionalized and, as a result, lose much of their previous freedom of choice, they are going to not only adjust to the new balance between internal and external forces; in doing so, they are also going to find other ways to be instrumental. This process of reappraising the forces and testing them to check the validity of the appraisal contributes to the experience of having control. *We need to learn more about the ways seniors either gain or retain the experience of control so that we can facilitate the process.* This Cognitive Social Learning Theory Of Control, contributing to a reconceptualization of psychological control, can be used to guide scientists and practitioners to look for the ways people respond to their age-related changes. This theoretically guided research may also help us to discern successful aging from non successful aging (Karuza, Rabinowitz, & Zevon, 1986).

Guided by this theory, we have begun research into ways seniors can adjust to changes brought upon by chronic illness and having to live in institutions such as hospitals. We hypothesized that an important factor in the adjustment to these changes is certain qualities of the relationship established between the senior and the health professionals on whom they depend for treatment and care. These certain qualities contribute to what we call participatory control.

Participatory Control

From our earlier research of applying concepts of psychological control to understand aging, we began studying ways seniors, who have undergone life experiences that lead to their loss of instrumentality, can retain the experience of control. We were particularly interested in how patients adjusted to chronic illnesses which are, by definition, incurable. For example, in one of our studies (Sangster, Blackwell, Quek, Reid, & Ziegler, 1981) specially trained graduate students undertook in-depth clinical interviews with hospitalized patients having a variety of chronic illnesses. The data (consisting of answers to 10 open-ended questions) were content analyzed carefully and extensively. From these data, we obtained our first discovery of how the better adjusted patients were more likely to differentiate those situations in which they had "control" from those they did not. The better adjusted were more likely to express acceptance of their situation. Besides conducting field research, such as the Sangster, et al., (1981) study we also extensively reviewed research on adjustment to chronic or life-threatening conditions such as cancer. (Reid, 1984).

It is remarkable how resilient humans can be under trying circumstances. It seems that even the most extreme stresses are typically transitory. In one way or another, people are able to regain control. We found a theme in the published research that also made sense of our own data. We found that victims of tragedies or persons accommodating to substantial changes in their condition often used others as a source for regaining personal strength, emotional forbearance and in regaining control over their lives. We refer to the process of gaining control via reciprocal interactions with others as participatory control (Reid, 1984).

The following discussion of participatory control is in terms of the working relationship between a patient and his/her health care provider. However, it is possible to apply the concept more broadly to include others with whom a person can gain control.

There are a number of components of participatory control. First, the person must come to the resolution that there are others who have more expertise, energy and/or resources to respond to his/her situation than he/she has. Making this conclusion is not always easy for it is both a concession of not being able to act upon one's situation and an acceptance of a need to depend on others to take care of one's health. One of the reasons that makes it difficult to come to this resolution is the doubt or mistrust that the others will operate with full interest in the individual's condition. By condition we refer not only to the person's health, but also his circumstances, emotional state and social position. Thus the individual's condition is a very personally relevant state of being. Unless one is socialized to completely trust in one's treatment by another, it is difficult to hand over control. It is unusual to have complete faith in the competence of another person to act effectively on behalf of oneself if the outcome is very threatening or personal.

To surrender one's situation to others is threatening because one realizes these others are also human, can make mistakes, fail to understand one's concerns and fears, and have their own invested interests, which might compete with the patient's wishes to not be harmed. The latter might be the patient's concerns that, as a result of his/her physician having more interest in keeping hospital costs down or serving many patients at once, his/her situation does not receive the thorough treatment it is entitled to. In order for the patient to depend on others, therefore, it is important for him/her to be able to be sure that the health professional will operate in the patient's best interest. In order for the health professional to benefit the patient, however, the health professional must also be given the power to undertake his/her professional functions.

To resolve this dilemma, of giving the necessary power to the health professional while at the same time not losing control over one's situation, patients can establish participatory control with the health professional. The underlying dynamics for the patient is that in giving over such powers to the health professional he/she is negotiating a better control over his/her condition than otherwise could be accomplished. With participatory control, the health professional becomes an agent of the patient in his/her acting upon the forces determining his/her condition. Consider, for example, a patient who is suffering considerable arthritic pain in her hip and has recognized her limits of endurance as well as the conditions (eg. being housebound) under which she lives because of the pain. Her striking a working partnership with a more competent other can help her respond to the situation; to do something about it.

To come to the resolution that there are others who are more powerful and ought to be given the power to take care of the patient, the patient will have had to appraise the degree to which the illness, environment and the staff are contributing to her/his condition. This requires, therefore, a recognition of these factors in order to respond. These factors, however, are not very predictable and to respond to them is difficult. It is here where the role of others is so useful in enabling the patient to experience control. But before these others can facilitate this control, they also have to recognize the forces contributing to the patient's condition. This recognition, which requires a sensitivity and observance, will come from open communication with the patient and a willingness to work with the patient. For participatory control to operate there also needs to be a reciprocal involvement by the other with the patient.

This partnership is like being a member of a team with its members working together to deal with the circumstance the patient *and* the other members are in. There is no denying the greater competence of the health professional to assist, but there is an involvement of the patient in the treatment that is substantive and genuine. There has to be a trust and a form of interaction between the patient and the health professional that facilitates the patient to be involved in the treatment/care.

The way that participatory control is enacted will differ from patient to patient and from situation to situation. However, there are a number of features needed to facilitate establishing participatory control. First, the patient needs the skills to express his/her concerns, to ask questions and to communicate his/her displeasure or encouragement to the health professional. These behaviors will be more likely if the others model these behaviors among themselves and with the patient. It helps to have a social environment where the patient's involvement in his/her care is encouraged. It should be a common expectation that the patient will and should test the health professional to assure that the health professional is indeed responsive and working to the best of his/her ability. Thus a frank and open communication is critical for the patient to retain an experience of control over her/his condition. In cases of extreme distress, the patient may want to imbue the health professional with considerable power or competence, but in doing this, serves to retain the experience of control because he/she feels the best possible actions in light of his/her condition will be done.

By establishing a working relationship with a health professional, the patient's anxiety about not being able to respond to his/her condition can be reduced. By establishing participatory control with another, the patient may be able to divert some of his/her energies to other activities. Furthermore, the establishment of participatory control should lead to better care, for under such conditions, communications and patient compliance should be optimized. And if mistakes do occur, there should be less anger vented towards the staff, if the staff are seen to have been in close communication with the patient and doing their best. Conversely, there should be less anger directed towards patients by staff.

Participatory control explains situations where an observer would consider a geriatric patient as not having much control because of the severity of the patient's disability or illness and his/her dependency on hospital staff. But the observer does not realize that, for the patient, the staff are very important for his or her control. The patient may recognize that without the staff s/he has less control. The patient, while acknowledging the severity of the disability, still operates with the experience of control. The reason is the control gained through others. What is critical, however, is that the power to act is not entirely given over to others; it is shared. In short, the other person, such as a physician, can help the patient appraise the situation by determining what internal (e.g., physiological status) and external forces (e.g., the recommendations and the effectiveness of the surgeon willing to operate) are determining the patient's condition and then make the best possible decision.

Research Guided By Participatory Control

There are two studies recently completed that were guided by participatory control. They are summarized here to illustrate using the concept to study aspects of aging. In both studies we were interested in studying the role of the interactions of health care professionals with geriatric patients in facilitating the well-being of their patients. It should be mentioned that, in both cases, the studies were not designed to directly measure the concept. Rather the concept was used to study particular behaviors. Participatory control was used to generate working hypotheses to investigate the issues being studied.

The purpose of the first study was to determine whether the interactions of nurses with their patients can be altered so as to benefit the well-being of their patients. Participatory control, along with the Cognitive Social Learning Theory Of Control, was used to develop the design and strategy of the study. The strategy was to work *with* nurses to influence their experience of control and problem-solving vis-à-vis undertaking the care of their patients. By doing this, we expected to facilitate participatory control, and this would affect improvements in the nursing unit "atmosphere" for the patients. This improvement was expected to positively affect the patients' sense of well-being. Nursing unit atmosphere was operationalized using the *Ward Atmosphere Scale* (Moos, 1974).

Nurses were randomly assigned to three groups consisting of (1) an intervention group, (2) an attention placebo group, and (3) a no contact group. The intervention consisted of 14 one-hour sessions given over a seven-week period.

The findings were that the nurses in the intervention group showed an increase in internality on the appropriate dimension of the multidimensional I-E scale (Reid & Ware, 1974). The patients in the intervention group perceived less Staff Control and greater increases of Spontaneity and Autonomy at post-testing than did patients in the other groups. Furthermore, the patients in the intervention group showed a greater increase in positive self-concept than did patients in the other two groups.

Of additional significance in this study was that the intervention, while experimentally controlled, was done within the dynamic social system in which the nurses and patients lived. The interventions were not a matter of mechanistically *making* another have control. Rather, the entire model was one of facilitating control in a way that was natural to the setting. The intervention addressed both the external forces of the hospital and the internal forces of the nurses and patients. The intervention involved interactions of the experimenter with the nursing staff and the nursing staff with their patients, respectively. The experimenter did not directly work with the patients, with the exception of interviewing them pre and post the seven-week intervention. The staff were not given mini lectures on control theory. Rather, the sessions that were undertaken were done to be representative of the issues as the nurses (and the patients as learned by the nurses) saw them. But the experimenter's understanding of participatory control was used directly in guiding the intervention. By undertaking research in an applied way, we also avoided some of the ethical problems that field research on psychological control has faced (Schulz & Hanusa, 1978).

The second study was about male geriatric patient preference for alternative ways physicians can behave towards their patients. This research was spurred by the supposition that the quality of the physician's behavior can have a strong influence on how the patient responds to treatment. Assuming that most medical advice is of value, it seemed important to discover which forms of doctor-patient interactions would optimize the likelihood of patients seeking the doctors' advice and abiding by it. Furthermore, if the well-being and comfort of the patient was influenced by the way the physician responded to him/her, we wanted to know which way was preferred.

The study was an analogue experiment where physicians were thrice videotaped acting in three differing ways towards a patient. There were three physicians portraying all three physician-patient styles of interaction and the presentation of these portrayals were counterbalanced according to a latin square ANOVA design. The male geriatric patients viewed, by random selection, one of three possible sets of 3 portrayals. The geriatric patients viewed each physician once, with each physician portraying a different style of behavior. After each portrayal, the patients rated the physician on a number of scales assessing their impressions of the physician. These included the perceived competence of the physician, how approachable he was and the patient's willingness to comply with the recommended treatment.

The presentation of doctor-patient interactions was controlled across portrayals on a variety of factors, including the patient's diagnosis, recommended treatment, duration and angle of the camera. With the doctor speaking directly into the screen, the geriatric patient was asked to respond as if he were the patient to whom the doctor was giving the diagnosis and advice.

The portrayal of the doctor-patient styles was systematically manipulated to differ along three related dimensions on which a doctor might act in order to facilitate a patient's gaining participatory control. Manipulation checks confirmed the distinction of the portrayals along these dimensions. The first dimension was the degree to which the doctor acted so as to necessitate the patient's active involvement in discussing his disease. The second was the degree to which the doctor acted so as to direct or control the patient's treatment. The third was the degree to which responsibility for patient care was in the hands of the doctor in contrast to being shared between the doctor and the patient. While the tapes differed along these dimensions we referred to the most participatory oriented style as the negotiator style. The least participatory oriented was the expert style and the mid-dimensional style was called the consultant style.

The results showed the negotiator style--where participatory control was most likely--was the most preferred style and the one patients would most comply with, visit again, etc., even though there were no differences among styles in perceived competence. These differences held for all three physicians.

Studies Addressing Participatory Control

Affleck, Tennen, Pfeiffer and Fifield (1987) recently used a partial operationalization of participatory control in a study of patients' adaptation to having rheumatoid arthritis. This study also addressed the multidimensional compensational model that patients will make distinctions between what they can and cannot influence as part of their adaptation. Ninety-two patients between the ages of 20-65 years received 90-minute interviews covering a broad range of topics involving their adaptation to their illness. Included in the interviews were questions of disease severity, appraisals of the patients' personal control, including control over symptoms, control over long-term course of the disease and control over treatment of the illness. Patients also answered parallel worded questions about the control that health care providers have over their symptoms and the course of their disease.

Of the different measures of control, the perception of control over treatment processes (as distinct from control over disease) was the form of control most consistently correlated with measures of adaptation. The authors stated that "Several patients volunteered that following the advice of their physicians and nurses provided them the means of gaining control over their illness" (p. 278). They also stated their findings are ". . . consistent with Reid's (1984) contention that optimal adaptation to a chronic disease depends on the patient's ability to come to terms with what she or he can and cannot control" (p. 278).

Cicirelli (1987) conducted a correlation study of 105 senior patients (mean age = 71.9 years) hospitalized in a high constraint situation. Nursing staff ratings of patients on items assessing patient adjustment were correlated with the patients' scores on (1) the multidimensional *Health Locus of Control Scale*, and (2) a measure of perceived constraint and distress over loss of independence in the hospital situation. More positive adjustment ratings and reports of less distress were correlated with beliefs that health outcomes were controlled by powerful others. Patients who believed that they controlled their own health outcomes reported greater distress and were rated as less effectively adjusted. Cicirelli reports that these findings are consistent with the notion of participatory control.

Meta-Sensitization--A Model For Facilitating The Interactional Control Experience

The reconceptualization of control presented in this chapter is one that is process oriented and emphasizes the interaction of the person with his/her situation including both internal and external forces. What is necessary is a means to understand how the experience of control may be facilitated in light of this conceptualization of control. As noted earlier, the experience of control is a phenomenological perspective that benefits from being able to stand back and evaluate the situation so that one can act upon it. Piper and Langer's mindfulness construct, discussed earlier, has also been described as a process oriented model of control that emphasized that increased cognitive activity would promote more control. Although we can appreciate their intention, we feel their model is inefficient for applied research because the necessary components of such a process are not defined.

As an adjunct to our research on participatory control and the institutionalized elderly (Stirling & Reid, in preparation) we posed the following question: How can individuals be assisted in best utilizing their existing personal control to most productively accommodate themselves? We feel that simply creating a greater perception of control, while it may be initially motivating, can be potentially harmful to individuals if their subsequent experience does not corroborate such beliefs. It can leave them environmentally vulnerable and, consequently, contribute to experiencing the loss of control. Therefore, the experience of control must have a reality base.

We also realized that while one can talk to individuals about their options, contingencies, abilities, etc., they are not always able to apply what they hear.   It is somewhat like the expected parents who are told in detail what to do as parents and what it is like.   But until they are parents, they do not know what it is like and what it means.   To influence only beliefs is to risk only influencing the persons' cognitions and not the affective and be- havioral components of their attitudes that may be necessary to have a lasting impact.   From this standpoint we assume that it is more effective to influence beliefs by having persons experience control. The question is: How does one do this?   The following is a guide which stems from our research on assisting senior patients.

Responding to both developmental and therapeutic models of adjustment, we concluded that both *cognitive* and *emotional* components of experience are essential if control is to be facilitated.   Along with these components, we described a four stage process consisting of *recognition, definition, acceptance,* and *action.*   For example, in a psychotherapeutic process, the first stage, recognition, would involve an active awareness that there is a problem (Something is wrong, I'm not happy, etc.).   This stage would include both thinking and feeling components (cognitive and emotional).   In stage two, definition would involve mentally defining the problem (What is it that is causing me to feel this way?).   This is mainly a cognitive component.   Acceptance, in the third stage, would involve the emotional acceptance (internalization) of the problem (emotional component).   Stage four, action, would involve active problem-solving in order to accommodate a more satisfying/copeable state (cognitive and emotional components).   This process is not, however, limited to the pathology inherent in psychotherapeutic experiences.

We attempted to develop the empathic potential of nurses in a geriatric institution, so that they would be able to demonstrate a greater appreciation/insight into their personal control in relation to their patients' personal control and their joint environment (the institution).   We felt that it would be necessary to sensitize the nurses to their own general needs, their environmental experiences and to the fact that such sensitization was necessary.   We called this process meta-sensitization.   In order to achieve the highest degree of participatory control (i.e., the most reciprocally productive interactional control between these nurses and their patients) nurses would need to internalize this sensitivity.

Consistent with our earlier-described process, we implemented a program that addressed the first three stages, namely: recognition, definition and acceptance.   For stage one, nurses were encouraged to become more sensitized to themselves and their environment.   To help them pick out stress areas at work and in other areas of their lives, they completed assignments that included dividing a circle into a 24- hour schedule and shading in each section the degree to which work encroached on other activities.   On another circle, they divided up a day's work into the different tasks involved and shaded in the degree to which each task was stressful.

The second stage of definition was dealt with by using the technique of self-remembering. This involves having individuals take time to cognitively attend to themselves and their environments in the course of carrying out any activity without altering the activity per se. In so doing, they develop an "objective" awareness of themselves. They are "standing back" and appraising their situation, as described in an earlier section on compensation.

Acceptance, the third stage, was accomplished by using the areas defined as stressful by the nurses. For example, nursing stations were described as high stress environments because of the multitude of activities and responsibilities that occur there. As a result, nurses were encouraged to accept these as stressful environments and not to expect them to be otherwise. Therefore, to feel stressful in this environment was realistic. Only with such an acceptance could they then direct their energies to effectively accommodate this environment instead of consuming energy in fighting against the environment. As the fourth stage, action, is the outcome of the first three stages, there was no intervention here.

The criterion we used in determining whether or not the process we attempted to implement was successful, was the spontaneous feedback from the nurses. The following is an example of the feedback we received. A nurse reported this incident that occurred during the course of a work day. "It was a hectic day, and I was really annoyed because I felt that I was doing more than my share of work. The others (nurses) were nowhere in sight, and Mr. R. needed to be hoisted from the chair onto his bed. Since no one else was around, I decided to do it by myself. While I was trying to get him on the bed, two family members of another patient were asking me about their father. They weren't rude, but I was so upset that I was really short with them. I don't know why, but I decided to self-remember, and I realized just how tense and angry I was. And I thought: 'What am I doing?' Here I was trying to do a job that takes two people and snapping at my patient and these other people because I couldn't manage. So first I lowered Mr. R. back into the chair and told him I'd be back in a few minutes with help. Then I told the relatives that what I was doing needed my full attention, but that if they could wait for 20 minutes in the lounge, I would be happy to answer any questions I could. Next I found another nurse and asked him to help me hoist Mr. R. into his bed. Then I talked with the relatives. Then I told another nurse that I would be in the quiet room (nurses' lounge) if anyone was looking for me and went and had a break to relax. I felt I deserved it."

Such examples demonstrated to us that the process was indeed occurring. In the above example, it was only after the nurse was able to understand her situation and give into the fact that the control she was trying to maintain was not effective in that situation, that she was able to realistically, and effectively accommodate her environment and have a genuine experience of control.

Conclusions

A major point in this chapter is that advances in psychological control and aging research require the reconceptualization of control, so that control can be better applied to social-psychological aspects of aging. Many of the control constructs were not developed for the study of aging and their application has been problematic and limited.

In the field of psychological control research, there is a trend towards developing concepts that are more interactional in focus and this chapter underscores some of the contributions to this trend. To add impetus to this trend, this chapter presents a reconceptualization of control that emphasizes a phenomenological perspective that is more readily applicable to the study of aging phenomena. This expanded notion of psychological control is described within the Cognitive Social Learning Theory Of Control and the associated concept of participatory control. The utility of this re-interpretation is presented in terms of examples as well as empirical studies. One of these studies was a controlled experiment to show how, from the systems oriented perspective of participatory control, nurses can become involved in ways that could alter both their own appraisals and those of their patients. These are practical ways for facilitating the experiencing of control.

The recommendation of this chapter is that while better theory is required, we also should realize that the theory needs to be applicable. The value of the theory is in the ease with which it can be used to study aging phenomena. The issues of whether one theory differs from another theory, or has construct validity or is based on false assumptions are very important. These issues, however, should be examined not in contrived demonstrations (which at best are merely pilot work to more substantive investigations) but in the study of psychological phenomena in the field. It is possible that, when applied in the field, the apparently differing control constructs are more similar than different. Thus Schulz's (1976) attempt to manipulate predictability from choice or decision making made no difference in outcome, although both manipulations benefitted the senior patients when compared to patients in a no treatment control group. One of these (predictability) was a confound of the other. It is possible, in behavioral science, to continue to conceptually divide phenomena (ie., control) into ever finely distinguished parts, and fail to add them back together. By rooting the development of control theory on data obtained in field settings, we may be able to keep the refinement of our conceptualizations consistent with the phenomena studied.

Footnotes

1. Researchers on aging are placing increasing emphasis on the
    role of "meaning in life," reminiscence and beliefs about
    the world for adjustment to aging (cf. Lazarus & Delongis
    1983). The suggestion here is that these beliefs, by
    helping the person to appraise their situation (particularly
    under ambiguous circumstances), facilitates their being able
    to act and gain control.

2. Rotter (1966) makes a similar point with the exception that
    he refers to beliefs in either complete internal or external
    locus of control as non-adaptive. Krause and Stryker (1984)
    provide data on middle-aged men to show that extremes of
    either internal or external control beliefs are maladaptive.
    Having a balance of internal and external beliefs buffered
    the negative effects of job and economic events on well-
    being.

3. During the 1970's there was an outgrowth of research into
    the multi-dimensionality of Internal-External locus of
    control (Lefcourt, 1976, 1982; Reid & Ware, 1974). In
    addition there has been the publication of research into
    population specific and situation specific I-E scales
    (Lefcourt, 1981, 1984). Rotter emphasized that expectations
    will differ according to the situation (Rotter, 1975). All
    of this research indicates that persons will differentiate
    so-called external sources of control.

References

Affleck, G., Tennen, H., Pfeiffer, C., & Fifield, J. (1987).
  Appraisals of control and predictability in adapting to a chronic
  disease. *Journal of Personality and Social Psychology, 53,* 273-279.

Averill, J. R. (1973). Personal control over aversive stimuli   its
  relationship to stress. *Psychological Bulletin, 80,* 286-303.

Baltes, M. M., & Baltes, P. B. (1986). *The psychology of control
  and aging.* Hillsdale, NJ: Lawrence Erlbaum Associates.

Bandura, A. (1977). Self-efficacy: Toward a unifying theory of
  behavioral change. *Psychological Review, 84,* 191-215.

Bandura, A. (1982). The self and mechanisms of agency. In J. Suls
  (Ed.), *Psychological perspectives on the self (Vol. 1)* (pp. 3-
  39). Hillsdale, NJ: Lawrence Erlbaum Associates.

Bandura, A. (1986). *The social foundations of thought and action: A social cognitive theory*. Englewood Cliffs, NJ: Prentice Hall.

Bulman, R. J., & Wortman, C. B. (1977). Attributions of blame and coping in the "real world": Severe accident victims react to their lot. *Journal of Personality and Social Psychology, 35*, 351-363.

Cicirelli, V. G. (1987). Locus of control and patient role adjustment of the elderly in acute-care hospitals. *Psychology and Aging, 2*, 138-143.

deCharms, R. (1968). *Personal causation*. New York: Academic Press.

Deci, E. L. (1975). *Intrinsic motivation.* New York: Plenum Press.

Deci, E. L., & Ryan, R. M. (1987). The support of autonomy and the control of behavior. *The Journal of Personality and Social Psychology, 53*, 1024-1037.

Gergen, M. M., & Gergen, K. J. (1986). The discourse of control and the maintenance of well-being. In M. M. Baltes & P. B. Baltes (Eds.), *The psychology of control and aging* (pp. 119-138). Hillsdale, NJ: Lawrence Erlbaum Associates.

Hoff, E. H., & Hohner, H. U. (1986). Occupational careers, work, and control. In M. M. Baltes & P. B. Baltes (Eds.), *The psychology of control and aging* (pp. 345-371). Hillsdale, NJ: Lawrence Erlbaum Associates.

Karuza, J. Jr., Rabinowitz, V. C., & Zevon, M. A. (1986). Implications of control and responsibility on helping the aged. In M. M. Baltes & P. B. Baltes (Eds.), *The psychology of control and aging* (pp 373-396). Hillsdale, NJ: Lawrence Erlbaum Associates.

Krause, N. (1987). Understanding the stress process: linking social support with locus of control beliefs. *Journal of Gerontology, 42*, 589-593.

Krause, N., & Stryker, S. (1984). Stress and well-being: The buffering role of locus of control beliefs. *Social Science Medicine, 18*, 783-790.

Kuhl, J. (1986). Aging and models of control: The hidden costs of wisdom. In M. M. Baltes & P. B. Baltes (Eds.), *The psychology of control and aging* (pp. 1-33). Hillsdale, NJ: Lawrence Erlbaum Associates.

Lachman, M. E. (1986). Locus of control in aging research: A case for multidimensional and domain-specific assessment. *Journal of Psychology and Aging, 1*, 34-40.

Langer, E. J., & Rodin, J. (1976). The effects of choice and enhanced personal responsibility for the aged. A field experiment in an institutional setting. *Journal of Personality and Social Psychology, 34,* 191-198.

Lazarus, R. S., & DeLongis, A. (1983). Psychological stress and coping in aging. *American Psychologist, 34,* 245-254.

Lefcourt, H. M. (1976). *Locus of control: Current trends in theory and research.* Hillsdale, NJ: Lawrence Erlbaum Associates.

Lefcourt, H. M. (1981). *Research with the locus of control construct (Vol.1).* New York: Academic Press.

Lefcourt, H. M. (1982). *Locus of control: Current trends in theory and research* (2nd. ed.). Hillsdale, NJ: Lawrence Erlbaum Associates.

Lefcourt, H. M. (1984). *Research with the locus of control construct (Vol. 3).* New York: Academic Press.

Lumpkin, J. R. (1986). The relationship between locus of control and age: New evidence. *Journal of Social Behavior and Personality, 1,* 245-252.

Magnusson, D., & Endler, N. S. (1977). *Personality at the crossroads: Current issues in interactional psychology.* Hillsdale, NJ: Lawrence Erlbaum Associates.

Moos, R. H. (1974). *Ward atmosphere scale.* Palo Alto: Consulting Psychologist Press, Inc.

Piper, A. I., & Langer, E. J. (1986). Aging and mindful control. In M. M. Baltes & P. B. Baltes (Eds.), *The psychology of control and aging* (pp. 71-89). Hillsdale, NJ: Lawrence Erlbaum Associates.

Reid, D. W. (1977). Locus of control as an important concept for an interactionist approach to behavior. In D. Magnusson & N. S. Endler (Eds.), *Personality at the crossroads: Current issues in interactional psychology* (pp. 185-191). Hillsdale, NJ: Lawrence Erlbaum Associates.

Reid, D. W. (1984). Participatory control and the chronic-illness adjustment process. In H. M. Lefcourt (Ed.), *Research with the locus of control construct (Vol. 3)* (pp. 361-389). New York: Academic Press.

Reid, D. W., & Ware, E. E. (1973). Multidimensionality of internal-external control: Implications for past and future research. *Canadian Journal of Behavioral Science, 5,* 264-271.

Reid, D. W., & Ware, E. E. (1974). Multidimensionality of internal-external control: Addition of a third dimension and nondistinction of self versus others. *Canadian Journal of Behavioral Science, 6,* 131-142.

Reid, D. W., Haas, G., & Hawkings, D. (1977). Locus of desired control and positive self-concept of the elderly. *Journal of Gerontology, 22,* 441-450.

Reid, D. W., & Ziegler, M. (1981). The desired control measure and adjustment among the elderly. In H. M. Lefcourt (Ed.), *Research with the locus of control construct (Vol. 1)* (pp. 127-159). New York: Academic Press.

Rodin, J., & Langer, E. J. (1977). Long-term effects of a control-relevant intervention among the institutionalized aged. *Journal of Personality and Social Psychology, 35,* 897-902.

Rothbaum, F., Weisz, J. R., & Snyder, S. S. (1982). Changing the world and changing the self: A two-process model of perceived control. *Journal of Personality and Social Psychology, 42,* 5-37.

Rotter, J. B. (1966). Generalized expectancies for internal external control of reinforcement. *Psychological Monographs, 80,* (1, Whole No. 609).

Rotter, J. B. (1975). Some problems and misconceptions related to the construct of internal versus external control of reinforcement. *Journal of Consulting and Clinical Psychology, 43,* 56-67.

Sangster, S. L., Blackwell, J. E., Quek, J., Reid, D. W., & Ziegler, M. (1981). *Adjustment in the chronically disabled elderly.* Paper presented at the joint meeting of the Gerontological Society of America and the Canadian Association on Gerontology, Toronto, Canada. November 8-12.

Schulz, R. (1976). The effects of and responsibility on the physical and psychological well-being of the institutionalized aged. *Journal of Personality and Social Psychology, 33,* 563-573.

Schulz, R., & Hanusa, B. (1978). Long-term effects of control and predictability-enhancing interventions: Findings and ethical issues. *Journal of Personality and Social Psychology, 36,* 1194-1201.

Seligman, M. E. P., Maier, S. F., & Geer, J. (1968). The alleviation of learned helplessness in the dog. *Journal of Abnormal and Social Psychology, 73,* 256-262.

Slivinske, L. R., & Fitch, V. L. (1987). The effects of control enhancing interventions of the well-being of elderly individuals living in retirement communities. *The Gerontologist, 27,* 176-181.

Shanfield, S. B. (1980). On surviving cancer: Psychological considerations. *Comprehensive Psychiatry, 21,* 128-134.

Skinner, B. F. (1983). Intellectual self-management in old age. *American Psychologist, 38,* 239-244.

Stirling, G., & Reid, D. W. (In preparation). *The application of participatory control to facilitate patient well-being: An experimental study of nursing impact on geriatric patients.*

Weiner, B. (1982). The emotional consequences of causal attributions. In M. S. Clark & S. T. Fiske (Eds.), *Affect and cognition* (pp. 185-209). Hillsdale, NJ: Lawrence Erlbaum Associates.

Weiss, J. M. (1972). Psychological factors in stress and disease. *Scientific American, 226,* 104-113.

Weiss, J. M., Glazer, H. I., Pohorecky, L. A., Bailey, W. H., & Schneider, L. H. (1979). In R. A. Depue (Ed.), *The psychobiology of the depressive disorders* (pp. 125-158). New York: Academic Press.

Weisz, J. R., Rothbaum, F. M., & Blackburn, T. F. (1984). Standing out and standing in: The psychology of control in America and Japan. *American Psychologist, 39,* 955-969.

White, R. W. (1959). Motivation reconsidered: The concept of competence. *Psychological Review, 66,* 297-323.

Ziegler, M., & Reid, D. W. (1979). Correlates of locus of desired-control in two samples of elderly persons: Community residents and hospitalized patients. *Journal of Consulting and Clinical Psychology, 47,* 977-979.

PART IV

RECONSTRUCTIONS OF CONTROL

Psychological Perspectives of Helplessness
and Control in the Elderly, P.S. Fry (ed.)
© *Elsevier Science Publishers B.V. (North-Holland), 1989*

Chapter Nine

LOSS OF CONTROL AMONG THE AGING? : A CRITICAL RECONSTRUCTION

Mary GERGEN

The Pennsylvania State University, Delaware County Campus

Abstract

An issue of relatively long-standing in the literature on aging in social psychology has been that of the effects of personal control or its absence on well-being. Theorizing and research by psychologists such as Rotter, Seligman, Bandura, Langer, Rodin and Schulz in general conclude that the risk of physical decline and death are increased as personal control is diminished. In addition psychological distress and impairment are also seen to increase with greater loss of control. This chapter briefly reviews the work of the major contributors mentioned above. The positivistic approach of this work is then criticized from a contemporary philosophy of science position. Research that avoids these limits is then presented. This study relies on discourse analysis, and is within a social construc-tionist paradigm. Sociological critiques that impugn the value of the self-controlled autonomous individual are then offered. These criticisms emphasize the limitations of the rhetoric of personal control and well-being. Special emphasis is given to feminist arguments that highlight the valuational biases adherent in the preferences given to high internal control. The advantages of reconceptualizing people as socially embedded and interdependent are advanced.

Introduction

Among the most intriguing topics of study in social psychology in the past twenty years has been that of personal control. Various theorists and researchers have discussed the topic, in texts too numerous to cite here, and subject populations from cradle to grave have been examined for traces of the valuable ore. In general the foci of these investigations of personal control have been: who's got it, how much, under what conditions, and to what end.

Why has this variable attracted so much attention, one might ask? A common sense answer is that personal control is at the core of our society's value system.   In order to have a stable, rational and effective political order with a democratic governmental structure, we must have citizens who are able to exercise their public duties as lawful and self-directed members of the social order.   If, however, the participants in such a system are without the power of self-direction necessary to carry out their functions, the system would deteriorate.   In a system constituted by people without personal control, no one would be responsible for personal conduct; no one would be able to work towards personal or societal goals; and, no one would be able to enjoy the fruits of such labors.

Such observations are not unique.   Max Weber first equated the ideology of internal control with the Protestant Ethic (Furby, 1979). Based on the belief that hard work, skill and ability are important determinants of success, this ideology took root in the fertile soil of the United States.   Weber (1930) described the United States as "a culture that emphasized the unique, independent and self-reliance of the individual . . . [a country that] places a high value on personal output of energy for solving problems . . . [and where] status is achieved through one's own efforts" (p. 122).

It is this same ideology of control that appears to inform the profession of psychology.   With little doubt or exception, researchers have endorsed the values of control for personal well-being.   To illustrate:

"With the strengthening of the perception of control comes a variety of beneficial effects including an increase in motivation, a decrease in stress, and facilitation of problem solving" (Perlmuter, Monty & Chan, 1986, p. 92).

"Interventions aimed at enhancing a sense of control and developing coping strategies appear to mitigate environmental challenges to the older person's adaptive resources, thus reducing harmful physiological reactions and lessening the chances of disease development" (Rodin, 1986, p. 160).

"We expect that the observed decrease in perceived 'personal control over development' should be accompanied by a corresponding increase of a depressive attitude toward one's development" (Brandtst-ädter, Krampen, & Heil, 1986, p. 288).

The value of personal control is associated with energy, robustness, achievement, health and high hopes--major values within the humanist tradition.   A person who failed to favor personal control might risk the danger of seeming anti-American, anti-democratic, and anti-humanist!

While the vast majority of studies concerning personal control have used youthful research subjects, this field has also attracted the interests of gerontologically-oriented psychologists. This focus of concern has been based on the assumption that the aging process is one of general decline with a concomitant loss of personal control. Older people have been thought to experience lessening personal control over their physical environment, social and economic circumstances, bodily resources and psychological functions (e.g., loss of intelligence, memory, and sensory-motor processes). Various social psychologists, for example Rodin (1986), Langer (1983) and Schulz (1976) have studied the impact of personal control on measures of well-being and mortality among aged populations. The basic theme of their research endeavors has been that if older people increase their actual or their perceived personal control, they will slow the aging process, be more vigorous, have greater social integration and consequently accumulate fewer social costs. Volumes such as this one and Margret and Paul Baltes' edited volume, *The Psychology of Control and Aging* (1986), indicate the importance of this body of theory and research, especially in improving the lives of older people.

And what will this chapter contribute to this vast array of texts on personal control and the aging person? What do I have to add to all of this? My general plan for this chapter is to first review rather sketchily the foundations of contemporary theory and research in this vast field of personal control related to the aging. After a brief perusal of these bases, I plan to offer a critique of the existing literature from a philosophy of science perspective. Then I will present a research project on personal control that will be analyzed from a perspective that is different from previously mentioned research. The study attempts to avoid some of the pitfalls of a traditional empiricist science paradigm. After presenting this research, I will summarize a group of critiques that have unsettled for me the value of these data, as well as those of many other researchers. These critiques will encompass sociological and feminist writings regarding contemporary research on personal control. This last portion of the chapter will particularly emphasize the importance of recent writings of feminist scholars who have developed arguments against the cult of the self-reliant (i.e., internally controlled) individual.

Theoretical Background to the Study of Personal Control

In terms of theoretical contribution, a triumvirate of major figures steps to the fore. Beginning with Rotter (1966), who became well-known for his work developing the I-E scale, then followed by Seligman (1975), whose work spans the shift from actual to perceived personal control and capped by Bandura (1977), whose theory of self-efficacy is highly regarded, the history of theory revolves around these men. Additional inputs to the study of personal control comes from the common sense vernacular, as well as from attributional theorists' formulations regarding personal versus situational attributes of causation (e.g., Heider, 1958; Jones & Nisbett, 1971; Kelly, 1967; Weiner, 1974). After defining the central concept of the field, we will explore the approaches of the major theorists in greater detail.

While the exact definition of this field of study varies, depending on the theoretical source, one such definition states: "A high level of control is indexed by behaviors and beliefs that characterize an individual as someone who knows about his [sic] agency and exhibits actions (or behaviors) that result in anticipated consequences" (Baltes & Baltes, 1986, p. xviii). This statement highlights the significant elements of most definitions of personal control: awareness of personal agency; freedom to act; ability to plan and pursue self-determined goals; foreknowledge of consequences; and an awareness of the relationship of one's actions to their consequences. While people high in personal control are characterized by these qualities, people low in personal control, or externally controlled, believe that powerful others and external forces shape their destinies. Researchers, in general, explore ways in which various levels of personal control influence aspects of an individual's life (e.g., levels of motivation, well-being, and achievement).

Julian Rotter: Parent of the IE Scale

Julian Rotter may be seen as the progenitor of research into the area of personal control. In the forties and fifties, Rotter (1954) theorized that the likelihood of a person engaging in a particular behavior was dependent on two variables: 1. the degree to which the person expected the behavior to bring about a certain endpoint, and 2. how much the endpoint was valued. Rotter argued that the higher the expectation and the more valued the outcome, the more likely it was that the person would act in a particular fashion. This hypothesis was built on a social learning approach to behavior, and was at that time strongly situationally driven, as well. Rotter included in his formulations not only a person's generalized expectancies, but also specific context-dependent ones. While early formulations were interactional, (i.e., person and situational variables together were vital) the situational variables tended to be overlooked in latter years. In 1966 Rotter developed the *Internal-External Scale*, which still remains a basic research tool for many psychologists. As most readers know, the scale is composed of a series of 23 paired statements, one of which must be selected by subjects as the statement with which they most strongly agree. For example: "Many times I feel that I have little influence over the things that happen to me" versus "It is impossible for me to believe that chance or luck plays an important role in my life." Generalized expectancies for control had evolved into a personality trait, with causal influence on subsequent action.

Rotter and his colleagues studied the effects of this locus of control variable within many different contexts (cf. Lefcourt, 1976; Rotter, 1966; Rotter, Chance & Phares, 1972).   Their work inspired many others.

Martin Seligman: Coiner of "Learned Helplessness"

The second major contributor to the theoretical side of personal control is Martin Seligman.   In the tradition of behaviorist psychology, Seligman's work began with animal studies.   Seligman studied the responses of dogs presented with inescapable shock, a situation of noncontingency between response and outcome.   The later refusal of the experimental dogs who had undergone the uncontrollable shock to make any response to avoid further shock encouraged Seligman (1975) to create the notion of learned helplessness.   Learned helplessness was the state in which the animal has learned that its actions were ineffective, and the shock was inescapable.   Once the dogs fell into the learned helplessness condition, they were said to become lethargic.   Arguing by analogy, Seligman traced the parallels between his lethargic dogs and mental patients suffering from depression.   He posited that depressed patients also suffer from the lack of personal control or learned helplessness.   He suggested that experiences of noncontingency in their pasts had lead these victims of depression to their malaise.   Earlier formulations of learned helplessness emphasized the lack of contingency between response and reinforcements; later Seligman and his colleagues emphasized that the *perception* of helplessness was the crucial component in producing poor coping strategies and depression (Abramson, Seligman & Teasdale, 1978).   This transition marked the shift from a behavioral to a cognitive psychological approach to learned helplessness for Seligman.   However, this alteration did not modify the basically deterministic causal model or empiricist methodology, which is part of the cognitive psychology paradigm, as well as the behavioral one.

Albert Bandura's Self-Efficacy Model of Personal Control

Albert Bandura (1982) advocates the importance of self-efficacy in the examination of personal control variables.   Along with Seligman, Bandura is interested in *perceptions* rather than actual experiences. "Perceived self-efficacy is concerned with judgments of how well one can execute courses of actions required to deal with perspective situations" (Bandura, 1982, p. 122).   The distinctions of interest to Bandura are between perceiving oneself as skilled or unskilled at a relevant activity, and perceiving the environment as rewarding or withholding of reward.   People whose sense of personal control is low due to a lack of confidence in their own behavioral abilities are seen as less likely to try to control their environments than those who are confident.   Bandura believes that those low in self-efficacy require different interventions for change than those who see themselves as capable, but the environment as unyielding.

In his emphasis on environmental variation, Bandura's theory supports Rotter's earlier distinctions. Like Rotter and Seligman, Bandura works in the mainstream of the empiricist metatheory. His work revolves around discovering lawful relationships between antecedent and subsequent events, using a combination of behavioral and cognitive variables.

Several other theorists have created similar models of personal control, among them are, Heinz Heckhausen (1980), Jochen Brandtstädter (Brandtstädter, Krampen & Heil, 1986), and Julius Kuhl (1986). Each works within a form of the expectancy-value framework established by Rotter. Kuhl's work is strongly influenced by the cognitive movement in psychology, and computer metaphors in particular. His information processing model of action control deals with propositional networks representing intentions relevant to the self, one's personal commitment to action, the situation and the intended action. While more heavily weighted emphasis on cognitive variables occurs in these theoretical orientations, they remain within the traditional empiricist framework of science.

The Empiricist Tradition of Personal Control Research

The research tradition that has developed within the personal control domain has been strongly influenced by the attendant empiricist metatheory and methodology of social psychology. Using a deterministic causal model, an experimental methodology and a mechanistic model of persons, researchers attempt to produce lawful regularities. A brief perusal of this enterprise follows.

Highlights of Research on Personal Control and the Aged

Any comprehensive review of the empirical work related to personal control would necessarily cover a vast territory. Over 1500 published studies on personal control are available in the psychological literature in the English language alone (cf. Lefcourt, 1976, 1981, 1982; Perlmuter & Monty, 1979; Phares, 1976; Rotter, Chance & Phares, 1972). In the more specific area of control and old age, Baltes and Baltes (1986) and this volume brings to light hundreds of studies either directly or indirectly related to this topic. Because of the wealth of empirical evidence, any attempt to encapsulate this work in a brief summary is impossible to do with sufficient balance or comprehensiveness. Interestingly, despite the voluminous literature, certain research projects have been taken as "classics" in the field, and are almost always referred to regardless of context. They are studies by Ellen Langer and Judith Rodin (cf. Langer & Rodin, 1976; Rodin & Langer, 1977) and Richard Schulz (cf. Schulz, 1976; Schulz &

Hanusa, 1978). The work done by these researchers shares the characteristic of having been done with residents in nursing homes. Also the basic design of these studies share a similarity: the researchers try to evaluate the level of internal locus of control and well-being among the residents before and following an experimental intervention of inducing greater personal control.

More recent writings of Langer (Langer, Blank & Chanowitz, 1978; Piper & Langer, 1986) indicate that she has turned away from her commitment to locus of control and has reinterpreted her earlier work, and that of many other psychologists concerned with personal control, as related to mindlessness, rather than control. She has argued that the process by which older people improve in their life satisfactions and longevity is through renewed activation of their minds, or mindfulness, rather than simply by increasing contingencies or perceived contingencies in the external world. She has also criticized personal control theorists for concentrating too much on the external outcomes of actions, and too little on the meaning of events and internal processes to the actor. As Piper and Langer (1986) have summarized their view: "The mindless individual is caught in a cycle that is quite vicious, even deadly: When s/he is in various ways told that s/he is no longer competent . . . the individual mindlessly accepts this negative image, loses feelings of self-worth, and consequently, makes little or no attempt to disprove the label. Instead s/he supports the notion of incompetence by becoming unduly helpless and ill, often terminally so" (p. 71).

While Langer and her colleagues have shifted attention from the "personal control" variable to "mindlessness," the basic experimental foundation and causal explanatory model has remained basically unmodified. However, Langer's growing emphasis on the importance of a subject's interpretation of events, as well as her emphasis on the importance of process rather than product or outcome suggests a turning away from a strict empiricist tradition (Piper & Langer, 1986). We shall return to the significance of interpretation in more detail later.

Rodin has remained more faithful than Langer to the traditional formulations of personal control in explaining positive outcomes, especially as related to health issues among the older population. In general she has found that the elderly are more vulnerable to various threats of illness and loss, but are benefitted by increased feelings of personal control. Her recent data indicate that uncontrolled stress has negative consequences for the immune system among older people. Rodin also has indicated some reservations about regarding internal personal control as a panacea for older people. As she has said, "Feelings of control may be stress inducing for some, especially when individuals believe that there are actions they ought to be taking but are not" (Rodin, 1986, p. 159). She has suggested that the desire for excessive control can create problems of the same type as increased control can ease. Rodin also is more optimistic about the aging process than most other researchers. She does not assume that aging is the inevitable slippery slide into oblivion that so many researchers in their field seem to accept as *a priori* fact. Among the aspects that Rodin argues give buoyancy to the process of aging are having a sense of personal control and the necessary coping strategies for the problems that arise.

Rodin's work tends to adhere to an empiricist framework of science. However, her questioning of the value of personal control, and her reluctance to accept the stereotypes of aging that frequently undergird the rationale of gerontological studies suggest ways in which Rodin has deviated from the traditional path of scientific practices within this realm.

The clarity of the findings of the original research by Langer and Rodin were clouded somewhat by similar research by Schulz and his colleagues. While Langer and Rodin found that their subjects seemed to benefit over a year's time by interventions to increase their personal control over a detail of their lives, Schulz found that these effects were actually reversed for some of his subjects. In his studies nursing home residents were allowed various degrees of control over visits they were to receive from undergraduates. Later, when the visits ceased, the subjects were found to experience detrimental effects (Schulz, 1976; Schulz & Hanusa, 1978). Various explanations have been found for these seemingly contradictory findings. Sufficient differences in the experimental conditions occurred, such that each project provided a different perspective on the problem. Kuhl (1986), for example, has suggested that the favorable long-term results for the subjects in the Rodin and Langer experiments may have occurred because the subjects learned new coping strategies that generalized to other aspects of their social environment, while Schulz's subjects were left without any increment in personal control strategies. A later study by Rodin (1983) supports this line of thinking. Schulz and Hanusa (1978) have also suggested that subjects in the Rodin and Langer studies had made stable changes in their self-attributions, while their own subjects saw their experience of control as temporary. This interpretation may be substantiated by recalling the abruptness with which the researchers and "visitors" took their leave when the study was over, probably without asking the residents what they wanted to have happen. It must have been clear to the residents that they really did not have much say in the process at the termination point.

These descriptions of the experimental results and the adjudication of findings for these studies are entirely "within paradigm." That is, the type of controversies raised and the types of resolutions made are part of the empiricist tradition. They do not focus on issues of a different scope - for example, the underlying values and assumptions substantiated by these experimental manipulations. We will look at these issues later.

Margret Baltes and her colleagues (cf. Baltes & Reisenzein, 1986; Baltes & Skinner, 1983) have considered the same setting and set of problems as the researchers previously mentioned. Taking a behaviorist position, their perspective on personal control has been from a somewhat different angle (Baltes & Barton, 1977, 1979). They see patient behaviors in terms of their reinforcement values, and they do not presume to judge whether or not they *seem* to be under personal control or not. From their analysis, dependent behaviors, such as asking for help or service, are the most effective strategies for producing a contingent response. Thus, somewhat ironically, those behaviors that appear to signal circumstances of external control (i.e., dependent behaviors) are those that produce the most internally controlled outcomes. Thus, one might conclude that highly dependent behaviors are the most internally controlled behaviors. In addition, independent behaviors prove to be ignored by the caretakers, and thus, people who "help themselves" end up with no rewards, and are often punished for their efforts. Their research draws attention to the further complexity of the apparently straightforward notions relating personal control to positive outcomes, often assumed by others.

Baltes' research emphasizes the fragile web of verbal conventions upon which much personal control research is built. The potential for a close analysis of "key terms," such as *personal control*, to disclose serious problems in conceptualization is clear. Such a possibility is found by Lachman (1986), who has surveyed both cross-sectional and longitudinal studies on personal control among the elderly. Her review indicates that contradictory results accrue concerning how the elderly perceive their level of personal control, depending on how they are assessed. For example, elderly people are more likely to reveal decrements in perceived personal control over issues like health and intelligence, but maintain or increase their sense of personal control for other things, such as personal efficacy. These and other findings show that the field of personal control among the aged is not as concise and clearly established as the promises of an experimental methodology might lead one to expect.

Critiques of the Personal Control Literature

Criticisms of the concept of personal control have been offered by many psychologists in the past decade. Within this portion of the chapter I will summarize and embellish on illustrative critiques based on certain philosophic questions. Taking these criticisms seriously leads one to questions concerning the coherence, utility, and moral value of the notions of personal control.

Philosophical Criticisms of the Study of Personal Control

My remarks about philosophical criticisms focus on three major questions: What defines the internal versus external locus of

control?   How does one escape the mind/body dualism implicit in
various aspects of the problem? And how can one have personal control
in a deterministic world?   Naturally one can hardly expect social
psychologists to solve age-old problems of such stature as the
mind/body problem.   However the blithe manner in which the problem is
glossed over in the experimental literature does deserve a word of
commentary.

Defining the Internal Versus External Locus of Control

The seemingly simple issue of how one defines the concept in question
has interested John Sabini and Maury Silver.   In a recent paper
(Sabini & Silver, in press) these authors have attacked the multitude
of meanings that have accrued to this seemingly obvious dichotomy of
internal and external control.   They describe the distinction as
follows: "'internal-external' is not a dimension, but a congeries of
disparate contrasts relating to: dispositions, responsibilities,
wills, diseases, hallucinations, errors, and courtesy" (p. 1).   In
support of Sabini & Silver, one might look more closely at various
definitions of personal control in the theories of Rotter, Seligman
and Bandura, as well as at the theoretical and operational definitions
of various other experimenters to find that many different conceptions
are clustered about the same descriptive phrases.   The importance of
perceiving oneself as a causal source of one's actions, and the
positive value attached therein lead to other philosophical issues
concerned with the mind/body problem and the dilemma of free will and
determinism.

There are several implications for older people of definitional
vagueness concerning the concept of internal versus external control.
Overall, the thrust of most research in the gerontological field is to
find that older people experience reductions in personal control, to
their detriment.   The more general and amorphous the definition of
control, the more debilitating and derogatory the "old age" syndrome
becomes.   For example, if a group of older people agrees that they
have less control over children's actions as they grow older, this
would probably not constitute a derogating finding.   However, if the
summary definition of the results implies a generalized loss of
control (perhaps including less competent decision-making abilities),
then a vague and comprehensive definition of what control means is
potentially harmful to these subjects.

The Mind/Body Problem in the Research on Personal Control

The mind/body problem always haunts the interstices of cognitive
causes and physical action.   For example, the notion of "perceived
control," which can be manifested in various definitional forms within
Rotter, Seligman and Bandura's theoretical frameworks, is regarded as
a mental state, more or less stable within the individual.   This

mental state is then viewed as a causal component for such behavioral variables as "working steadily at a difficult task," "fighting against social inequities," "developing good coping strategies for survival," "behaving in a vigorous and healthy manner," and even "staying alive." Fortunately for purposes of daily life, our discourse practices sweep the contradictions inherent in such formulations under the rug of common parlance as much as possible. As psychologists interested in both mental states and behavior, we avoid confronting the question of how and to what extent mental perceptions of personal control interact with bodily entities such as muscles and bone. Because this problem is normally considered intractable, I will not dwell upon it, except to note that its presence within the control literature is rife. For example, our "expectations of control" somehow interact with our bodily parts as we "move in the direction of the goal." Thus our wishes, wants and will interact with neuron firings. More is at stake, however, with the philosophical problem of free will and determinism because moral issues related to the "double dealing" among incompatible concepts must be noted. An expansion of what I mean by this remark will follow.

Free Will and Determinism in Research on Personal Control

The corpus of gerontological work that supports personal control as a significant variable in determining the mental (and physical) health and well-being of a person is experimental. Taken from the natural sciences paradigm, the experiment is regarded as the chief methodological tool for discovering causal sequences. (Pick up the latest foundational textbook in psychology to read this fact in the methodology section at the end of the introductory chapter). The power of the experiment is that the experimenter can introduce controls into the experimental situation so that the variations that occur can be analyzed for causal properties. A publishable study is able to isolate causal factors that produce subsequent behaviors. Thus within the mechanistic framework of the traditional experiment, the notion of voluntarism and free will is irrelevant. The language of the natural sciences that has been borrowed for the social sciences tends to be rather strict in excluding humanistic notions such as free will from the experimental context.

The notion of studying personal control within an experimental setting is paradoxical. Perhaps it is for this reason, in part, that the trend for experimenters has been to talk about "perceived locus of control." In this manner the experimenter alludes to the possibility that personal control is an illusion to be handled as such. In fact, we may all be operating as ciphers in a systematic calculus, but we pretend more or less that we are free. At least this would be a sensible metaphor within a deterministic framework. Some gerontological experimenters go on to advocate that even when circumstances are very clearly constrained, "subjects" should be encouraged to believe that they are operating under their own power because it is a health-

giving illusion.   Perlmuter, Monty and Chan (1986) state the control
strategy of the experimenter baldly:

> "The outcome of these studies on choice and environmental
> control add new information to a growing body of literature
> that shows that the perception of control can be effectively
> manipulated and studied in laboratory as well as in applied
> settings.   More importantly, these studies show that an
> increase in the perception of control can have a variety of
> benefits for the individual, ranging from an improvement in
> learning and memory to the enhnacement of the quality of
> life itself . . . .   However, the researcher in studying
> control as opposed to choice or, the clinician in awarding
> control must be mindful that the perception of control can
> be established only with effort on the part of the subject,
> that is, *ars est celare artem* (It is true art to conceal the
> art) is a critical ingredient in the recipe for harvesting
> the benefits of control" (p. 116).

To emphasize my point, note that the authors, in this last
sentence, remind the experimenter that to truly succeed in getting the
subjects or clients to believe that they are perceiving personal
control one must make the subjects or clients work for it a little.
That is, the effective "con artist" must not show the hand behind the
scenes or the trick is up!

This fascinating quotation is representative of a general view
expressed less clearly in much personal control work with older
populations, especially, that is, that subject or client populations
should be deceived into believing that they have control (for various
benigned purposes, such as to enhance their life circumstances).
Philosophically, it is a rather contorted situation, with externally
controlled subjects being "suckered" into believing they are in
control by presumably free willed experimenters and clinicians.   The
moral issues at stake here have parallels with the "behavioral
engineer" problems stirred by B. F. Skinner's (1948) well-known
Utopian fantasy, *Walden Two*.   These problems have a moral component
because the control-givers have placed themselves in a dominant
position with regard to their subjects and have decided that they know
best what their subjects need, without the knowledge or permission of
the subject group.   Because the subjects are elderly and seen to be in
danger of losing essential resources, researchers have taken a
"benevolent dictator" approach, which allows for practices of
deception that would be less acceptable if recommended for less
subordinated or more powerful groups.   (This technique, enhancing
perceived if not actual control, has been suggested for minority
groups, depressed people, women and hospital patients, as well as the
elderly, all relatively low-status groups).   Clearly the notion of
researcher superiority is exemplified by these practices, and, in
addition, the political order is preserved.   The resulting ontology
remains confused, as one is uncertain whether or not the experimental

world is construed by deterministic causal laws or by some form of voluntarism. The logic of the situation suggests (somewhat incoherently) that the researchers have free will, and the subjects do not.

Beyond Determinism: A Research Demonstration

Overall social psychological studies in the field of personal control research are produced within a deterministic causal framework; however, I would like to describe an investigation that shifts the focus from a causal exploration to a linguistic one (Gergen, 1980). From this perspective, dependent variables, such as scores on an attitude measure, which were formerly regarded as the causal product of prior manipulations of states or of personality traits, are seen as socially constructed integers in a contextualized dialogue between persons. Thus discourse analysis regards statements made by respondents concerning personal control as performative statements within a social interaction (Potter & Wetherell, 1987). As such, we regard them as forms of social practices rather than as indicators of dispositions, feelings, beliefs, or as representing other cognitive states resulting from experimental conditions. What these statements mean depends on how the speaker uses them within the social arena. Different forms of statements, for example, "I chose this for her" versus "I had to take what I could get" serve as integers for different interpersonal scripts. Using a linguistic analysis avoids the mind/body problem and the deterministic/free will dilemma, two horns on the realist beast.

This particular study (i.e., Gergen, 1980) revolved around explanations of personal control made by aging people. There are many ways to behave as one ages, and it seems likely that different styles of language use might be embedded into different self-projections in later adulthood. While there are some choices, in general all socialized members of a society have to adhere somewhat to the social scripts of their groups. The range of possibilities for behaving are constrained rather powerfully (Hagestad & Neugarten, 1984). Forms of explanation, like other behavioral forms, are under social control. Aging is a time of transition, and not a very positive stage for the person who is passing from middle-age to old-age. Because there is an expectation within the culture that older people are losing control, influence and power as they age, the aging generations tend to follow scripts that give them appropriate expressions for the occasion. Thus, they begin to describe themselves as "getting old," which they never did under similar circumstances five years before. Saying "My memory is slipping" becomes an apt way to explain why one made a mistake to a younger person. This does not make it true or false, however. Personal control statements are integers in a socially engineered script, not a reflection of the true state of affairs.

        To shift to the linguistic analysis does not change the data from
any given study, but it does change the ways one might look at their
significance.   Questions may be asked about nature of the self-
presentations that are evoked with various linguistic tropes and about
how language practices might stabilize or change within various
contexts.   For example, do people develop preferred styles of
responding, and how do these styles affect other performance patterns?
One might also look at the reflexivity of the linguistic patterns of
individuals.   Do people who consistently use negative statements, such
as "I cannot handle the situation anymore," also describe themselves
in a manner more in keeping with the stereotype of the elderly person
than those who emphasize their personal control over matters? Beyond
this, do people who often use statements emphasizing personal control
also feel and act in a more youthful manner?   The approach toward
linguistic analysis that informed this study is favorable to these
connections.   Within this study, we sought the relationship between
styles of verbal performances, life satisfactions and engagement in
activities.

        As an analytic device, self-explanations concerning control were
divided into two polar dimensions: Internal versus External locus;
and Determined versus Voluntary force.   The locus is the source of the
influence over the behavior, whether it is within the person or
outside of the person.   Traditionally, personal control theorists have
assumed that if a locus of control was internal, the person was "in
control" of the situation.   However, where conditions or influence
such as infirmity and aging are concerned, the sense of personal
control might be very low despite the internality of the locus of
power.   A second polar dimension was thought to be needed.   The second
dimension, determined versus voluntary, specifies how the influence is
interpreted, as uncontrollable or as under one's control.   For
example, respondents who said they never remarried because they were
"too old" were credited with an Internal-Determined form of explanation; being too old is an internal state over which they have no
control.   Those who answered that they did not want to change their
life styles through marriage were credited with an Internal-Voluntary
form.   They emphasized their own personal control over this decision.
Others' responses highlighted the influences and constraints of the
external world.   For example, one woman said, "Gordon spoiled me for
other men."   This explanation was defined as External-Voluntary.   Her
comment emphasized that she had some control over her options in this
regard (And, as a matter of fact, this woman did remarry sometime
later).   Another woman who said, "There are no men for an old woman
like me" was making an External-Determined explanation.   Table 1
illustrates these dimensions with prototypical examples.

        The form of explanation one uses fits into conventions of
language.   Each form is allowed into the conversation by certain
practices and thwarted by others.   In turn people create certain
opportunities for others by some forms, and close them off by others.
People also create impressions of themselves for others through their

TABLE 1
Forms of Explanation

Locus	Force	
	Determinant	Voluntary
Internal	"I was too old."	"I didn't want to."
External	"No one asked me."	"Most men aren't worth the trouble."

speech acts, gestures, non-verbal expressions and physical actions. These forms have been explored in more detail in other work (cf. Gergen & Gergen, 1982; Gergen & Gergen, 1986). It is of central import to underscore the nonobjective character of these choices.

How Do Aging People Explain Their Behaviors?

The basic goal of the study described above (Gergen, 1980) was to examine the relationships between various forms of self-attributions and well-being measures. The major hypothesis was that people who gave Internal-Voluntary explanations as to why they behaved in a particular way would feel more in control of their lives, and consequently more satisfied with themselves, their life situations and their health than those who chose forms that gave Determined explanations indicating little or no personal control.

A group of 72 adult men and women, ages 62 to 93, served as research participants. Unlike many studies of personal control among the elderly, which use nursing home patients, these people were all self-sustaining people, either living in their own homes or in retirement villages. Within the context of a semi-structured interview they were asked to talk at length about their lives. The interviewer took notes concerning attributions made by the respondents about changes in their life activities. Embedded in the interview schedule were questions about the change in frequency of such activities as going to church, travelling, going out to social activities, working, being involved with intimate relationships, and pursuing hobbies. The expectation was that in the vast majority of cases where activity level had changed, the involvement was less than it had been five years earlier. This view was supported by the data. Reduction in activities was sought in order to facilitate explanations that were Internal-Determined, such as "I am too old." When changes were mentioned the interviewer probed for an explanation of why these had occurred. For example, the interviewee might mention that she had stopped working for the Democratic party as a committee-woman. The interviewer would then ask her why she had stopped. The response was recorded, and then later evaluated as to form of explanation.

Each respondent was given a rating based on the proportion of each form of explanation he/she chose to mention to the total number of explanations. For example, a rating of .33 on Internal-Voluntary attributions meant that one-third of the respondent's self-attributions were in this form. Respondents also filled out questionnaires regarding their feelings of life satisfaction, self-esteem and health, as well as other daily life and demographic information.

Results indicated that with passing years older people used more Internal-Determined explanations than younger people did. That is, they said things like, "I am too old," more often than younger people in the sample did. This might be expected given the relevance of age

and aging to appropriate activities in the culture.   More interestingly, those who described themselves as "young at heart," regardless
of age, were more likely to give Internal-Voluntary explanations than
those who described themselves as "elderly."   Thus, the "young at
heart" were not as likely to say, "I am too old," regardless of
chronological age, as those who were "elderly" at heart.   Multiple
regression analyses were performed to assess the effects of various
styles of explanation on self-reports of esteem, life satisfaction and
activity level.   Among the correlates of self-esteem the tendency to
use Internal-Determined explanations (such as "I am too old") was
negatively related to self-esteem.   People with higher levels of self-
esteem tended not to explain their behaviors by saying they were too
old, or physically unable.   Table 2 illustrates the multiple regression analysis for self-esteem.

A similar analysis was conducted with a life satisfaction self-
report.   Feelings of well-being were positively related to making
Internal-Voluntary attributions.   That is, people who tended to
describe changes in their life activities as under their own self-
control were more likely to be satisfied with life than others.   Note
in Table 3 the relationship of this variable to feelings of well-
being.

Respondents reported the extent to which they engaged in a
variety of activities outside the home.   People who were more active
tended to use more Internal-Voluntary attributions than less active
people.   Table 4 indicates these results.

The study supports previous work concerning the relationship of
personal control and well-being; it also suggests that self-esteem and
a more active life style are also related to self-attributions of
personal control.

As was previously mentioned the guiding viewpoint within which I
perceived the study was linguistic.   Whatever people said about the
origins of their behavior is based on social conventions and the way
in which people perceived themselves as fitting into the society.   In
order to appear consistent, people may often make similar types of
explanations.   The linguistic interpretation of this study would
suggest that this sample of aging people had access to four different
forms of explanation for their daily lives, and respondents who chose
those explanations higher in personal control were more satisfied than
those who chose explanations rated as low in internal control.

The emphases on societal expectations and stereotypes of the aged
are very important in understanding how to conceive of forms of
explanations.   The social world puts stringent limits on what is
sayable.   For example, an eighty-year-old woman who explained she was
studying for the law school entrance examinations in order to become a
Supreme Court judge might engender fears for her mental health among
family members.   Yet, in general, people who consistently choose an

M. Gergen

TABLE 2
Explanatory Performance and
Self–Esteem

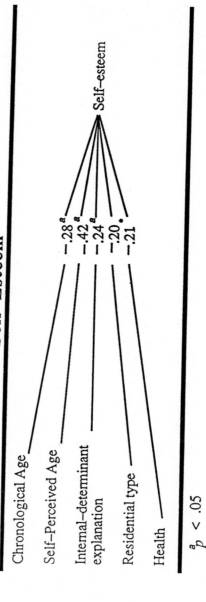

Chronological Age

Self–Perceived Age

Internal–determinant
explanation

Residential type

Health

Self–esteem

−.28[a]
−.42[a]
−.24[a]
−.20
−.21

[a] p < .05

TABLE 3
Explanatory Preference and Feelings of Well–being

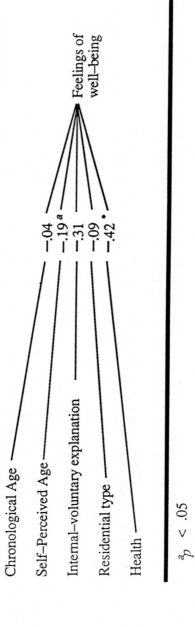

Chronological Age   −.04

Self–Perceived Age   −.19 [a]

Internal–voluntary explanation   .31

Residential type   −.09

Health   −.42 *

Feelings of well–being

[a] $p < .05$

M. Gergen

TABLE 4
Explanatory Preference and Activity Level

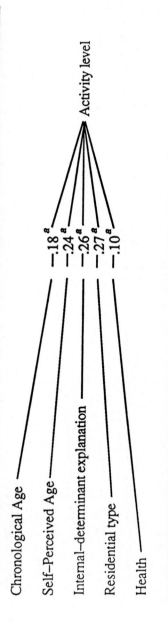

Chronological Age —————— $-.18^a$

Self–Perceived Age —————— $-.24^a$

Internal–determinant explanation —————— $.26^a$

Residential type —————— $.27^a$

Health —————— $-.10^a$

Activity level

$^a p < .05$

Internal-Voluntary form of discourse and who avoid Internal-Determined explanations are likely to declare themselves more satisfied and involved in life than others. And others around them, who see this type of behavior may be convinced that the person is more like a younger person than some more negativistic and dependent peers. In this respect, the aging person can avoid some of the stigma of old age by talking like a more youthful person.

The trick then becomes to train people in the importance of using "control" speech, it would appear. Is this the solution then? Or are there other issues to be taken up, once the problem of empirical reality is overcome? I think there are.

Critiques of Theories of Personal Control

Sociological criticism of the study of personal control

The central sociological critique of the personal control literature focuses on the decontextualized nature of the research. Henderikus Stam (1987) has argued that personal control indicators seem to be effective descriptors of behavioral variability because subjects have been extracted from their generative social contexts, and then reconstituted in a laboratory setting, where interactions, if any, are controlled in almost mechanical fashion by the researcher. Any relationship between the ordinary social structure and social behaviors is disrupted. This has the effect, according to Stam, of disrupting the normal behavioral patterns as well.

Stam's other criticisms concern the lack of attention researchers pay to the relationship of individuals to institutions. For example, a researcher may disregard the power of nursing home administrations to evoke obedience when evaluating the reluctance of patients to express "personally controlled" behaviors. In fact, what may seem like a lethargic attitude toward personal outcomes may be a patient's realistic strategy for avoiding unpleasant confrontation and even punishment. This contextual feature cannot be contained in most simple experimental or observational designs. Stam also argues that researchers overlook the specificity of personal control as a social value popular during this period of history and within western culture, especially among the upper-middle class. He argues that researchers have assumed that internal personal control has always been and always will be a highly desirable personal trait, and not a temporally dependent value. Lastly Stam suggests that psychologists tend to assume that we live in a smoothly working social order based on rational principles. The sense of conflict, class domination, and power relations that constitute the world of a Marxist, for example, has no place in the *a priori* conditions of society assumed by the American and European theorists and researchers identified with the personal control literature.

Other critics of the decontextualized study of personal control (Furby, 1979; Wexler, 1987) also tie their commentaries to the political realities assumed by most personal control researchers. Wexler, who advocates a "critical social psychology," argues that the value placed on personal control allows those who are in control to maintain it. When researchers verify that powerful positions are the just rewards for a life well-planned and well-executed they provide a rationale for the power inequities of the "late capitalist" period (Wexler, 1987). Lila Furby (1979) argues that the extent to which people have actual control over events in their social worlds varies greatly, contrary to what most psychologists working in the field of personal control believe. Thus the dialectic between actual control and perceived control requires more thorough study than it has been given by current personal control researchers.

The major thrust of the sociological critiques is to insist that societal arrangements and processes, of which one is a part, create powerful channeling effects upon people's behaviors and their beliefs about the world. To ignore these controlling influences, regardless of whether one is an elderly person confined to a wheelchair in a nursing home or a tenured MacArthur Foundation professor studying personal control is to be blinded to significant aspects of the environment. This insensitivity to social institutions and their influences on individuals lead to theorizing that overestimates the freedom of individuals to control their own destinies.

Feminist critique of the study of personal control

Previously, I have raised philosophical and sociological arguments against traditional empiricist research in social psychology as part of a feminist critique (Gergen, 1988). Within this chapter, I wish to segregate one particular area of concern as especially relevant to feminist theory. This is the problem of what constitutes the image of the ideal person, which is a necessary background to work on personal control. Within the rhetoric of the personal control literature the ideal person is assumed to be an autonomous, self-determined in-dividual, that is, one who has a high level of personal control. (For specific citations of texts that support this view and for additional critical commentary, see Furby, 1979; Kitzinger, 1987; Sampson, 1988; Stam, 1987; Wexler, 1987). And as mentioned in the first section of this chapter, the notion of free individuals who are accountable for their deeds is basic to western democratic societies. Personal control and thus personal responsibility for our deeds is a corner-stone in the major systems of reward and punishment from the kinder-gartens to the courts. Much is invested in maintaining this aspect of the existing ideology. It may be difficult for us to give up this image.

An alternative theoretical perspective on personal autonomy has been created and elaborated by several contemporary feminist writers (cf. Dinnerstein, 1977; Flax, 1983; Gilligan, 1982; Harding, 1986;

Keller, 1982; Martin, 1987). On this account, the ideal person is seen as an interdependent, socially embedded individual. These arguments have several strands, but a central thread is that autonomy is predicated on separation. Nancy Chodorow (1979), for example, has argued that male children are required to develop their personal identities by separating and differentiating themselves from their mothers. While mothers tend to regard daughters as continuations of themselves, they see their sons as separate. With continuous social reinforcement, the male child grows up to value his separated self, seemingly free and independent of his authoring kin. This form of self-definition creates the ideal personality to fit into the external world of affairs, where one is rewarded and punished according to how well one plans and controls one's own fortunes, with little regard for others.

The girl grows up in an ethos of connectedness and caring support. Her rewards are garnered by continuing and extending her relational ties with others. As a result of these socialization practices, women are less likely to experience themselves as detached, autonomous, and free to control their own destinies. They are subject to many demands that evolve from their interdependencies with others, and find greater difficulty than men in reaching autonomous goals. While it may be argued that men are also enmeshed in relational ties, the myths of the culture tend to disguise this view. Joseph Campbell (1949), for example, has argued that the basic myth of western culture concerns the lone hero who staves off his enemies until he is victorious, (and wins the prize) is vanquished. In addition, the connective tissue of many male ties is contractual in nature rather than affective or duty bound. Thus, for example, a computer consultant contracts with a company to do basic research for 1600 hours a year. Mothers, on the other hand, rarely engage in contractual relations with their off-spring. (The meeting of these twain in the 1987 Mary Jane Whitehead surrogate mother trial has caused considerable grief on all sides. The final outcome of the litigation indicated the reluctance of the patriarchal court system to allow women to enter into contractual arrangements vis-à-vis the mother-child relationship.)

It is not necessary to adopt the reasoning of feminist scholars on the origins of autonomy to consider the ramifications for non-autonomous individuals with regard to levels of personal control. Logically, if one is autonomous, one is likely to have a higher level of personal control than if one is interdependent with others. Yet, the relationship may not always hold. Sometimes dependent others also are able to control others. As Baltes and Reisenzein (1986) have found in a nursing home population, personal control may be expressed through the judicious use of dependency requests. When one begins to argue that dependency conditions can foster certain forms of personal control initiatives, then the concept of control can become quite murky. Helplessness and control begin to merge.

A fresh glance at these problems may lead one to suspect that the image of the ideal person, independent, free, and with a high level of personal control is part of the necessary underpinnings in the rhetoric of the patriarchal social order. If the cardinal goal of a social system is to reproduce its status quo, then the dominant order within it would do well to exemplify and ratify the features of the ideal person within it. In a meritocracy it is fitting that the "best" should reach the top. Women, girls, the elderly, the poor and other oppressed minorities reveal themselves as less than ideal people by not exhibiting the proper levels of personal control. It is no wonder they do not attain positions of authority.

The underside to this fantasy of omnipotence and control is that certain insecurities, fears of failure, and a sense of loneliness may prod those at the top of the pyramid. Many realize that they do not feel as much in control as they are supposed to feel. Yet, the socialization runs deep. To admit to a loss of control is to experience a critical loss of manhood. As Engel (1968) describes the sense of loss of control, it is "a sense of psychological impotence." Men, thus, become committed to the virtues of personal control in order to sustain their hold on their masculinity. It is a privilege and an obligation that allows them to keep their place.

Where is the happy ending to such a tale? What can we do to rescue the fair damsel in helpless distress or our tragic hero burdened with the thorny crown of personal control? Writing is much simpler than living, and we can dive out of our dilemma with a few optimistic words about futures beyond the rainbow. Whether what is written will ever become realized is another matter. The option that must evolve in order to solve our dilemma concerns relinquishing the idealize image of human beings as autonomous individuals. Instead of looking to an isolated individual as the agent of action, we must find new ways of describing the world. Kenneth Gergen and I (in press), for example, have written about the "relational self," which conceptualizes the self as an organized and dynamic matrix of relationships. A similar definition of self is made by M. B. Lykes (1985), who describes the self as "an ensemble of social relations" (p. 364). Sampson (1988) espouses an "ensembled individualism," as distinct from "self-contained individualism," in which the ensembled self has "more fluidly drawn self-nonself boundaries and field control" (p. 16). Field control, in contrast to personal control, refers to locating power and control in a field of forces that extends beyond any one person. These examples are only illustrative of this new and exciting work.

Once the notion of selves independent of environments and each other begins to dissolve, shifts in attributions of responsibility and personal control must inevitably occur. A social constructionist perspective on interactions that emphasizes the multiply interactive sets of relationships that influence behaviors will (ideally) emerge. Forecasts of this perspective can be noted among a certain vanguard of psychologists (cf. Gergen, 1985; Henriques, Holloway, Urwin, Venn, & Walkerdine, 1984; Kitzinger, 1987; Steele, 1986; Young, 1988). Within the area of personal control among the aged, Gatz, Siegler, George and Tyler (1986) note, "We are convinced that there is a relational and interactist quality to control, with person and environment influencing one another in the course of any event" (p. 261). Research on the adjustment of people to the changes that aging can bring should focus less on the variable of personal control, and more on how interdependent connections can be facilitated among various generations, support systems, and physical resources. Rather than urging the elderly to "get a hold on themselves," it might be more fruitful to instigate pathways that would help people work in interdependent relations with others to the enrichment of their lives.

Conclusions

The notion of personal control is part of our everyday discourse of explanation and is also used as a theoretical tool within the social sciences. Within this chapter my hope has been to unsettle the conventional acceptance of this term in science and in society, as well as the underlying assumptions about human nature that are necessitated by this term. I am also suggesting that scientists and social change agents shift their attention from trying to force a version of autonomy on others to recognizing that each of us - young, middle-aged and elderly - is embedded in interactional networks, which provide us with life sources, to a greater or lesser extent. As gerontologically focused researchers and scholars we need to attend to the shifting balances of resource distribution within social networks and to understand how to regulate our interdependencies for the benefit of all.

So the happy ending of the story is that the fair damsel in distress and the lonely self-determined hero recognize that they are interdependent selves, embedded in a social world, and that theories that describe their actions are socially construed, along with everything else. In addition they realize that "personal control" is a form of traditional rhetoric reproduced throughout society for the not altogether incidental benefit of maintaining the status quo. Together they will work to form a new language that will reduce their distress and improve their lives and those of others with whom they are attached. They will grow old happily, caring and cared for by those with whom they have lived.

References

Abramson, L. Y., Seligman, M. E. P., & Teasdale, J. D. (1978). Learned helplessness in humans: Critique and reformulation. *Journal of Abnormal Psychology, 87,* 49-74.

Baltes, M. M., & Baltes, P. B. (Eds.) (1986). *The psychology of control and aging*. Hillsdale, NJ: Lawrence Erlbaum Associates.

Baltes, M. M., & Barton, E. M. (1977). New approaches toward aging: A case for the operant model. *Educational Gerontology: An International Quarterly, 2*, 383-405.

Baltes, M. M., & Barton, E. M. (1979). Behavioral analysis of aging: A review of the operant model and research. *International Journal of Behavioral Development, 2*, 297-320.

Baltes, M. M., & Reisenzein, R. (1986). The social world in long-term care institutions: Psychosocial control toward dependency? In M. M. Baltes & P. B. Baltes (Eds.), *The psychology of control and aging* (pp. 315-343). Hillsdale, NJ: Lawrence Erlbaum Associates.

Baltes, M. M., & Skinner, E. A. (1983). Cognitive performance deficits and hospitalization: Learned helplessness, instrumental passivity or what? *Journal of Personality and Social Psychology, 45*, 1013-1016.

Bandura, A. (1977). Self-efficacy: Toward a unifying theory of behavioral change. *Psychological Review, 31*, 65-110.

Bandura, A. (1982). Self-efficacy mechanism in human agency. *American Psychologist, 37*, 122-147.

Brandtstädter, J., Krampen, G., & Heil, F. E. (1986). Personal control and emotional evaluation of development in partnership relations during adulthood. In M. M. Baltes & P. B. Baltes (Eds.), *The psychology of control and aging* (pp. 265-296). Hillsdale, NJ: Lawrence Erlbaum Associates.

Campbell, J. (1949). *The hero with a thousand faces*. New York: Pantheon.

Chodorow, N. (1979). *The reproduction of mothering: Psychoanalysis and the sociology of gender*. Berkeley, CA: University of California Press.

Dinnerstein, D. (1977). *The mermaid and the minotaur: Sexual arrangements and human malaise*. New York: Colophon.

Engel, G. L. (1968). A life-setting conducive to illness. The giving-up, given-up complex. *Annals of Internal Medicine, 69*, 293-300.

Flax, J. (1983). Political philosophy and the patriarchal unconscious: A psychoanalytic perspective on epistemology and metaphysics. In S. Harding & M. B. Hintikka (Eds.), *Discovering reality* (pp. 59-73). Dordrecht: Reidel.

Furby, L. (1979).   Individualistic bias in studies of locus of
control.   In A. Buss (Ed.), *Psychology in social context* (pp. 169-
190). New York: Irvington Press.

Gatz, M., Siegler, I. C., George, L. K., & Tyler, F. B. (1986).
Attributional   components   of   locus   of   control: Longitudinal,
retrospective, and contemporaneous analyses.   In M. M. Baltes & P.
B. Baltes (Eds.), *The psychology of control and aging* (pp. 237-263).
Hillsdale, NJ: Lawrence Erlbaum Associates.

Gergen, K. J. (1985).   The social constructionist movement in modern
psychology. *American Psychologist, 40,* 266-275.

Gergen, K. J., & Gergen, M. M. (1982).   Form and function in the
explanation of human conduct.   In P. Secord (Ed.), *Explaining social
behavior: Consciousness, human action and social structure* (pp.
127-153). Beverly Hills, CA: Sage.

Gergen, K. J., & Gergen, M. M. (in press).   Narrative and the self as
relationship.   In L. Berkowitz (Ed.), *Advances in Social Psychology,
Vol. 21.* San Diego: Academic Press.

Gergen, M. M. (1980).   *Antecedents and consequences of self-attribu-
tional preferences in later life.*   Unpublished doctoral dissertation. Temple University.

Gergen, M. M. (1988).   Toward a feminist metatheory and methodology
in the social sciences. In M. M. Gergen (Ed.), *Feminist thought and
the structure of knowledge* (pp. 87-104).   New York: New York
University Press.

Gergen, M. M., & Gergen, K. J. (1986).   The discourse of control and
the maintenance of well-being.   In M. M. Baltes & P. B. Baltes
(Eds.), *The psychology of control and aging* (pp. 119-138).
Hillsdale, NJ: Lawrence Erlbaum Associates.

Gilligan, C. (1982).   *In a different voice.*   Cambridge, MA: Harvard
University Press.

Hagestad, G. O., & Neugarten, B. L. (1984).   Age and life course.   In
E. Shanas & R. Binstock (Eds.), *Handbook of aging and the social
sciences* (pp. 35-54). New York: Van Nostrand.

Harding, S. (1986).   *The science question in feminism.*   Ithaca:
Cornell University Press.

Heckhausen, H. (1980).   *Motivation und handeln.*   Lehrbuch der
Motivations-Psychologie. Berlin: Springer-Verlag.

Heider, F. (1958). *The psychology of interpersonal relations.* New York: Wiley & Sons.

Henriques, J., Holloway, W., Urwin, C., Venn, C., & Walkerdine, V. (1984). *Changing the subject.* London: Methuen.

Jones, E. E., & Nisbett, R. (1971). *The actor and observer: Divergent perceptions of the causes of behavior.* New York: General Learning Press.

Keller, E. F. (1982). Science and gender. *Signs: Journal of Women in Culture and Society, 7,* 589-602.

Kelly, H. H. (1967). Attribution theory in social psychology. In D. Levine (Ed.), *Nebraska Symposium on Motivation, 16* (pp. 192-240). Lincoln: University of Nebraska Press.

Kitzinger, C. (1987). *The social construction of lesbianism.* London: Sage.

Kuhl, J. (1986). Aging and models of control: The hidden costs of wisdom. In M. M. Baltes & P. B. Baltes (Eds.), *The psychology of control and aging* (pp. 1-33). Hillsdale, NJ: Lawrence Erlbaum Associates.

Lachman, M. E. (1986). Personal control in later life: Stability, change and cognitive control. In M. M. Baltes & P. B. Baltes (Eds.), *The psychology of control and aging* (pp. 207-236). Hillsdale, NJ: Lawrence Erlbaum Associates.

Langer, E. J. (1983). *The psychology of control.* New York: Sage.

Langer, E. J., Blank, A., & Chanowitz, B. (1978). The mindlessness of ostensibly thoughtful action: The role of "placebo" information in interpersonal interaction. *Journal of Personality and Social Psychology, 36,* 886-893.

Langer, E. J., & Rodin, J. (1976). The effects of choice and enhanced personal responsibility for the aged: A field experiment in an institutionalized setting. *Journal of Personality and Social Psychology, 34,* 191-198.

Lefcourt, H. M. (1976). *Locus of control: Current trends in theory and research.* New York: Wiley & Sons.

Lefcourt, H. M. (Ed.). (1981). *Research with the locus of control construction: Vol. 1. Assessment methods.* New York: Academic Press.

Lefcourt, H. M. (Ed.). (1982). *Locus of control: Current trends in theory and research* (2nd ed.). Hillsdale, NJ: Lawrence Erlbaum Associates.

Lykes, M. B. (1985). Gender and individualistic vs. collectivist bases for notions about the self. *Journal of Personality, 53,* 356-383.

Martin, E. (1987). *The woman in the body: A cultural analysis of reproduction.* Boston: Beacon Press.

Perlmuter, L. C., & Monty, R. A. (Eds.). (1979). *Choice and perceived control.* Hillsdale, NJ: Lawrence Erlbaum Associates.

Perlmuter, L. C., Monty, R. A., & Chan, F. (1986). Choice, control, and cognitive functioning. In M. M. Baltes & P. B. Baltes (Eds.), *The psychology of control and aging* (pp. 91-118). Hillsdale, NJ: Lawrence Erlbaum Associates.

Phares, E. J. (1976). *Locus of control in personality.* Morristown, NJ: General Learning Corp.

Piper, A. I., & Langer, E. J. (1986). Aging and mindful control. In M. M. Baltes & P. B. Baltes (Eds.), *The psychology of control and aging* (pp. 71-89). Hillsdale, NJ: Lawrence Erlbaum Associates.

Potter, J., & Wetherell, M. (1987). *Discourse and social psychology: Beyond attitudes and behavior.* London: Sage.

Rodin, J. (1983). Behavioral medicine: Beneficial effects of self-control training in aging. *International Review of Applied Psychology, 32,* 153-181.

Rodin, J. (1986). Health, control and aging. In M. M. Baltes & P. B. Baltes (Eds.), *The psychology of control and aging* (pp. 139-165). Hillsdale, NJ: Lawrence Erlbaum Associates.

Rodin, J., & Langer, E. J. (1977). Long-term effects of a control-relevant intervention with the institutionalized aged. *Journal of Personality and Social Psychology, 35,* 897-902.

Rotter, J. B. (1954). *Social learning and clinical psychology.* Englewood Cliffs, NJ: Prentice-Hall.

Rotter, J. B. (1966). Generalized expectancies for internal versus external control of reinforcement. *Psychological Monographs, 80* (1. Whole No. 609).

Rotter, J. B., Chance, J. E., & Phares, E. J. (1972). *Applications of a social learning theory of personality.* New York: Holt, Rinehart & Winston.

Sabini, J., & Silver, M. (in press). Internal-external--dimension or congeries? *International Journal of Moral and Social Studies*.

Sampson, E. E. (1988). The debate on individualism: Indigenous psychologies of the individual and their role in personal and societal functioning. *American Psychologist, 43,* 15-22.

Schulz, R. (1976). The effects of control and predictability on the psychological and physical well-being of the institutionalized aged. *Journal of Personality and Social Psychology, 33,* 563-573.

Schulz, R., & Hanusa, B. (1978). Long-term effects of control and predictability-enhancing interventions: Findings and ethical issues. *Journal of Personality and Social Psychology, 36,* 1194-1201.

Seligman, M. E. P. (1975). *Helplessness: On depression, development, and death.* San Francisco: Freeman.

Skinner, B. F. (1948). *Walden Two.* New York: MacMillan.

Stam, H. (1987). The psychology of control: A textual critique. In H. Stam, T. Rogers & K. Gergen (Eds.), *The analysis of psychological theory: Metapsychological perspectives* (pp. 131-156). Washington, DC: Hemisphere.

Steele, R. (1986). Deconstructing histories: Toward a systematic criticism of psychological narratives. In T. Sarbin (Ed.), *Narrative psychology: The storied nature of human conduct* (pp. 256-275). New York: Praeger Press.

Weber, M. (1930). *The Protestant ethic and the spirit of capitalism.* London: Unwin University Books.

Weiner, B. (1974). An attributional interpretation of expectancy-value theory. In B. Weiner (Ed.), *Cognitive views of human motivation* (pp. 1-23). New York: Academic Press.

Wexler, P. (1987). *Critical social psychology.* Boston: Routledge & Kegan Paul.

Young-Eisendrath, P. (1988). The female person and how we talk about her. In M. M. Gergen (Ed.), *Feminist thought and the structure of knowledge* (pp. 152-172). New York: New York University Press.

Psychological Perspectives of Helplessness
and Control in the Elderly, P.S. Fry (ed.)
© *Elsevier Science Publishers B.V. (North-Holland), 1989*

Chapter Ten

THE IMPLICATIONS OF GENDER AND SPEECH FOR THE EXPERIENCE OF CONTROL IN AGING

Adrienne HARRIS and Naomi MILLER
Rutgers University

Abstract

In this essay we review literature on sex differences in aging, concentrating on differences in adaptive capacities, differences in life continuities, and differences in men's and women's reactions to loss, separation and dependency. Implications for men and women in coping with increased dependency and helplessness are considered. The Soviet perspective on language use and the regulatory function of speech is reviewed, focusing on the work of Luria, Vygotsky and Bahktin. The capacity for speech to regulate both discrete activity and extended streams of behavior and experience is considered. These concepts are compared to similar treatment of speech and its role in self-regulation in the work of D. Winnicott on transitional objects. It is argued that these speech functions are potentially adaptive in mediating experiences of helplessness and loss of control. We argue that there are selected advantages to women in respect to the aging process and to increasing feelings of loss of control and helplessness. Finally, we suggest a reconceptualization of the concept of 'control.' We argue against the idealization of that term and of models of psychological functioning in which autonomy and separateness is stressed at the expense of relational models of functioning.

Introduction

Growing old male. Growing old female. In this essay we will consider the impact of gender on certain processes in the experience of aging. Specifically, we want to explore the interdependence between gender, aging, communicative competence and helplessness. We begin by posing a series of questions. How much of this 'helplessness' among older

persons is a socially arranged attribution? How much is the loss of
power or efficacy an internal and inevitable part of growing older?
Our culture reads older persons as helpless, increasingly powerless,
and often desexualized. How does gender impact on this reading? If
helplessness comes in part from externally originating attributions,
how are these cultural constructions internalized and how are they
resisted?   Do men and women go through this process of acculturation
and resistance differently? What is the role of speech in augmenting
or shaping experiences of relative control and helplessness in aging?
How might models of verbal regulation articulated in the study of
early development map to the experience of aging?

In this paper we bring together research and writing on gender
with the analysis of speech and self regulation which has been
developed primarily in the Soviet Union through the work of Luria and
Vygotsky and articulated in North America in the work of Meichenbaum,
Cole and Scribner and others. (See Zivin, 1979 for a review of the
Soviet and North American work on speech for self and see Wertsch,
1985 for a consideration by American psychologists of the impact and
important contributions of Vygotsky).   Self-management and self-
control are processes in which language and speech appear to play a
powerful regulatory and sustaining role. Seen through this perspective, language is a prosthetic for activity and planned behavior. How
will speech activity, which we will construe here in both a micro and
macro sense, impact on the self-regulatory and sustaining practices of
older people?

The treatment of language and speech which we will pursue in this
chapter owes much to the newly emerging models in psychology and the
social sciences, namely the hermeneutic method with its focus on the
constitutive importance of narrative and symbolic activity carried in
speech.   Freeman (1984, 1985) places this theoretical development
under the rubric of organismic theories. He uses the schema proposed
by Reese and Overton (1970) who oppose organismic theories with the
more mechanistic models of functioning, studied through more conventional methodologies. In promoting the hermeneutic approach, with its
focus on text and discourse and on social events as texts to be read
and interpreted, Freeman (1985) also considers the power of the
concept of narrative as construct. "For at least a portion of the
task of a life span psychology, the explication of human change can be
nothing short of a narration founded not only on the dialectic of
influences contributing to the formation and reformation of the
experiencing subject, but the dialectic ... of the researcher and the
researched" (p.12).

Narrative activity characterizes both the work of the researcher
and the primary activity of individuals in constructing and maintaining themselves and their life histories. Handel (1987) has noted the
potency of self-narratives for older persons and the power of personal
narrative and autobiography as an organizing experience in self-
representation.

We will begin by reviewing two areas of research relevant to this analysis - the intersection of aging with gender socialization and verbal regulation. In thinking about the complex interactions and interdependencies between these areas we will draw on selected interview and observational data from elderly persons we have been studying. Taking a phenomenological approach, we will be using older persons' self-descriptions to illuminate the theoretical perspective we are developing (Honey, 1987).

Gender and Aging

To begin we want to develop an analysis of sex differences in the aging process. What do we know of the strengths and liabilities of gender differences in the middle aged and elderly person? Gender is, of course, not a simple construct. We intend, in the term 'gender,' to mean, at the simplest level of analysis, roles and traits given some attribution of 'masculinity' and 'femininity' in particular cultural and personal settings. This concept owes much to the analytic work of the feminist anthropologist Gayle Rubin (Rapp, 1975) who used the term 'sex-gender system' to name the process of assignment of individuals to particular roles and expectations on the basis of biological sex. On the other hand, gender is a deep and complex set of internal representations, both conscious and unconscious, which form a profound and primary experience of self. Gender is treated here both as social attribution and as an aspect of depth psychology. That is, every individual, by the force of social, familial and cultural processes, comes to take up a position as a gendered subject, and to feel that position as a core part of self. Gender, as a set of roles, traits and stereotypes, is a crucial and central focus for attribution over the entire life span. Gender is also a primary internally lived form of identity. Like 'aging,' the phenomenon of gender is an inside and an outside experience. The social definition and the internal lived sense of self operate in a dialectical dynamic, shaping and changing each other reciprocally.

An inventory and detailed discussion of all the sources and aspects of sex role socialization and gender differences in aging is beyond the scope of this essay. We have concentrated, therefore, on those aspects of gender socialization which appear to have particular relevance for issues of control, self control and regulation. We looked at the importance and meaning of social support, the continuities and discontinuities in men's and women's aging experience, sex differences in dependency behaviors, the history of men and women with respect to the management of loss and separation, and sex differences in attributions.

One quite systematic finding in gender research and lifespan functioning is that flexibility in gender roles is highly adaptive (Lowenthal, 1977; Neugarten, 1964, 1968; Sinott, 1977). For individuals and couples for whom gender is not such a rigid category of behavior and social meaning, the process of aging is less severe. Put another way, the lighter the mantle of gender, the greater the prospects for successful aging. Bart's research on middle aged women (Bart & Frankel, 1976) and the work of Markides and Vernon (1984) on Mexican-Americans suggests that in cultures or sub-cultures where sex role is highly traditional (and this usually means particularly rigid and defining for *women*), the impact of gender upon aging is negative. It is the most traditional women in various cultures who are most at risk for midlife depression. Seen in this light, the power of sex role socialization as a self-percept may put women at particular risk in aging. One model for understanding depression has been to see it as a manifestation of learned helplessness - in this instance, the absorption by the middle aged woman of the life long lessons of passivity and social definition. We will see, however, that looked at somewhat differently, womens' social practices, separate from the psychological experience of role, perhaps may facilitate the aging experience and militate against primary feelings of loss of control and helplessness. In the Bart studies women were depressed in the process of aging through the loss of role, in particular the role of mothering. But there are many aspects of women's social life and practices which are persistent and unchanging.

One crucial variable, then, in assessing the impact of gender upon aging is role flexibility. So we may then ask, what are the conditions - interpersonal, internal, social or historical - which promote sex role flexibility. Flexibility, as a general personality trait, is important for aging, so it is not surprising that gender flexibility is important. What we must include in our model of gender and aging is the cultural and historical context which variously expands or contracts the possibilities for individuals. Flexibility is not merely a personality construct, but a trait shaped and influenced by the surrounding culture. Bart's research focused on middle-aged women of the post war generation who became middle-aged in the 1960's and 1970's. This cohort thus entered middle-age at a time of dramatic social change for women, social changes that for the most part had not included them. These women are much more closely identified with conventional sex role traits and with the idea of sex role traits as relatively fixed.

At the same time as we note the importance of flexibility and adaptativenss to change, we also must note the profound importance in aging of the *sustaining* of self and self-awareness. An abiding strength in the aging process is a coherent experience of self and self in relation to others (Butler, 1963). The capacity to maintain this continuity of self and self-image into old age is central to successful adaptation (Lieberman, 1975; Lowenthal & Robinson, 1976; Tamir, 1979). Later in this chapter we want to make a connection between self-continuity and language or verbal regulation. For the moment, however, we explore the various forces and situations which promote such self-continuity.

Despite such phenomena as disengagement, alienation and increasing inwardness or self-reflection in aging, the primary realm in which a continuity of self is maintained is the social. In thinking of the social realm we include both ongoing social experience and the individual's social history, which is carried as a complex set of internal object relations. This construct - internal object relations - is developed from the post Freudian psychoanalytic theories of Winnicott, Fairbairn, Balint and Klein (see Guntripp, 1973 for general introductory review of this work). From this perspective, the individual carries (in internal representations including images, verbal echoing, auditory imaging or dialogues) the experience and the history of social interactions. These relational experiences shape and influence the current social relations, and would also provide a source of rich reflection and engagement which is perhaps such an important part of the older person's turning inward.

Recently, the empirical work of Daniel Stern (1985) has provided sound empirical evidence in support of the early registration and representation of social experience in the infant. A central interpretation of Stern's data has been that there is a primacy of shared experience, and that early in life the infant begins to build up a rich mixture of representations - in symbolic and presymbolic form - of the shared interaction with the caregiver. These coalesce in a schema of self-presentation in which what is called the self is the residue of social interactions and relational positions and experiences. Coherence is thus built up over time in the infant's experience, and what is termed the self is in fact the relational history as it exists in sensory and cognitive-linguistic representation. Applied to the social and interactional experience in adulthood and therefore also in aging, this model speaks to the power of past dialogic history as the constructor and shaper of ongoing experience, and an essential aspect of the coherence of self.

Whether or not the social structure remains the same, the capacity to behave towards others in a way that reflects one's view of oneself is central. It allows for continuity with and ongoing development of internal object relations, as well as for a meaningful relatedness to the current social world. The ability to maintain access to fulfilling relationships and ego-syntonic roles, then, is crucial. The ways in which older men and older women do this are, on the whole, quite different from one another.

Lowenthal and Haven (1968) found that the presence in an elderly person's life of a 'confidant' significantly curtailed the negative effect of most later life stressors. Social support - and an ongoing social interaction in which one is regularly experienced and known - is both adaptive for aging and implicated in the experience of control and self-control. Persons with whom one has a history and ongoing interaction provide one arena for feelings of regularity and predictability, as well as for common interpretation. Berger and

Luckman (1967), along with other social theorists, point to the power of social interpretation in the construction and maintenance of the experience of reality. Attention to and attunement with the social matrix is thus one element in the maintenance of continuity of personhood and self control.

In this regard the social practices of women may be a decided advantage in the aging experience. Women, in general, find confidants and social support among friends and relatives. Lipman and Longino (1984), in a study of the support systems of older women, found that the general tendency is for the older woman to view her own support network as an extension of an ongoing life-long exchange system in which she relies on help from those to whom she has given or will give help in return. Social support is thus, for women, bound up in a system of empathy and reciprocal involvement. In this sense, the strongly 'feminine' traits of empathy, caregiving and nurturance, noted by Chodorow (1978) and Dinnerstein (1976) and others as the hallmark of female socialization, continue to be the sustaining traits and activities of women in aging. Empathy, and cognitive style differences associated with a more relational style of thinking, moral judgment and processing seem a pervasive outcome for female socializ-ation. Gilligan's (1982) work on cognitive functioning in moral judgment tasks for men and women, and Belenky et al.'s (1986) work on women's ways of knowing, document these traits as among the most systematic and enduring sex differences in personality and cognitive functioning. To the degree that male socialization robs men of experience and practice in the maintenance of a social matrix, older men are disadvantaged in activities and social practices which provide continuity and an experience of social efficacy.

In addition to these cognitive and personality traits, women's relatively more active role in the extended family and in childrearing may offset the lessening of control and social power in other domains. In new situations, beyond the network of extended family and long term relationships, women traditionally find it easier to develop new intimacies in which personal and emotional concerns are verbalized and controls are achieved. Men, on the other hand, come to such watershed experiences as retirement with a life-long pattern of looking to the structured situation of work to provide a common ground for companion-ship. The loss of that structure through retirement undermines male patterns of interaction and self-maintenance quite profoundly.

Traditionally, men rely much more thoroughly on a spouse for social and emotional support. Those men who do retain ongoing social relationships in the course of aging still do so in the context of 'instrumental' roles (Kaye & Monk, 1984), sustaining contacts through part time work, etc. To do this may also require reliance (not always consciously acknowledged) on wives to meet the more emotional needs in social support networks. Men, as a group, are very reliant on their larger option for remarriage to sustain the intimate social support which is so highly adaptive for aging. Maintaining social cohesion, and the impact of this on a sense of efficacy and self-control, is solved by men, for the most part, through a change in personnel, an external shift and new partner. For women, on the other hand, social support and social and self-cohesion flow from long-standing and relatively more flexible styles of sociability and functioning.

Interlude

Mrs. D. is a 68-year-old woman who has been widowed for two decades. She has maintained an active work life and relations with friends, children and extended family. She misses her husband's company but feels she has done well. She articulates, however, some concern as to what her husband would have done if she had died first.

> "I can't imagine--oh, I think he would have taken care of himself. But they would have had to pry him out of his house or he would have spent the rest of his life reading, and not ever dealt with people. I think the kids would have worried more about him than about me. Even though I don't have a whole lot of friends, I maintain contact. I keep a life going. I'm not sure he would have done that. I'm more in touch with the world... although he was, too... I don't know. I don't think he would have fared as well. He was a good person. But he really needed to lean on somebody a little, without actually knowing it himself."

Gender and Dependency

The prescriptive suggestions from studies of adaptation and adaptive functioning in the aging experience point to this interesting paradox, the need for a balance between continuity of self and flexibility, the mediation between internal self-image and external reflections of self. Success in this phase, then, relies heavily on individual capacity to negotiate increasing dependence while maintaining independence in realms that are close to the person's core sense of self. In this light, we may consider the different implications for men and women.

Dependence is one of the central traits around which strong sex differences develop (Maccoby & Jacklin, 1975). There are clearly powerful negative stereotypes in respect to this trait. The term evokes ideas of submission, weakness and vulnerability. Polarized in opposition to the more affirmatively viewed concept of autonomy, dependence seems to be less developed, less evolved, and more regressive a state of being and feeling. There is, however, a more salutory way of defining this term, extracting from it such concepts as capacity for intimacy, attunement to others, an awareness and sensitivity to the social or environmental matrix, and a commitment to

a relational perspective. We want to argue that this trait aids in
some adaptive functioning in the aging process, and further that it is
a trait with which women are more comfortable and which men are
decidedly more in conflict over. To summarize briefly the findings of
sex differences, we note the research literature on the construct
field independence and field dependence, a construct examined in
domains of perceptual, cognitive and social functioning. The
relatively stable finding of field independence as a mode of functioning for males and field dependence as a form for women is mirrored in
much clinical literature on the relative differences in developmental
patterns towards autonomy in male and female children (Mahler, Pine &
Bergmann, 1975). Perhaps the most appropriate way to summarize this
research is to say that women, throughout the early part of the life
cycle, are encouraged to be comfortable with many experiences of
dependency - empathy, social intimacy, perspective taking, etc. -
activities or traits which Chodorow has summarized as 'the reproduction of mothering.'

Developmental research provides documentation of the relative
power of male socialization in respect to autonomy and independence,
which we might see as traits of questionable value in flexible aging
and the acceptance of increasing dependence. But the clinical
literature goes further, providing evidence and theory to suggest that
male socialization involves some powerful inhibitors to dependence.
Dependency behaviors may be quite toxic for men, not merely under-
developed. That is, dependency is not merely deemphasized in male
socialization, it is discouraged and prohibited. In the internal life
of many men it comes to be dangerous. This argument is not, it should
be noted, a statement in support of the notion that sex differences
yield up some odd division of labor in which women have feelings and
empathy and men do not. The argument is rather that the dependency
behaviors and needs which may play a vital role in aging are relatively unavailable to men, or constitute such a radical shift in self-
image and attribution that they are not easily taken up or manifested.
For men, dependency and gender appear in contradiction. The heart of
this argument rests on the pervasive social fact that the primary
figure through early socialization is the mother, almost always a
woman. As many developmental psychologists have noted, this means
that women have an easily accessible model for self, while male
identity is worked through in interactions with fathers who remain
rather abstract figures (Lynn, 1959).

In the conventional contemporary family, fathers are often not so
accessible, remaining more involved in work and activity outside the
home. Hence, Lynn argued, male identification may be based on a model
who remains more an imaginary and abstract figure than the mother who
for the little girl is a more concretely present and available source
of identification.

In addition to the relatively inaccessible male model there is
another dilemma which male identity formation poses. Current research

and theory on early interaction (Stern, 1985; Winnicott, 1971) stresses the cultural fact that early relatedness arises in the company of the mother. So for the young boy, his masculine identity is also a process of disidentification, an undoing of the earlier tie to the mother. For men, then, dependency seems often frightening. It is a reminder of early patterns of connection to a maternal figure. Dependency then evokes a relation prior to gender identity for the boy and thus is a reminder, often visceral and intense, of experiences of infant vulnerability and helplessness and also experiences before gender is a stable self-construct. Dependency in male experience may seem to undo gender, may evoke fears of a loss of gender.

These ideas are helpful in making sense of Guttman's work on reciprocal sex role development in aging (Guttman, 1976). During middle age, for both sexes, previously polarized roles are vicariously or directly absorbed. For some men, a new preoccupation with what has traditionally been the sphere of the feminine takes the form of turning towards community service and sometimes to religious observances. These choices, rather than direct expressions of dependency and nurturance, may minimize the sense of danger in dependency behaviors by mediating them in public social process or alternatively in private, even secretive religious practices. In sum, the personal, interpersonal and social benefits of sustained dependency may not be so available to aging men.

Women, unless or until they become seriously disabled, retain their long term relation to household management and care, food preparation, the social cohesion within the family and relational network - activities likely to be helpful in the maintenance of social coherence and social meaning and stability of self and self-concept. Retirement for men usually entails some move to a social structure centered around the family, a move which robs older men of arenas of effective activity and a move in which the adaptive skills of social intimacy and dependence may not be readily available.

Interlude

As a measure of how devastating this loss of context may be for women and how specific and practical the sense of context is, we cite a clinical example from our study. Mrs. E. at 74 was experiencing memory loss and considerable deterioration of her cognitive skills and general functioning. She had a fall and was hospitalized. When she returned to her home, a health aid worker was employed to cook and look after her. This other woman's presence in her own kitchen proved too deep a disruption in Mrs. E.'s sense of the continuity of her self and her context. This change, unlike many previous changes, she was unable to integrate. She developed a belief that this was not, in fact, her apartment but rather what she called 'a clever replica.' For weeks she begged her children and grandchildren to take her home.

Mrs. A. (aged 70) watching both father and husband after retirement: "Its as though controlling us was the only thing they had left, the only thing they could do to not feel completely helpless."

Mrs. B. (aged 66) speaking about her husband after retirement. "He follows me from room to room. The man couldn't fry an egg to save his life, but he stands there telling me how to make ravioli."

In the case of Mrs. B., where the maintenance of rigid gender roles created an untenable shift in the balance of power in the marriage after the husband's retirement, balance was restored at enormous cost to the wife: a woman who had previously been very independently active in her extended family, she developed serious agoraphobia in the first year of her husband's retirement, making it impossible for her to go anywhere without her husband driving her. Like the increasing frequency with which couples of retirement age seek marital counselling, this marital dilemma - and its complex interactional solution in which the wife takes on the burden of pathology - points to an emerging difficulty for older couples. This difficulty stems both from gender-role rigidity (compounded by some of the rigidity often associated with aging) and from the dialectical conflict between gender arrangements which remain rigidly structured, while social, historical and economic frameworks around marriages - i.e., patterns of work, social isolation, etc. - have eroded and altered.

Aging then must entail some accommodation to the experience of relatively more dependency. Increased reliance on the attunement of others must coexist with earlier patterns of self-reliance and autonomy. Here we focus on the positive aspects of dependency for aging and the relatively greater access that women have to this trait and its related behaviors. Dependency involves a balance between two forces: trust on the one hand and on the other hand an ability to demand what one needs without alienating the giver.

Since women rely for support on those to whom they have offered or will be able to offer support in exchange, women have a sounder, experiential basis for trusting in the efficacy and availability of support. Additionally, for women throughout their life cycle, there is a strong social learning in respect to personal vulnerability. Many women are financially, and all women are physically, in a position of vulnerability in relation to men. This vulnerability is intimately entwined with the process of becoming a gendered social being, while male gender identity stresses becoming invulnerable to others' whims. The centrality of autonomy in male sex role socialization places strong emphasis on maintaining boundaries, differentiating oneself from others, holding one's ground, etc. A similar difference emerges in gender styles of interpersonal negotiation. Straightforward contest and argumentation appear to offer an advantage to men by virtue of their greater comfort with aggressive and assertive

behaviors.   Kressel (1987) has studied the impact of this difference
in conflict resolution and divorce mediation.   This capacity may not
be so useful in negotiations from positions of relative powerlessness.
For women, negotiation appears to involve more interpersonal management, a polite term for manipulation, perhaps.   This skill is an
essential survival tactic for anyone in a dependent position.   For the
aging woman, an increase in the use of this form of interaction can be
assumed to be relatively ego-syntonic, to be in seamless continuity
with her social role as a female person.   For the aging man, this may
present a difficulty; if he develops these skills, he uses them only
at a loss to his sense of self-continuity.   Taking the other route and
maintaining self-continuity may lead to a shift in the social attributions manifest towards such men, and a cost in the support and
sympathy from the social surround.

Aging, Gender and Separation Issues

One factor with great potential relevance to an individual's experience of control and efficacy is the handling of experiences of
separation and loss.   The management of separation reactions are, of
course, potentially troubling throughout the life span.   We consider
now the particularity of separation and loss experiences in aging.
There is evidence, both in clinical psychology (Mahler et al., 1975)
and in social psychology (Tamir, 1979) that men and women often have
different experiences and successes with this rite of passage.   Tamir
points out that in traditional families, the husband's role of primary
economic producer undergoes no significant shifts until the abrupt
loss associated with retirement, whereas the social role of mothering
and caregiving undergoes numerous transformations that may act as
rehearsals of separation.   Women's social identities and social
experience undergo radical shifts when they become mothers.   Daily
life alters dramatically when children reach school age.   Adolescent
ambivalence and rebellion, often directed primarily towards mothers,
evokes in many women a very painful experience of loss of intimacy
and validation.   In traditional families, the empty nest syndrome
means a loss of primary identification for women.   For all women in
this culture which restricts feminine attractiveness and sexual power
as a phenomenon of youthfulness, the aging experience forces a
confrontation with loss of yet another type.   These stereotypic
standards are variously resisted and struggled with by many women.
Yet powerful social attributions of attractiveness and potency and
sexual power are more age-linked for women than for men.   These
experiences of separation and loss are thus ongoing throughout the
life cycle for women, whereas many men must face a first primary
identity shift only upon retirement.

Since the experience of living through and integrating loss is in
itself a process which leads to a greater sense of internal control,
efficacy and acceptance, as well as continuity of self, it is
significant that women have so much more experience with this before

old age. It might also suggest that men's tendency to remarry is not
only a function of their greater economic and social power, but also a
reflection of their lack of practice and experience in integrating
loss. Remarriage may ward off and appear to undo an earlier loss,
rather than to allow a full integration of the experience.

The Concept of Control

One outcome of the current study of gender differences in social,
personal and cognitive functioning is an increasing dissatisfaction
with the whole concept of 'control.' Through some contemporary work
in gender studies, we can interrogate this concept. In developing a
more precise model for a person's assessment of control and drawing
on Rotter's concept 'locus of control,' Gurin and Gurin (1972) tried
to specify the relative meaning of internal and external locus of
control in particular settings, and for particular groups. Belief in
internal locus of control in certain contexts may be variously
masochistic and distorted (a child's belief that he or she may have
caused the parent's divorce; a woman's belief that she deserves abuse)
or illusory. This work, along with the study of gender differences in
cognitive functioning and moral judgment (Gilligan, 1982: Ruddick,
1982) allow us to examine the idealization in psychology of such
concepts as autonomy and control. These concepts have been hitherto
rather uncritically accepted as the hallmarks of effective functioning. Several alternatives can be mentioned. First, there are
situations, and aging may well be one, where internal control and
assumptions of autonomy along with the privilege of independence and
separateness are counterproductive. There may be situations where the
illusion of control - what Jessica Benjamin (1988) has termed
'instrumental rationality' - may be dangerous, may render the individual rather less effective than someone who accepts limits and can
acknowledge the interrelational bedrock of what is. thought of as
purely autonomous functioning. In this light, male socialization may
hold a particular disadvantage in respect to aging and helplessness.
The distorted power of the idea and ideal of autonomy and independence
may place unrealistic burdens on aging men in regard to judgments of
their own functioning, and deny them the aid of social contacts and
dependency behaviors.

Aging and Gender Attributions

Turning to the area of social attributions, the data present a
murkier picture. Mitchell, Wilson, Revicki and Parker (1985) report
greater positive attributions towards older women than towards older
men. Damrosch (1984) ties positive attributions of the elderly, by
young adults, to whether the older person is seen as sexually active
or not. Since older males, both by cultural stereotype and by the
higher incidence of remarriage to younger partners, project active

sexuality later in life, they may receive positive feedback and positive attributions more regularly than women.

Perhaps the most important point to make about social attributions is that they are likely to be highly sensitive to social and historical change. Tavani (1984) and others have noted that the aging process is now spread over a longer period and that a larger proportion of elderly people live into their 80's. A larger cohort is thus living longer and experiencing the cognitive deficits associated with very advanced age. The argument, then, is that this relatively new cohort may contribute to negative social attributions and attributions of increased helplessness. These attributions then have the potential to operate as self-referential social markers, as newer cohorts of aging persons reach towards their 70's or 80's. At the same time, an alternative force upon social attributions arises from the changes in work experiences, the legal challenges to mandatory retirement, economic pressures that may compel elderly people to remain in the work force, social and recreational changes which may lead to altered patterns in diet, exercise and social or self-presentation. These social changes may well undermine attributions of helplessness and diminished control. The other powerful press on social attributions may be the demographic shifts and the presence currently of a large aging cohort. These changes apparently register differently for men and women. There has been a tremendous range of rehabilitative projects with regards to women's image and self-image and a challenge to traditional representations of women which has touched many aspects of social and personal life, spurred by the second wave (i.e., twentieth century) of feminism.

Speech and Regulation

The second theoretical focus in this essay is on the role of language and speech in mechanisms of regulation, planning and control. This focus arises in the tradition of work on verbal regulation and speech for self, emanating from the Soviet research and theoretical paradigms developed by Luria (1961, 1971), Vygotsky (1963, 1975) and others (Harris, 1979).

A central idea in this work, which appears both in Vygotsky's writing and in the research tradition of Luria and his co-workers and students, is that individual and internal mechanisms of regulation and planned activity arise first on a social or dialogic basis. The paradigm for internal regulation and management is, then, the dialogic relation arising in the speech between adult and child (in the developmental context). Instructional and interpretive dialogues (dialogues that tell you what to do and dialogues that tell you what things mean) provide the material for internal representations of self-structuring plans and regulation.

Vygotsky, in particular, suggests the power of language in the constitution of self and self-consciousness (Wertsch, 1985). Signs are best treated as tools, objects imbued with historical specificity and transformatory power for their users. It is through the materiality of language, its connection to and reflection of practical activity, that mind is constituted as a historically specific and not essentialist structure. Signs thus are crucial aspects of a dialectical process of mutual structuring, whereby the subject and his or her relation to the world is created by a constant interaction in which language is the necessary mediation. Through the basic functional unit in Vygotsky's theoretical system, verbal thought, a mental representation is developed that is simultaneously social and individual, in which the social dynamic is reproduced as an internal form of self-instruction and self-management.

The presentation of inner speech and the internal representation of verbal thought as essentially the remnant of a dialogic experience is consistent with another important Soviet thinker, the formalist and linguist Bahktin (1981). Bahktin capitalizes on a distinction from Saussurean linguistics, that between *langue* and *parole*. He was less interested in language as a formal system and more concerned to describe parole, speech and its functioning. He was more interested in what we might recognize as pragmatics, the study of language in use, and he assumed that any human speech carried the surrounding ensemble of social relations, crucial aspects of ideology and belief, and the specificity of the context. Any speech event is imbricated with power vectors, social practices and the history of the use of that sign in social life.

Speech is thus a practice open to social and historical forces; in Bahktin's terms, the sign - i.e. the word or utterance - is 'pregnant with possibilities.' The situation surrounding any speech event enters into the utterance as a necessary constitutive element. Speech has always this character of dialogue. Monologue is, in Bahktin's terms, rather an illusion. Our speaking provides a text, a discursive socially mediated event which is open to interpretation.

This commitment to the inherent sociality of the utterance, of any speech event, is the hallmark of Soviet work on language. This view is elaborated in the research tradition of Luria, which traces the internalization of the social dialogue into internal representation. The essentially dialogic and instructional or interpretive character of social discourse is thus the format for self-regulation. The bulb press experiments chart the growing control of the child over the inhibitory and semantic features of language (Luria, 1961). These studies were focused on the capacity of language and speech use to exert a managerial effect on motor activity. The observational studies of speech for self in problem solving (Luria & Yudovich, 1971) and the application of these instructional discourses for self-planning in therapeutic contexts (Meichenbaum, 1979) attest to the power of social speech as a self-regulator.

It is customary to think of the regulatory role, a prosthetic role for language, in a micro-process context. That is, language operates in the orchestrated management of discrete events and actions. Planned action is thus conceived in a cybernetic framework as a process sustained by feedback loops and error corrections which maintain various actions in a coherent and ongoing format (Harris, 1979).

We want to extend this conception of the regulatory function of language from micro- to macro- process, to consider the role of internal dialogue in the maintenance of self-structures in more extended streams of behavior. This would be to propose a connection and potential mutual influence between the experimental study of self-regulation and the more hermeneutic study of narratives. The regulatory function of speech in the service of sustaining and controlling activity in the broader sense would involve speech practices of two different types. On the one hand, the social discourse is seen as a process whereby, in collaborative talk and social interpretive practices, individuals make and maintain meaning. In this idea, the social skills and interpersonal strategies and experiences of individuals would be highly adaptive. Participation in social experience is thus one powerful mechanism for the management of feelings of powerlessness and helplessness. Coherence and continuity offset feelings of loss of control through the sustaining and structuring power of social discourse.

Secondly, speech may provide regulatory focus for individuals through the use and evolution of narratives. This capacity might be independent of social discourse and social practices and might therefore provide a source of continuity and coherence even in individuals relatively more isolated and detached from social life. Since language skills remain relatively more intact in the aging process than a number of other cognitive processes (Botwinick, 1983), narrative skills and structures might provide a strong source of self-control and cohesion. That is, even in older persons with relatively few social contacts, some abiding language capacity for story-telling and meaning-making may continue to enhance the older person's feelings of self-control, even if not of social control.

Narratives as Devices for Self-Maintenance

The role of narrative in social and personal processes is currently being studied in various domains (Bruner, 1986). In the study of broad social and historical forces, narratives gain social power as they become part of a centralized literary tradition (Foucault, 1982). An example of this process is the codification of sin into a scheme of Seven Deadly Sins, creating a coherent set of ideas in medieval theology which offered to individuals in that period a useful mnemonic and precis available for 'narratizing' or understanding one's own life.

It is interesting to note that these devices of self-understanding, these schemes of sin and narratives of confession, replaced earlier external forms of social control and social management. This process of the internalization of motive and management mirrors, on the social and cultural plane, the process of internalization in the individual, noted by Luria and others. Narratives are thus socially, institutionally and interpersonally developed structures with a powerful constitutive effect on individuals. Bruce Chatwin's account of the musical narratives in aborigine culture (Chatwin, 1987) is a marvelous explication of the use of narrative as cognitive map, mnemonic device and planning instrument.

Narrative skills rely both on internal representation and social context. This is a central tenet in the anthropological studies of Geertz (1983), who proposes interpretive activity as a primary social process. Geertz and others (Giddens, 1976, 1979) construe the power of interpretive activity as a constituent element in social life and social interactions. Language, in Giddens' analysis, is a skilled performance, providing a world of words which specify, as Geertz notes, "the way the world is talked about, depicted, charted, represented, rather than the way it intrinsically is." In this skilled production, meaning and interpersonal context is managed and sustained. Language, in this view, occupies a dual position. Speech is used to read the world but also to double back and interpret (or read) itself. This property of reflexivity means that language not only serves as the medium for social and self construction, but also provides what Giddens has termed 'the accounting' procedures for what is meant. Bateson (1972) makes a similar point in talking about discourse as a basic site for the adjudication of what is happening, what has just happened, what is meant, and how the world is to be read. This hermeneutic position in language studies , developed in philosophy and social theory, is an increasingly powerful tool in psychological research and in our understanding of the function of language and speech in individual functioning (Ricoeur, 1970).

We may summarize these intellectual traditions as follows. Language as a formal system and speech as a social practice may function as a prosthetic for action and for self maintenance. In a micro sense, speech may become the spine for streams of motor action or regulated behavior, providing a sequencing and organizational structure for the maintenance and performance of activity. Also, speech as internal dialogue, the residue of social dialogue, provides a representational source for self-coherence. In thinking of the telling and retelling of internal dialogues or narratives in a dyachronic process, we must probably rely on work like Bartlett's (1932) to stress that the memory structures for narrative are profoundly influenced by social context. We are thus making no claims for accuracy or verisimilitude in narrative. The coherence provided by lifelong narratives, or life narratives, may be distorted as part of the ongoing demand for self-coherence experienced by people attempting to interpret and thus to know and gain some measure of control over their own lives (Handel, 1987).

Finally, inner narratives and dialogues interact with social process in a complex two-way manner. Story-telling may be a profoundly powerful experience for older persons, as it often allows increased participation in social interaction. It may be a factor in their continued sociality. Social contexts, to the degree that an older person can make use of them in collaborative story-telling, may contribute to a more powerful sense of control and self-control for the aging individual. As an underlying assumption, we are claiming that the making and maintaining of stable meaning structure is a powerful individual tool for experiencing control and a lessening of helplessness.

In sum, the dialogic and narrative properties of speech, and the inherent discursive and narrative structure of inner verbal thought, are important sources of agency and efficacy in any individual, and thus hold powerful possibilities as a way of understanding relative experiences of control and helplessness in aging persons.

Interlude

Miss C. was observed over a 15 year period in a private nursing home to which she was confined after increased physical disability, though with initially no diminished social and cognitive functioning. As sensory functioning deteriorated over the last five years of this period, she began to be increasingly socially isolated. This social isolation in conjunction with some physiological deterioration began to contribute to increasing episodes of dementia and senility. The trajectory we want to follow here is in the changing shape of narrative structures in the social interactions with this aging woman.

Early in the nursing home period, social visits were structured often by individual and socially produced narratives. During this time, much rich narrative history was produced. Childhood memories, usually in narrative structure, were brought forth in the context of the social visits. These stories were produced in characteristic format, what language researchers have termed the story grammars (Mandler & Johnson, 1977) in which locale, setting, character and dramatic structure are presented in a quite structurally stable manner. These stories, as Handel (1987) and others have noted, are both highly salient to the elderly and form an ongoing part of a life review process. They also maintain in living working memory some representation of the life cycle of the individual and thus provide primary experiences of self-coherence. In this period there were *work narratives*, extended narrative discourses in which her work history, a history of domestic service and child care, was reviewed. In these narrations chronological order was preserved, a working life review in the sphere of work was maintained. These narratives also contained and summarized belief systems regarding personality and character development, stressing also the abiding quality of character. Since her work was child rearing, these stories focused on good and bad parenting and tended to promote the idea of permanence and cohesion in character. Stories and reminiscences were often tailored for particular visitors. A 10-year-old boy was told the stories of wartime Scotland, the presence of military ships in the Glasgow harbor. Adults who had been children under her care were treated to the narrative history of their childhoods under her supervision. These stories were repeated, altered, polished like some favorite much handled stone. These stories carried narrative schemas - i.e. had the formal properties of story structure (Propp, 1968) - and also summarized and organized primary experiences of self and self in relation to primary social others.

In addition to work narratives, certain stories emerged to be told in a social setting after long periods of secrecy and silence. These were what we might term *'crisis' narratives*, again preserving the format of narrative structure, but containing difficult personal material and memory. In Miss C's case, this involved two different episodes, an extended period of sexual molestation by an older relative and a year long work experience of extreme cruelty and harshness. In the context of this woman's strong religious feelings, these narratives summarized strongly her experience of self, always focusing on moral or spiritual conclusions and interpretations. These were exemplary moral tales in the narrative form, inevitably initiated in the story-telling format 'Did I ever tell you how I became a Christian...' .

As her sensory capacities deteriorated, her potential for social engagement lessened. Hearing loss clearly altered the potential for social interaction and the give and take of conversation, so that visitors were increasingly reduced to the role of listening. Verbalizations for Miss C. were gradually reduced to structurally simpler forms, functioning primarily to indicate and maintain attention, and to confirm to the speaker the continued presence of the listener. Psycholinguists studying adult language to children, the baby register, have noted the use of this language form for the elderly (Reich, 1986). The simplified syntax, slower speech, use of diminutives, and reduction in lexicon characterize this register. We might see this as one aspect of the diminishing sociality for older persons, in the reduction of their treatment as fully competent adult speakers. Speech to Miss. C became increasingly restricted, mainly providing attention, maintenance, and simple probing or confirmation. Characteristically, in this period her language capacities were relatively undiminished. Her comprehensive and communicative competence was altered, but not the productive capacities and not the production of narratives. Narratives gradually simplified to a structured and often ritualized repetition of family members, what we might call *narratives of genealogy.* Relatives were named, relations characterized, persons were noted as alive or dead. These narratives seemed to function both as self-cohering and social-cohering devices. In the absence of social communicative devices and practices, conversation was maintained as a pseudo-dialogue while the narrative monologue was sustained. Story-telling was a way of preserving the fabric of social connection.

Narrative performance in this case preserved a social space in a relatively isolated setting and in interpersonal situations in which dialogue transactions were relatively impoverished. In this instance the internal coherence in this individual survived her diminished sociality. It is also possible that the deterioration in sensory functioning (deafness and loss of sight) by leading to diminished social contact, also led to the diminishing and simplifying of narratives. Any model for the relative efficacy of speech and self-maintenance and control experiences would need to include complex interactions between the social and internal representation spheres.

Words as Transitional Objects

There is another aspect of language use with relevance to the issue of control and helplessness. We will develop an analysis of speech functions drawn from the clinical and developmental theory of D. D. Winnicott, a tradition with strong compatibility to the basic paradigm of Vygotsky and Luria. Winnicott's idea was that in the course of development a child must rely on the structuring activities of the parent for an experience of security and ongoing experience. This idea computes well with the current use of Vygotsky's idea of the zone of proximal development as a scaffolding device whereby the child was led to higher levels of functioning through an interaction with an adult who provided a bridge, by way of instruction support or elaboration, towards a more advanced functioning. Winnicott's idea of the developmental necessity of a 'transitional space' is quite close to the Vygotskian concept of the zone of proximal development. More specifically, Winnicott thought of the child as using this space to develop stable representations of self and other. This structuring activity, in which the parent's participation was crucial, was, for Winnicott, a creative moment in which the child produced through play and the familiar objects of his world a set of representations and structures which came to be endowed with animate properties and personhood. These forms, which he termed 'transitional objects', could be toys, stuffed animals, a blanket, in some cases an imaginary friend or companion of quite elaborated form and character. These objects were used by the child in activities of self-soothing and self- structuring as the focus of dramatic play and enactments in the service of self-understanding and self-presentation. Horton (1985) has recently begun to extend this analysis of transitional objects to include - as a crucial exemplar of this construct - words and speech. Speech is particularly powerful as a transitional object by virtue of

several interesting properties.   It is symbolic and thus capable of
absorbing and displaying complex representations and metaphors.
Speech is also a material form and here Horton means to indicate the
prosody, rhythm, and sound of speech as a powerful evocation of early
caretaking.   Transitional objects are transitional in several ways.
They are transitional devices to enable development and more elaborate
cognitive and social structuring.   They are also transitional in the
sense of occupying an intersubjective space, capturing aspects of the
parent and aspects of the child.   The emotional intensity of the
childs' attachment to and use of these objects speaks to the strong
evocation of the parental figures these objects represent.   Again,
speech carries this mix of material and symbolic features, providing
emotional evocation in the melodic pitch and shape of speech as well
as symbolic capacity in the semantic and syntactic structure.

      This theoretical development which Winnicott brought to bear in
clinical work and in his writing on development maps well to the work
of Luria and Vygotsky, who also stressed the motoric and impulsive
aspects of speech in the service of regulation.   We thus would look to
the capacity of speech to regulate and manage difficult experiences.
In childhood these objects are particularly important in the management of anxiety and affect in experiences of separation and loss.   In
conceiving of speech as an adaptive form in mediating feelings of
helplessness and uncertainty, its function as a transitional object
should be noted.

      While the clinical work and theory of Winnicott has stressed the
power of transitional objects in early development, Horton (1985) and
others have suggested the power of speech in its function as a
transitional object across the lifespan.   Speech may be a source of
soothing and self-maintenance, in the sense that Winnicott indicates
for the transitional object, and as such speech would have preservative and regulatory impact upon the elderly.

                              Conclusions

Can we now map some of this work on speech and control to the question
of gender and aging?   Are there sex differences in the relative use
men and women might make of these language processes in aging?

      On the one hand, language skills, in terms of productive and
comprehensive capacities, are relatively gender neutral and somewhat
robustly resistant to age changes (Botwinick, 1983).   The implication
then is that language capacities offer for men and women a rich set of
possibilities for the maintaining of structures which aid in experiences of control and coherence.   In particular, narrative structures may
provide abiding and evolving systems of self-explanation and self-
representation with great adaptive value for aging.

Looking at language functions and speech practices in the context of sex differences suggests that current sex role socialization patterns may offer to women an advantage in the maintenance and honing of speech practices which serve this adaptive functioning. Women, by virtue of their wider and more interactive social networking, their social and empathic skills and their less problematic relationship to dependency, may be better able to use these narrative and speech practices in the service of sustained functioning over the aging process.

The way in which we converse with others as much as the content of the conversation affects the nature of our social ties. It also affects our sense of self and therefore addresses various levels of self with which we feel in continuity. In this light, it may be important to consider the differing ways in which men and women use language and the differing meaning it holds for them (Harris, 1986).

Sherman, Ward and LaGory (1984), in a study of gender factors in the choice of confidants among older people, found that 47% of the men in their sample of persons over 60 cited women as primary confidants, while only 19% of the women cited a man in this capacity. Most people regardless of gender rely on women to sustain intimate conversation, and this has perhaps to do with both women's use of language and the experience of speaking to a woman.

As we noted earlier, the degree to which one feels oneself to be helpless is in part a function of the ease with which one negotiates the interplay between dependency and autonomy. All older people face at least the possibility and often the reality of an increase in their dependence on others. One way of seeing the outcome in terms of perceived and self-perceived helplessness might be the relative capacity of the older person to maintain autonomy within a situation of dependence. We will argue that this is likely to be more easily facilitated for women. We will also argue that communicative competence and social discourse is one context in which this balance is worked out.

Two aspects of our earlier discussion can be brought out. One, there are sex differences in the comfort, acceptability and recognition of dependency as an aspect of personal identity. Men throughout their lives struggle against the anxiety and distaste associated with dependency. We might say then that men and women may have a quite different experience of helplessness and dependency with men, in general, more unsettled by dependency. Men may indeed have profound needs for dependency and contact but fewer social and linguistic resources to deal with the experience. Secondly, we have argued that speech practices contain a complex mix of emotionally charged and cognitively elaborated forms. Developmentally, our emergence from the real helplessness of early infancy coincides with the emergence and mastery over language forms. As Winnicott suggests, the emerging use of language is tied to separation experiences and may come to represent both loss and linkage. From this perspective, the act of speaking is this curious mix of autonomy and connectedness.

If one function of intimate conversation for older people is to negotiate autonomy within dependence, it may be important to use speech in conversational formats which tap both experiences of dependency and of autonomy. Narrative structures with the mixture of regularity and creative reframing may constitute such a format. Another way of seeing this would be to stress the importance of the non-instrumental use of language, the pragmatic rather than purely the mathematic functions, in Halliday's terms (1975).

Several factors may make this function more enabling and adaptive for women. In the structure of women's conversation, the social practices of networking and relational activity, women make more use of these non-instrumental formats. They may be able to experience the soothing and structuring effects of speech more easily and in a more ego-syntonic way than men. Women's ways of talking are often trivialized as 'gossip', an underestimation of the preserving power of speech.

Finally we examined sex differences in aging in respect to helplessness and in examining a potentially adaptive role for speech, as narrative, as transitional object and as prosthetic for planned activity. We have found it necessary to (critically) examine the very concept of control and the personal styles and attributes which intersect with it. Control as a conceptual term standing for independence and autonomous functioning, for the rigid management of experience and the idealization of individualism at the expense of relatedness, may need redefinition. The illusory and irrational aspects of 'control' and 'instrumental rationality' may be counterproductive for aging. The implication of this discussion is that social practices, narrative structures and experiences which facilitate the experience of dependency may play an important role in the older person's management of feelings of helplessness. A further implication is that even though men and women have quite equivalent patterns of language competence in aging, the gender-linked differences in language use, in communicative competence, in social functioning and in the meaning of speech may play a greater role in women's adaptation to aging.

References

Bahktin, M. (1981). *The dialogic imagination* (M. Holquist, Trans.). Austin, TX: University of Texas Press.

Bart, P., & Frankel, L. (1976). *The student sociologist's handbook*. Morristown: General Learning Press.

Bartlett, F. (1932). *Remembering*. Cambridge: Cambridge University Press.

Bateson, G. (1972). *Steps to an ecology of mind*. New York: Ballantine Books.

Belenky, M. F., Clinshy, B. M., Goldberger, M. R., & Tarule, J. M. (1986). *Women's ways of knowing: The development of self, voice and mind*. New York: Basic Books.

Benjamin, J. (1988). *The bonds of love*. New York: Pantheon Press.

Berger, P., & Luckman, T. (1967). *The social construction of reality*. Garden City, NY: Doubleday & Co.

Botwinick, J. (1983). *Aging and behavior*. New York: Springer.

Bruner, J. (1986). *Actual minds, possible worlds*. Cambridge, MA: Harvard University Press.

Butler, R. N. (1963). The life review: An interpretation of reminiscence in the aged. *Psychiatry, 26*, 65-76.

Chatwin, B. (1987). *Songlines*. New York: Viking Press.

Chodorow, N. (1978). *The reproduction of mothering*. Berkeley: University of California Press.

Damrosch, S. P. (1984). Graduate nursing students' attitudes towards sexually active older persons. *Gerontology, 24*, 299-301.

Dinnerstein, D. (1976). *The mermaid and the minotaur*. New York: Harper & Row.

Foucault, M. (1982). The subject and power. *Critical Inquiry, 8*, 777-789.

Freeman, M. (1984). History, narrative and lifespan developmental knowledge. *Human Development, 27*, 1-19.

Freeman, M. (1985). Paul Ricoeur on interpretation. *Human Development, 28*, 295-312.

Geertz, C. (1983). *Local knowledge: Further essays in interpretive anthropology*. New York: Basic Books.

Giddens, A. (1976). *New rules of sociological methods*. London: Hutchinson.

Giddens, A. (1979). *Central problems in social theory*. London: Macmillan Co.

Gilligan, C. (1982). *In a different voice.* Cambridge, MA: Harvard University Press.

Guntripp, H. (1973). *Psychoanalytic theory, therapy and the self.* New York: Basic Books.

Gurin, P., & Gurin, J. (1972). Internal-external control in the motivational dynamics of Negro youth. *Journal of Social Issues, 28,* 79-82.

Guttman, D. (1976). Individual adaptation in the middle years: Developmental issues in the masculine mid-life crisis. *Journal of Geriatric Psychiatry, 9.*

Halliday, M. A. K. (1975). *Learning how to mean.* London: Arnold Press.

Handel, A. (1987). Personal theories about the life-span development of one's self in autobiographical self-presentations of adults. *Human Development, 30,* 83-98.

Harris, A. (1979). Historical development of the Soviet theory of self-regulation. In G. Zivin (Ed.), *The development of self-regulation through private speech* (pp. 51-77). New York: Wiley & Sons.

Harris, A. (1986). *Women in relation to power and language.* Paper read at the Washington Square Institute, New York, NY.

Honey, M. (1987). The interview as text: Hermeneutics considered as a model for analyzing the clinically informed research interview. *Human Development, 30,* 69-82.

Horton, P. (1985). Language, solace, and transitional relatedness. *Psychoanalytic study of the child.* London: Marsfield Press.

Kaye, L. W., & Monk, A. (1984). Sex role traditions and retirement from academe. *The Gerontologist, 24,* 420-426.

Kressel, K. (1987). *The book of divorce.* New York: Basic Books.

Lieberman, M. A. (1975). Adaptive processes in late life. In N. Datan & L. H. Ginsberg (Eds.), *Lifespan developmental psychology.* New York: Academic Press.

Lipman, A., & Longino, C. (1984). Support systems of women by marital status. *The Gerontologist, 24,* 291.

Lowenthal, M. F. (1977). Toward a sociological theory of change in adulthood and old age. In J. E. Birren & K. W. Schaie (Eds.),

Handbook of the psychology of aging (pp. 116-127).   New York: Van Nostrand Reinhold.

Lowenthal, M. F., & Haven, C. (1968).   Interaction and adaptation: Intimacy as a critical variable.   In B. L. Neugarten (Ed.), *Middle age and aging.*   Chicago: University of Chicago Press.

Lowenthal, M. F., & Robinson, B. (1976).   Social networks and isolation.   In R. H. Binstock & E. Shanas (Eds.), *Handbook of aging and the social sciences* (pp. 432-456).   New York: Van Nostrand Reinhold.

Luria, A. A. (1961).   *The role of speech in the regulation of normal and abnormal behavior.*   New York: Boni & Liveright.

Luria, A. A., & Yudovich, F. (1971).   *Speech and the development of mental processes in the child.*   London: Penguin.

Lynn, D. B. (1959).   A note on sex differences in the development of masculine and feminine identification.   *Psychological Bulletin, 66,* 126-135.

Maccoby, E., & Jacklin, C. (1975).   *The psychology of sex differences.*   Stanford: Stanford University Press.

Mahler, M., Pine, F., & Bergman, A. (1975).   *The psychological birth of the infant.*   New York: Basic Books.

Mandler, J. M., & Johnson, N. S. (1977).   Remembrance of things parsed: Story structure and recall.   *Cognitive Psychology, 9,* 111-151.

Markides, K. S., & Vernon, S. W. (1984).   Aging, sex-role orientation and adjustment - a three generational study of Mexican Americans.   *Journal of Gerontology, 39(5),* 586-591.

Meichenbaum, D. (1979).   Clinical use of private speech and critical questions about its study in natural settings.   In G. Zivin (Ed.), *The development of self-regulation through private speech.*   New York: Wiley & Sons.

Mitchell, J., Wilson, K., Revicki, D., & Parker, L. (1985).   Children's perceptions of aging - a multidimensional approach to differences by age, sex and race.   *The Gerontologist, 25,* 182-187.

Neugarten, B. (1964).   Summary and implications.   In B. L. Neugarten et al. (Eds.), *Personality in middle and later life.*   New York: Atherton Press.

Neugarten, B. (1968).   *Middle age and aging.*   Chicago: University of Chicago Press.

316 A. Harris and N. Miller

Propp, V. (1968). *Morphology of the folktale*. Austin, TX: University of Texas Press.

Rapp, R. (1975). *Towards an anthropology of women*. New York: Monthly Review Press.

Reich, P. (1986). *Language development*. New York: Prentice Hall.

Reese, H., & Overton, W. (1970). Models of development and themes of development. In L. R. Goulet & P. B. Baltes (Eds.), *Life-span developmental psychology* (pp. 19-46). New York: Academic Press.

Ricoeur, P. (1970). *Freud, and philosophy: An essay on interpretation*. New Haven, CT: Yale University Press.

Ruddick, S. (1982). Maternal thinking. *Feminist Studies, 8*, 82-97.

Sinott, J. D. (1977). Sex-role inconstancy, biology and successful aging: Dialectical model. *The Gerontologist, 17*, 459-463.

Sherman, S. R., Ward, R. A., & LaGory, M. (1984). Gender differences in role models and confidants. *The Gerontologist, 24*, 281.

Stern, D. (1985). *The interpersonal world of the infant*. New York: Basic Books.

Tamir, L. (1979). *Communication and the aging process*. New York: Pergamon Press.

Tavani, C. (1984). Self-determination: Constraints and frontiers. *The Gerontologist, 24*, 277.

Vygotsky, L. (1963). *Thought and language*. Cambridge, MA: MIT Press.

Vygotsky, L. (1978). *Mind in society*. Cambridge, MA: Harvard University Press.

Wertsch, J. (1985). *Culture, communication and cognition*. Cambridge: Cambridge University Press.

Winnicott, D. D. (1971). *Playing and reality*. New York: Basic Books.

Zivin, G. (Ed.) (1979). *The development of self-regulation through private speech*. New York: Wiley & Sons.

PART V

PSYCHOLOGICAL ANTECEDENTS AND SOCIOLOGICAL PERSPECTIVES OF CONTROL AND AGING

Psychological Perspectives of Helplessness
and Control in the Elderly, P.S. Fry (ed.)
© Elsevier Science Publishers B.V. (North-Holland), 1989

Chapter Eleven

POWER, CONTROL AND WELL-BEING OF THE ELDERLY: A CRITICAL RECONSTRUCTION

Prem S. Fry
The University of Calgary

Lee R. SLIVINSKE
Youngstown State University

Virginia L. FITCH
The University of Akron, Ohio

Abstract

*The question of an interface between the older adults' need
for personal autonomy and social power relationships and the
societal forces that work to deflate the power resources is
discussed.   Societal structures and forces which act as the
sources of powerlessness and power deflation in the later
years are identified and various social exchanges which
foster responses of compliance, approval and passivity in
old age are evaluated.   Ways and means for maintaining and
promoting the power resources and controls of older persons
are discussed both at the individual instrumental level and
at the level of governmental mediation.   Implications for
health and mental well-being of older persons are discussed.*

Introduction

Power and control are recognized by a number of gerontologically-oriented social scientists as being integral elements inextricably linked with the psychology of aging and interwoven with aspects of personal and social identity and well-being of older adults.

To understand the workings of power and control in the relationship of older persons with other individuals and social groups one must also consider the situation of older adults' perceptions of themselves as weak and powerless.   In the cradle to grave populations studied, older adults in the Western culture are perceived to be the most central group of individuals in the wide category of the knowledgeable but weak and dominated.   The adjustments that older adults have to make in their power relations and in their equal or subordinate partnerships illuminate the whole range of power situations which have implications for their psychological well-being.   So the stereotypic formula "To be old is to be powerless" is also associated with another stereotypic notion that "to be powerless is to be old." Power and powerlessness are thus factored into old age and youthful images quite explicitly. Traditional wisdom holds that older adults are more aware than younger adults of the need for interactions and their power influences. At the same time they are becoming increasingly aware also of the loss of power they must accept with increasing old age. If that is so, acceptance of the loss of power is something they have learned--learned in order to ease things in the families and the social and political groups and often times to head off emotional collisions.

It is the purpose of this chapter to analyze the relationship of power with skills, knowledge, self-controls, self-efficacy and identity components in old age. The relationship between power influences and the well-being of older adults will be traced and sources of powerlessness and power deflation will be examined. We will identify and define the methods by which younger individuals develop the power resources necessary to manipulate their environment satisfactorily. Simultaneously we will examine the forces which impel older individuals to readjust to reduced levels of power and in-fluence. Such an examination will provide insight into some of the ways some elderly persons are able to accumulate and maintain surplus power resources while others experience an undersupply. Classic studies examining aspects of power, control and well-being will be reviewed so as to provide a picture of the way older adults perceive the world of power relationships to be ordered.

The discussion will include explanations of older adults' perceptions of their competencies, skills and controls and how these influence their ability to cope with or adapt to the societal forces which work to reduce the amount of power aged individuals have, and the perceptual changes in control that may be experienced.

Finally, the potentialities for control-enhancing and power-enhancing interventions will be discussed both at the level of the individual and at the level of social agencies and governmental impact.

Key Definitions and Meanings of Power

An historical review of the literature on power reveals that the concept has been defined in a variety of ways. Although a universally accepted definition of power is lacking (cf. Olsen, 1970; Winter, 1973) an underlying commonality is that power is discussed in terms of the ability of a person or group to influence another person or group (Pollard & Mitchell, 1972; Turk & Bell, 1972). Tauney (1931) defined power as "the capacity of an individual to modify the conduct of other individuals or groups in the manner which he desires, and to prevent his own conduct being modified in the manner in which he does not" (p. 229). Similarly, Weber (1974) in his writings on social order, described power as the probability that one actor within a social relationship will be in a position to carry out his own will despite resistance" (p. 152).

The preceding definitions of power are *logically tied to the ability of people to influence their environment*. Power in these definitions, is conceived broadly as the 'power of the individual' confronting the society. Power in either a broad or restricted sense refers to *capabilities* and may be defined as the capability to secure outcomes of freedom and influence where the realization of these outcomes depends on the agency of *others*. Individual skills and power are often considered as one concept which may be termed outcome freedom (Steiner, 1979). The possession of skills is thought to be unequivocally positive in the individual's attempt to gain and maintain power. In this sense personal power is believed to increase during the course of human development, parallel to the development of skills although not synonymous with it. However, by the time individuals reach late adulthood they may experience a decline in personal skills, capabilities and controls, and these perceptions of declining controls and capabilities may contribute to the older persons' beliefs that they possess little power to influence the environment (Seligman, 1975). Such perceptions of loss of power can be stressful and have a negative impact on the psychological well-being of older individuals (Brim, 1974).

The values placed on the individual's sense of mastery, competence and self-control imply that skills, personal capability and power are all developmental in character and are often considered as one concept. The individual's capacity to regulate, direct and coordinate personal resources can itself be seen as a type of personal power, and it can serve to increase the individual's social power. The individual's beliefs in personal capability or motivations for competence and capability are referred to as self-efficacy expectations leading to power (Bandura, 1977, 1978). Self-efficacy expectations often involve change in the individual's perceived ability to control or to communicate power to other agents in the environment. In this sense control and power are synonymous concepts in determining the perception people have regarding how much they influence the environment or are themselves influenced by it.

When psychologists discuss power, it is usually along the lines of control that individuals have over their personal agendas and outcomes. Thus psychologists point to the relationship between individualized constructs such as locus of control and power (e.g., Ng, 1980). However, such control theories simply serve to contain and mask the power perceptions of individuals, and do not address the production of power relations.

The second task then in the definition and meaning of power is to move beyond the individualist frame of control and power and to examine the meaning of power in a wider social environment.

The discussion which follows relies upon the fundamental idea that power is individual but at the same time it is an integral element in the reproduction of systems of structuration and interaction. In this context power is a logical component of action and interaction where the latter refers to mutually oriented forms of conduct between the individual and plurality of other agencies or actors (Giddens, 1977). The use of power in interaction can be understood in terms of resources or facilities which participants bring to and mobilize as elements of its production, thereby directing its course. Thus these productions of power relations include also the skills and resources which a participant is capable of bringing to bear so as to influence and control the conduct of others who are parties to that interaction, including the possession of 'authority' and the threat or use of 'force' (Giddens, 1976). Our concern at this point is to offer a generalized conceptual scheme which integrates the notion of power and the production of power relations into the social life and social relationships of older adults. What it is necessary to do is to relate this notion of power in interaction to the older adults' possession of relevant types of power resources to secure outcomes. The power resources may take the form of skills, knowledge, self-efficacy expectation and ability to mobilize authority.

Action, Interaction and Power Relations

Power in this context then becomes an element of action, and refers to the range of interventions of which an agent is capable (Giddens, 1976). Power in this broad sense when applied to older adults is equivalent to their transformative capacity for action: the capability of these individuals to intervene in a series of events so as to alter their course. The use of power in interaction can be understood in terms of resources or facilities which participants bring to and mobilize as elements of its production (Giddens, 1979). When power resources are assessed in older adults these may include concrete resources such as saleable skills, wealth, and property, but could also mean other intangible resources such as wisdom, insights, meaningful relationships and valued experiences gained over a life time of interaction. As later discussion will show, the reflexive elaboration of these more intangible resources is characteristically imbalanced in relation to the possession of the former more concrete resources of power.

Power in interaction can be understood in a 'relational' sense, but power here also implies domination. Power according to these notions suggests that the individual must use his/her transformative capacities to interact with agents of power or to seek freedom from domination in systems of interaction. Used in this sense, power exists not necessarily at the individual level but at subindividual and supraindividual levels simultaneously (Foucault, 1980). It is assumed that the creation of a power system does not necessarily entail the coercive subordination of the wishes or interests of one party to those of others.   Nor is the use of power inevitably correlated with oppression, exploitation or conflict (Giddens, 1976). Quite clearly, the existence of a defined role, status or financial position does generate power which may be used to achieve aims and goals.   This aspect of power has specific relevance to older adults. The inevitable risk of loss of role, ambiguity in status, and instability in financial standing of older adults may lead to considerable "power deflation" causing a spiralling diminution of confidence in the older adults' agency of power.   The result is that those previously subordinate to them come increasingly to question their position and to use various typologies of means to obtain compliance and deflate self-confidence and assertiveness.

Although it is recognized that economic and other material factors play a key part in power deflation of older persons, we argue that inducements, as distinguished from power, are often used as a means of bringing about power deflation.   Inducements offering some definite rewards in exchange for compliance are used more often with frail older adults whose transformative capacities of action and interaction become limited.   In this sense the power or absence of power in older adults is closely bound up with the notion of *praxis* or customary practice or conduct of being polite and gracious toward the elderly but treating them with benign indifference.

The influence of the older person's possession of mobilized experiences, insights or wisdom is seldom explored and the influence is indeed seldom felt outside the subjective reality of the individual's personal environment or the most mundane levels of everyday interaction.

Knowledge, Skills and Power

Before examining the effectiveness of older adults as producers and victims of power relations it is important to inspect briefly the status of older adults with respect to knowledge, skills and transformative capacities which contribute to the production of power relations.   At any stage of human development beliefs about personal power and control may arise out of the interplay between the motivations for power, knowledge, skills and capabilities of the individual on the one hand and the organizational complexity of the social environment in interaction with the individual.

The development of personal control arises in its most basic and realistic forms from concrete accomplishments.   As individual maturation proceeds, the further development of this belief requires continued social accomplishments which are dependent on an increasingly diverse range of skills.   In later life, however, the skills learned earlier in life are less likely to be effective because of the potentials for rapid and increasing change in environmental conditions. If there is sufficient change, old skills may not only be ineffective but counterproductive especially for older individuals for whom every change represents a challenge to coping capacity. The reason for this lies in the complex relationship between social and biological change, environmental instability, decrements in personal control and increase in stress reactions of older persons.

One result of rapid social and environmental change in old age is the discontinuity between skills, transformative capacities and interactional resources that facilitated beliefs of power and control at one point in the life cycle and those found necessary but unavailable later. The degree of initiative necessary, the conditions under which the authority of powerful others may be challenged, and the boundaries of acceptable discourse are not frequently left to the discretion of older persons. So, too, in old age institutional control, and relationship with helpers and caregivers may frequently discourage rather than reinforce the symmetry of power that arises naturally from adult skills and perspectives. These and similar experiences combine to produce anomalous messages of power and powerlessness among older persons.

Whereas one set of culturally sanctioned exhortations stress action, mastery interaction and the production of power relations and power resources throughout the life cycle, many other experiences culturally produced, if not sanctioned, result in the development of a deep sense of confusion and helplessness in the later years. One plausible outcome of these incompatible directives is a pervasive feeling of powerlessness in the older person's interactions. Issues such as these have fundamental implications not only for beliefs in self-efficacy but also for estimations of power or powerlessness in the larger social contexts of older persons.

Sources of Powerlessness in Late Adulthood

A pervasive sense of powerlessness in old age may arise in a number of ways. The most obvious route is subordination to family members, institutional control and financial considerations. In these situations the sphere of negotiation is rather small for older adults. General goals, means of attainment, sequences of procedure and rates of accomplishment are constrained only by the conscience of employers or by a crude calculation of sufficient levels of physical well-being and cognitive functioning to ensure continued productivity in the market place. Where replacements of skills, competencies or knowledge are not in short supply, levels of physical energy or cognitive functioning of older adults may be considered to be at a low level. In many cases decisions about terminating the services of older persons or explanations about the procedures and criteria used to terminate services have not necessarily been subject to any consensual process (Prewitt & Verba, 1977). Employers and social agency administrators of welfare services for older adults have been permitted a fair degree of local autonomy and have sometimes attempted a policy of nonresponsiveness vis-à-vis older adults. Any extended period of benign neglect in the social sphere of interactions and relationships becomes a contradiction in terms, since even the highest levels of self-confidence and personal mastery beliefs cannot be sustained by older adults in the face of chronic ineffectualness (cf. Renshon, 1974).

However, the development of a sense of powerlessness need not arise from inaction or lack of skills and knowledge alone. A second route to powerlessness is organizational complexity and rapid technological change. These factors may themselves produce a sense of powerlessness at two levels. First, complexity may present comprehension and communication difficulties especially if certain sophisticated cognitive or sensory-motor skills are involved. Complexity may also give rise to difficulties associated with the acquisition of new technological knowledge, interpersonal skills or retraining in order to regain a foothold in social interactions.

It is perhaps the diffusion of responsibility in democratic Western society that presents the most difficult barrier to maintaining power relations in old age. As noted by Renshon (1974), in democracies, the necessity to explore and consider alternative points of view requires a certain tolerance and acceptance of delay in the development of power relations. In old age, however, it is seldom that older citizens are permitted opportunity for collective activity, visibility, accountability or the option of delaying decision making. Even among the affluent elderly where some measure of visibility may exist, power relations do not exist in the absence of readily identifiable power centers (Renshon, 1974). This is one reason why the administrators of nursing homes and institutional centers for older persons have enormous power significance in the relational structures of most older adults.

These mediating factors are sufficiently formidable by themselves to raise serious doubts about the capability of older adults to maintain a sense of personal or social control in interactions with other agents of power and control. Additionally, as discussed earlier, there are two other contextual elements (i.e., rapid environmental change in late life and cultural expectations for self-efficacy and transformative capacities for manipulating power relations) which present a difficult barrier to maintaining personal power and control beliefs in the later years of life. The operations of the cultural double-bind system present a serious dilemma for older adults. Even where institutional structures remain stable, the course of the older adults' biological, psychological and cognitive development will not remain fixed. Among the many questions raised under these circumstances are whether old skills can be made useful and whether new and more effective skills can be developed in order that a sense of self-esteem and power relations with others can be maintained.

According to gerontologically-oriented psychologists and sociologists, older adults must continue to cope with a cultural double-bind which arises from the injunction to participate actively in the social sphere. The underlying assumption is that social agencies will be responsive to the participation and social exchange of older adults who should and ought to feel efficacious and strong (cf. Brim, 1974). The media all exhort older citizens to exercise their participatory rights and to exert influence and power. However most institutional frameworks in democratic societies convey substantially contradicting messages of power and influence to older adults. Our purpose here is not to indict but rather to draw attention to the fact that contradictory messages of influence and control lead to further anomie and loss of interest in the late adulthood years.

The concern of the psychology of aging with questions of mastery, autonomy and control is in part a denial of this problem of the contractual nature of power. The psychology of control in aging continues to emphasize the individualist frame of control and does not move sufficiently to view the construct of control as a component of power relations.

Perhaps the most articulate statement of this position is found in Toffler's *Future Shock* (1970) where he argues that rates of social change, accompanied by high technology and exacerbated by declining energies ensure that most social environments will cease to provide stable structures within which personal control, power relations or power resources may be maintained. The implications of Toffler's position for the power, control and influence of older adults living in mass societies are enormous and grim. The sense of powerlessness is suggested to be a causative factor in the development of anomie (Merton, 1957). Especially when applied to late life functioning, it may also be a causative factor in interpersonal and cognitive impairment.

Power and Identity

The relationship between power and identity is of crucial significance in understanding components of personal development and power relationships in older persons.

By identity is meant the distinguishing characteristics that mark people as unique individuals and that are not attributable to normative characteristics of the self. According to Goffman (1961), identity is always expressed, even in highly normative environments, and it is often expressed as a distance from normative requirements which can either contravene norms or contribute to the smooth functioning of the social order. This definition implies that throughout the life cycle identity is socially constructed. In other words, identity similar to power, is not a property of the individual but a relationship. Identity also becomes the sphere in which power relations are played out (Apfelbaum & Lubek, 1976).

When this notion of identity development is applied to the psychology of aging and adulthood, it poses a number of problems related to domination-compliance or domination-resistance. On older adults especially, there are too many social pressures to comply to values and rules that control their social future. In old age "compliance is an attempt to avoid identity-damaging controls" (Knights & Willmott, 1985). Similarly withdrawal from the social sphere or from the active forces fosters an identity-damaging isolation which retards social interdependence. Yet that interdependence is vital to identity maintenance in old age.

When seeking to defend themselves against institutional control and domination by powerful others, older adults are more often prone than younger adults, to respond in a submissive manner, in which case the expression of their creative and transformative power and their wisdom and insights becomes a pale reflection of their potentials. Alternatively, they may try to defend a privately preferred identity by mentally distancing themselves or physically withdrawing themselves from the conditions of their subordination or from the powerful agents who are responsible for divesting them of their autonomy.

At this point it may be helpful to elaborate and draw out briefly some implications of our argument concerning the power-identity relationship in the later years. In contemporary society at least, youth's preoccupation with identity and power routinely involves a securing of self-esteem and self-enhancement through instrumental participation in social relations and the reproduction of power relations. In old age, however, people tend to become separated off from one another and from those in positions of power. As social support stemming from interdependence is weakened, the vulnerability of identity is paradoxically increased and the loss of power is correspondingly increased. The negation or distortion of interdependent relationship in the later years have the effect of impeding the reproduction of the forces of power and yet they offer no fundamental solution to the experience of anxiety and insecurity which results from a loss of social identity.

Faced with a loss of power and precariousness of identity implicit in the uncertainty of social relationship, older adults are constrained to maintain a *nomos* that offers a degree of protection from the existential anxiety and uncertainty of their social identity. Although one understands the source of the problem of identity disintegration in older persons there is no theoretical explanation for the effect it has on the emotional outlook of older persons. Lacking in the developmental or social psychology of aging is a descriptive or theoretical penetration or appreciation of how preoccupation with identity in old age may, unintentionally, contribute to the reproduction of conditions of compliance, passivity and depression. There is little theoretical penetration of how, through the problematic of identity formation and maintenance, older adults become victimized by their own lack of will or skill to transform the structures of control that reproduce the conditions of indifference. When reviewed in the light of this framework, the psychology of self-control in aging is seen not to appreciate sufficiently how older persons' preoccupation with securing or defending a particular sense of identity has the effect of undermining the productive potential of interdependence in power relations, and of unintentionally reinforcing the dominant structures of self-control through the process of self-restraint and control of self as a form of compliance (Knights & Willmott, 1985).

Our central thesis in this part of the chapter has been to argue that there are implicit social pressures on older adults to express their valued image of self or identity through individualistic self-restraint and compliance rather than through interdependence and power relationship. In the process, the development of the creative and productive power of interdependence is distorted and undermined. Similarly the control of self to dominate the environment (cf. Bandura's (1977, 1982) discussion of executive control) is also undermined. Either way an individualistic response of self-restraint or compliance directly frustrates and undermines the productive power inherent in the older person's need for social interdependence. More specifically, both in institutional settings and wider social settings, there are capitalist pressures to act in a restrained or constrained manner. These institutional and social pressures weaken the power of older persons to act collectively to transform the structural conditions of their subordination. The individualistic concern in old age about maintaining ego-identity, self-esteem and dignity leaves older adults vulnerable to manipulation by institutional forces. A psychology of control which encourages the pursuit of individual self-interest, personal control and personal mastery is eventually an identity-limiting discourse and diminishes the productive power of collective interdependence (Knights & Willmott, 1983, 1985).

Power, Its Distribution and Social Exchange

The study of power relationships, especially as these apply to adult interactions, are critical for understanding the process by which individuals perceive themselves to have influence over elements of their social, economic and political environment. As explicit in social exchange theory, the development of power relationships involves an exchange process through which people gain or lose power. Power is therefore derived from imbalances in social exchange which produce differentiated demands for compliance or resistance and independence or dependence. Barrow and Smith (1983) contend that older persons relative to younger persons have less power because of their greater dependency on others who command resources and services.

These exchange processes give rise to a differentiation of power in which certain agencies of intervention attain power by making the satisfaction of the older persons' needs contingent upon their compliance. Therefore, Blau (1964) refers to power as the kinds of influences exercised in social transactions or exchanges where one individual or groups induce others to accede to their wishes by rewarding them for doing so. Modern social scientists continue to use these and very similar definitions of power (cf. Coleman & Cressey, 1984; Doob, 1988; Stark, 1985).

According to these social scientists, various patterns of social interaction are maintained because they yield profit, are rewarding or because they are need-fulfilling. As long as the social exchange is perceived as being more rewarding than costly and leads to minimal loss of personal freedom, the probability of perpetuating the behavior increases (Byrne, 1971; Shaw & Costanzo, 1970). Power relationships and power differentiations are perpetuated in social exchanges as individuals who are more desirous of maintaining the relationship are often placed in inferior position. Individuals use their past experience or personal perceptions of control and effectiveness to predict the outcomes of similar exchanges in the present and for judging the adequacy of outcomes of the future exchange. The ratio of rewards to costs and the ratio of dependency and compliance to independence and resistance will determine if people will have an abundance or deficiency of power resources (Knights & Willmott, 1983, 1985; Renshon, 1974).

However, an important factor about the exchange relationship which cannot be ignored pertains to costs associated with the social exchange. First, there are investment costs that relate to the expenses involved in obtaining skills necessary for providing instrumental services and for acquiring the knowledge base, experience or status related to competent performance in the services. Second, there are direct costs and opportunity costs related to the satisfactory fulfillment of the exchange transaction. The net balance of these rewards and costs determines the extent to which power is possessed (Nichols & Beynon, 1977).

Power in the social exchange between agents or agencies is implicit as long as one agent has resources the other needs and is willing to enter into a relationship in which another's needs may be satisfied. As long as the agents do not extract more compliance than social norms dictate or permit, the interaction process will operate smoothly and continue to be legitimated (Apfelbaum & Lubek, 1976). In fact, the consensus that is maintained will reinforce the norms that are operating and will strengthen the power of those in command.

In summary, a positive balance of exchange is maintained when (1) services can be supplied in order to obtain other needed services; (2) services can be obtained from alternative sources providing similar services; (3) coercion or compliance can be used to force the supply of services; (4) services may be foregone or substituted.

When these basic principles of social exchange are applied to social transactions between older persons and other influential persons it becomes clear that there are a number of inequities in the social exchange with family members, caregivers and institutional agencies. Through forced retirement and the ensuing decreased income there is considerable reduction in the power resources of older persons who, in effect, become social dependents. Those without entitlements become dependent upon friends and relatives leading to further net losses of personal autonomy and power. Martin (1971) proposes that once past obligations have been estimated and paid, family members' feelings of obligation decline while the cost of additional interactions with the socially and economically dependent elders increases. Martin postulates that the "chances of loneliness in old age are in inverse proportion to the number of rewards older people can offer their children for paying attention to them" (p. 110). Under such circumstances social visits will decline considerably unless moral guilt is aroused by the older person's complaints about ill-health, pain or severe depression.

The general picture of social exchange may be somewhat more favorable for those elders who have other sources of power such as money, skills needed or attributes (e.g., pleasant personality, intelligence, social skills) that are in demand. They can use their power resources, in part, to buy some social interactions. But even money alone may not be an appropriate resource to be exchanged for friendship, loyalty, or commitment. However, those that desperately lack reward and attribute resources in social exchange may regain a measure of strength in the relationship by their willingness and capacity to give unquestioned approval and compliance (Dowd, 1975).

In economic social transactions between the old and young, the balance of exchange often favors the younger set who are in demand because of their vitality, current knowledge and technological expertise. Unless older persons are prepared constantly to update their skills and knowledge, the power of older persons is considerably diminished in the market-place. If older people's work history or performance capabilities in the past have been obscure, that is because the stereotypic labels attached to their performance have often caused older persons to act and to portray in accordance with the negative stereotypes (Snyder & Swann, 1977). Many employers expect older persons to be passive and to surrender control and society does not disapprove of these expected patterns. The patterned way of doing things that has been established tips the balance of the exchange relationship in society's favor (Press & McKool, 1972). Many exchange relationships, therefore, involving compliance with authority become legitimized by the normative structure. In many instances pressures are exerted and informal sanctions are levied against the older person to induce total compliance in individuals whose other power resources have been considerably diminished or consumed. An older person may ultimately exchange esteem or status needs for a lowered work load in the work place. The question raised here has clear bearing on the status of older persons. The relationship between power resources and control in later life is not directly patterned by a loss of personal controls or control beliefs in old age but more by normative sanctions and their legitimation in the social structures of the work place.

It is commonplace today to say that the negative labeling and stigmatization process that accompanies old age adversely affects the behavior of elderly individuals, reduces their self-esteem and other power resources (Gergen & Gergen, 1986). Like all generalities, it tails off without any specific recommendations for *how* to look at the power resources in old age and *what* to look for. What we need is a guide to the way in which the older half of humanity connects with and affects the other younger half, via differences and likeliness in motivations for power and influence, dependence and independence, control and self-efficacy. One of the first steps in this complex analysis is to examine the normative structures in power relations and their legitimation in the working world of older persons. We need also to identify the norms and structures that must be indicted, condemned or modified. As discussed earlier in the section on the sources of powerlessness, we know pretty much how the interests of the powerful social structures affect the older persons. To what extent do the interests of the older and weaker persons deprive the younger and more powerful persons with considerably greater power resources? As a first step toward answering this question we need to study the actual sanctions within the social contracts that permit dramatic decreases in the personal autonomy and self-esteem of older individuals as witnessed in a number of research studies (cf. Arling, Harkins & Capitman, 1986; Schulz, 1976, 1978; Schulz & Brenner, 1977). There are recently a number of studies to show that perceived loss of power relations and control are crucial factors in determining mortality rates of older individuals (Bourestom & Pastalan, 1981; Schulz & Brenner, 1977). Heavy demands for passivity or compliance in social exchanges lead to stern power deflation and have been found to be associated with greater physical and mental health impairment and higher rates of mortality in older adults (Krantz & Schulz, 1980; Lieberman & Tobin, 1983; Zweig & Csank, 1975).

To summarize, social control theory suggests that having control and a sense of influence over the environment produces more positive results in the social, emotional and cognitive functioning of older individuals. Conversely, losses in control or pressures for compliance, obedience and approval lead to mortality, depression and impairment in functioning.

Such conclusions are based mostly upon finding of studies done with younger populations and often in laboratory settings. More studies need to be undertaken, however, which address questions of

power deflation in the older persons and which examine the processes
and mechanisms whereby control-enhancing interventions can be designed
for older subjects.

Power and Control Concepts as the Basis
for Promoting Well-Being

The relationship of well-being to feelings of personal control and
influence has been discussed extensively. It has been shown that
perceptions of diminishing control and lack of power and influence in
the environment is associated with a variety of problems and deficits
in the physical, social and mental health functioning of older
persons. Conversely, those who have access to power resources and
perceive they have control and influence generally experience fewer
and less severe problems. What are the implications of these findings
for promoting the well-being of older adults in Western society?

   In a general sense it is not too difficult to design promotional
policies or to restructure environments of older persons to facilitate
the development of feelings of power, influence and vital participation. These statements are based on the assumption that older
people's more basic needs such as food, clothing, shelter, personal
security and self-respect have been satisfactorily met and that what
needs to be redressed are essentially deprivations in higher order
needs such as those of status, role, self-esteem and influence. In
order to increase perceptions of well-being control-enhancing
interventions are necessary at both the individual and societal
levels. Structurally, public policies are necessary which prohibit
the unnecessary reduction of power resources of the elderly. In the
wider social arena, too, it is possible to think of policies designed
to prevent power deflation and to decrease feelings of powerlessness.
In the work place, for example, forced retirement based solely on
chronological age should be discouraged if not prohibited. Comprehensive national health coverage and long-term pension plans would
discourage older adults' economic dependency on others and would
enable older adults to retain more power resources.

   In the area of social change, programs may be developed which
would provide encouragement and support of efforts based on older
individuals' initiative and choice. So too in the family settings,
institutional settings and long-term care settings, the value of
initiative, choice, responsibility and self-efficacy as a basis for
developing helping relationships could be made more widely known and
reinforced. Where expansion or intervention is necessary in the
social domain, Toffler (1970), for example, has recommended a series
of programs including continuing education for coping with social,
cultural and technological change. One may envision educational and
health centres where time and professional assistance are made
available to older persons to work through problems anticipated with
immediate or impending social and occupational transitions or health-

related concerns.   In the area of educational facilities, scholar-
ships, assisted leave period and tuition waivers would revitalize
elderly individuals whose employment skills and knowledge base have
become outdated.

Perhaps the best that can be done in the immediate future is for
governments and social groups to actively educate the public regarding
the significant personal, social and experiential resources which the
older adults have, with straightforward recognition and public
appreciation of the wealth of goods and services older individuals may
provide despite the decline in physical energies.   Here the major
interventive thrust must be on two levels:

(1) The expectations for personal control, influence and social
productivity of older persons must be raised in various spheres of
their social, economic and health-related functioning.   Especially
when diverse and frequently contradictory messages about the capabilities for control and influence are being communicated to older
persons, they are more likely to surrender control to others and to
accept the stereotypes that undervalue them.   Gerontologically-
oriented psychologists, sociologists, medical practitioners can play
their part in integrating elements of control, influence and power
which older adults are realistically capable of acquiring and/or
maintaining and to communicate these to older groups.   Not only must
control-enhancing interventions be designed for older persons but more
importantly, older individuals' initiatives, choices, and directives
must be supported and reinforced.   It should not be too difficult to
think of social policies designed to foster the sense of inclusion of
older persons in the economic, educational and health system, which
would provide their own kind of emotional satisfaction and sense of
self-efficacy.

(2) Beyond the immediate support of control-enhancing activities
lie some fundamental action that will be necessary on the part of
democratic governments to draw out the emancipatory potentials of
older citizens.   Public policies must be firmly articulated so that
older citizens are convinced that the government is responsive and
that citizens do have an impact.   Given the existence of structured
social inequality in the market-place, the structures of domination
used by employers do not exist independently of their continued
reproduction in social practice (Knights & Willmott, 1985).   Accordingly, the primary concern of democratic governments must be to study
the neglected connection between levels of structure (power) and the
surrounding networks of relationships (identity) which undermine or
inhibit the transformative potentials and capacities of older persons
to be independent and interdependent in the use of their power
resources.

Conclusions

The elderly in past times had high levels of perceived power and influence due to their recognized status, role and performance capabilities embodied in the social and religious tenets and mores (Martin, 1971). Today, older adults are not viewed as effective contributors to knowledge, labor or productivity. All too often older citizens are seen to be the most central group of individuals in the wide category of the weak, helpless and repressed (Schulz & Hanusa, 1980). The question raised here has a clear bearing on the power status and power resources of older adults in the society.

Societal pressures exist that reduce the level of the power resources of older persons. Mechanisms for bringing about power deflation also exist and are embodied in the social structures governing the lives of older individuals. Also, age norms that are established and legitimated further reduce the power resources of older persons in society. Evidence examined shows that power deflation and a sense of powerlessness in old age arise out of the complex interplay between the needs of older individuals for security, dignity, self-esteem and influence and society's needs for individuals to be capable, productive and in executive positions of control and influence.

In examining the relationship between power, control and well-being, it is becoming increasingly evident that older persons' perceptions of diminishing control and ability to influence the environment are associated with a variety of mental and physical health problems. What is being argued here is that older persons are being conditioned into becoming helpless and weak because of their generalized expectancies that their actions, efforts or resources cannot and do not influence social outcomes. The strands of these multiple messages combine to produce a widespread social belief system that older citizens cannot and do not exercise influence in their social environment. When individuals do not feel they have sufficient control over events, processes and agencies which are seen to affect their lives an outcome of satisfied acceptance and quiescence cannot be expected.

A review of the literature examining various aspects of control and power resources of elderly individuals shows that losses in power and control have substantially deleterious effects. However, on the positive side, there is evidence to show that older persons' negative perceptions of control and influence over themselves and their environment can be altered. It has also been shown that control-enhancing interventions which allow older persons to successfully manipulate the environment are associated with improved health and well-being. The results collectively suggest that declines in control and perceptions of influence formerly attributed to biological aging may actually be produced by environmental forces and the reactance of people to them. Such findings lead to the conclusion that democratic societies would benefit greatly by taking the older persons' need for autonomy, control and influence more seriously. Elderly citizens must be shown and convinced that they can impact their environment.

Future research needs to be conducted to further unravel the intricacies of these complex phenomena. The nature of specific conditions that contribute to age-related decrements and increments must be more clearly identified and examined more thoroughly. Also the exact combination of structural and individual factors must be determined as well as the relative importance of each.

Control-enhancing interventions primarily at the level of the family, community and social agency, and secondly at the level of governmental impetus are necessary to accomplish the goals which older citizens have to maintain power resources and power relations.

References

Apfelbaum, E., & Lubek, I. (1976). Resolution versus revolution? The theory of conflicts in question. In L. H. Strickland, F. E. Aboud & K. J. Gergen (Eds.), *Social psychology in transition*. New York: Plenum Press.

Arling, G., Harkins, E. B., & Capitman, J. (1986). Institutionalization and personal control: A panel study of impaired older people. *Research on Aging, 8*, 38-56.

Bandura, A. (1977). Self-efficacy: Toward a unifying theory of behavioral change. *Psychological Review, 80*, 191-215.

Bandura, A. (1978). The self system in reciprocal determinism. *American Psychologist, 33*, 344-358.

Bandura, A. (1982). Self-efficacy mechanism in human agency. *American Psychologist, 37*, 122-147.

Barrow, G. M., & Smith, P. A. (1983). *Aging, the individual and society* (2nd ed.). New York: West Publishing.

Blau, P. M. (1964). *Exchange and power in social life*. New York: Wiley & Sons.

Bourestom, N., & Pastalan, L. (1981). The effects of relocation on the elderly: A reply to Borup, J. H., Gallego, D. T., and Heffernan, P. G. The *Gerontologist, 21*, 4-7.

Brim, O. G., Jr. (1974). *The sense of personal control and life-span development.* Unpublished manuscript, Foundation for Child Development, New York.

Brand, F., & Smith R. (1974). Life adjustment and relocation of the elderly. *Journal of Gerontology, 29,* 336-340.

Byrne, J. J. (1971). Systematic analysis and exchange theory: A synthesis. *Pacific Sociological Review, 14,* 137-146.

Coleman, J., & Cressey, D. (1984). *Social problems* (2nd ed.). New York: Harper and Row.

Doob, C.B. (1988). *Sociology: An introduction* (2nd ed.). New York: Holt, Rinehart & Winston.

Dowd, J. J. (1975). Aging as exchange: A preface to theory. *Journal of Gerontology, 30,* 584-594.

Foucault, M. (1980). *Power/knowledge: Selected interviews and other writings.* (C. Gordon, Ed.). New York: Pantheon.

Gergen, M. M., & Gergen, K. J. (1986). The discourse of control and the maintenance of well-being. In M. M. Baltes & P. B. Baltes (Eds.), *The psychology of control and aging* (pp. 119-138). Hillsdale, NJ: Lawrence Erlbaum Associates.

Giddens, A. (1976). *New rules of sociological method.* London: Hutchinson.

Giddens, A. (1977). *Studies in social and political theory.* New York: Basic Books.

Giddens, A. (1979). *Central problems in social theory.* London: Macmillan Co.

Goffman, E. (1961). *Asylums.* Garden City, NY: Anchor Books.

Knights, D., & Willmott, H. C. (1983). Dualism and domination: An analysis of Marxian, Weberian and existentialist perspectives. *Australian, New Zealand Journal of Sociology, 19,* 33-49.

Knights, D., & Willmott, H. C. (1985). Power and identity in theory and practice. Sociological Review, 17, 22-46.

Krantz, D., & Schulz, R. (1980). A model of life crisis, control and health outcomes: Cardiac rehabilitation and relocation of the elderly. In A. Baum & J. Singer (Eds.), *Advances in environmental psychology, Volume 2* (pp. 25-59). Hillsdale, NJ: Lawrence Erlbaum Associates.

Lieberman, M. A., & Tobin, S. S. (1983). *The experience of old age, stress, coping, and survival.* New York: Basic Books.

Martin, J. D. (1971). Power, dependence, and the complaints of the elderly: A social exchange perspective. *Aging and Human Development, 2,* 108-112.

Merton, R. (1957). *Social theory and social structure.* New York: Free Press.

Ng, S. H. (1980). *The social psychology of power.* London: Academic Press.

Nichols, T., & Beynon, H. (1977). *Living with capitalism.* London: Routledge & Kegan Paul.

Olsen, M.E. (Ed.). (1970). *Power in societies.* London: Macmillan Co.

Pollard, W., & Mitchell, T.   (1972).   Decision theory analysis of social power. *Psychological Bulletin, 78,* 433-446.

Press, I., & McKool, M., Jr. (1972). Social structure and status of the aged: Toward some valid cross-cultural generalizations. *Aging and Human Development, 3,* 297-306.

Prewitt, K., & Verba, S. (1977).   *An introduction to American government* (2nd ed.). New York: Harper & Row.

Renshon, S. A. (1974). *Psychological needs and political behavior: A theory of personality and political efficacy.* New York: Free Press.

Schulz, R.   (1976).   Effects of control and predictability on the psychological well-being of the institutionalized aged. *Journal of Personality and Social Psychology, 33,* 563-573.

Schulz, R. (1978). *The psychology of death, dying, and bereavement.* Reading, ME: Addison-Wesley.

Schulz, R., & Brenner, G.   (1977).   Relocation of the aged: A review and theoretical analysis. *Journal of Gerontology, 32,* 323-333.

Schulz, R., & Hanusa, B. H. (1980). Experimental social gerontology: A social psychological perspective. *Journal of Social Issues, 36,* 30-46.

Seligman, M. E. P. (1975). *Helplessness: On depression, development and death.* San Francisco: Freeman.

Shaw, M. E., & Costanzo, P. R.   (1970).   *Theories of social psychology.* New York: McGraw-Hill.

Snyder, M., & Swann, W.   (1977).   Behavior confirmation in social interaction: From social perception to social psychology. *Journal of Experimental Social Psychology, 14,* 148-162.

Stark, R. (1985). *Sociology.* Belmont, CA: Wadsworth.

Steiner, I. D. (1979).   Three kinds of reported choice.   In L. C. Perlmuter & R. A. Monty (Eds.), *Choice and perceived control* (pp. 17-27). Hillsdale, NJ: Lawrence Erlbaum Associates.

Tauney, R. H. (1931). *Equality.* London: Allen and Unwin.

Toffler, A. (1970). *Future shock.* New York: Bantam.

Turk, J., & Bell, U.   (1972).   Measuring power in families. *Journal of Marriage and the Family, 34,* 215-222.

Weber, M.   (1947).   *The theory of social and economic organization.* New York: Oxford University Press.

Winter, D. G. (1973). *The power motive.* New York: Free Press.

Zweig, J. P., & Csank, J. Z.   (1975).   Effects of relocation on chronically ill geriatric patients of a medical unit: Mortality rates. *Journal of the American Geriatrics Society, 23,* 132-136.

Psychological Perspectives of Helplessness
and Control in the Elderly, P.S. Fry (ed.)
© *Elsevier Science Publishers B.V. (North-Holland), 1989*

Chapter Twelve

ENHANCING MEMORY BY MODIFYING CONTROL BELIEFS, ATTRIBUTIONS, AND PERFORMANCE GOALS IN THE ELDERLY

Elaine ELLIOTT
Center for Cognitive Therapy, Newton, MA

Margie E. LACHMAN
Brandeis University

Abstract

Fear of losing memory is a prevalent concern of the elderly. Most researchers seeking solutions to the memory problems associated with aging have focused on psychopharmacological interventions or traditional memory training programs, e.g. teaching the use of visual mnemonics or organizational strategies. To date, neither approach has been highly effective in producing generalized, sustained improvements. We present an alternative approach to intervention-- cognitive restructuring of self-conceptions about memory. Self-conceptions include a set of beliefs concerning one's memory capabilities, the degree to which one can exercise control over memory, and whether aging results in irreversible memory loss. We present evidence that these self-conceptions affect memory performance and that the elderly are especially vulnerable to maladaptive self-conceptions; i.e. a belief that memory capacity shrinks with age and is irreversible. We describe a framework in which self-conceptions of memory and goals result in adaptive and maladaptive constellations of cognition (e.g., attributions), affect (e.g., anxiety, depression), and behavior (e.g., use of effective strategies, persistence) that impact on memory performance. We present two cognitive restructuring interventions designed to modify dysfunctional self-conceptions of memory, and thus, promote adaptive thought, affect, and behavior to cope with memory problems. This approach could be used in conjunction with psychopharmacological treatments or memory strategy training programs to ameliorate memory loss in older adults.

Introduction

Along with fears of losing health and independence, the fear of losing memory is one of the most prevalent concerns of the elderly in our society. In fact, for many, memory loss is equated with senility or Alzheimer's disease. Often images of devastating and irreversible cognitive deterioration are conjured up at the instant an elderly individual misplaces shoes or forgets a name. While there are losses in memory functioning that accompany the natural aging process, not all memory problems are irreversible.

Solutions to the problems associated with memory loss seem imperative if we are to optimize functioning in later life. Much attention and research monies have gone into psychopharmacological solutions, but to date there are no highly effective drug treatments (Eisdorfer & Stotsky, 1977; Reisberg, Borenstein, Franssen, Shulman, Steinberg, & Ferris, 1986; Reisberg, Ferris, & DeLeon, 1981; Riesberg, Ferris & Gershon, 1981). Other researchers have devoted attention to developing training programs to ameliorate memory loss. Most of these have focused on helping the elderly develop mnemonic strategies (e.g., method of loci). As will be seen, these training programs have failed to produce generalized, sustained improvements in memory.

In this chapter we will present a third area of intervention-- cognitive restructuring of self-conceptions about memory-, which could be used in conjunction with psychopharmocological or memory strategy treatments. Self-conceptions include a set of beliefs concerning one's memory capabilities, the degree to which one can exercise control over one's memory, and whether aging results in irreversible loss. We present evidence that these self-conceptions affect memory performance and suggest that the elderly are especially vulnerable to maladaptive self-conceptions of memory, e.g., a belief that memory capacity shrinks with age. We propose cognitive restructuring interventions designed to modify the elderly's dysfunctional beliefs about the uncontrollability of memory and its inevitable deterioration.

We propose that restructuring maladaptive self-concepts of memory could be beneficial regardless of the underlying cause of the deficit. That is, even in some cases with an organic etiology, an adaptive self-concept of memory will facilitate the implementation of strategies that will ameliorate the impairment. Moreover, those with non-organic memory deficits may, as a result of their self-concepts of memory, appear very similar to those with organically based problems. The focus of this chapter is how to prevent and remediate memory problems associated with normal aging and not those losses associated with major organic brain syndrome. We do, however, suggest that cognitive restructuring could be used in conjunction with more traditional pharmacological interventions for early stages of Alzheimer's disease.

In overview, we will review traditional memory training treatments, discussing progress and limitations in ameliorating memory loss in the elderly. We will then present a rationale for another area of intervention, cognitive restructuring of self-conceptions of memory. This intervention is rooted in research which demonstrates that control beliefs and attributions are important mediators of cognitive performance. First, we will review this literature and studies illustrating that the elderly are especially prone to maladaptive control beliefs and attributions. We will then present a theoretical framework in which self-conceptions of memory ability and goals set up adaptive and maladaptive constellations of cognition (e.g., beliefs about control over memory, attributions), affect (e.g., anxiety, depression), and behavior (e.g., use of effective strategies, persistence) that impact on memory performance. Next we present a rationale and plan for a research program that involves training of memory strategies in conjunction with cognitive restructuring of beliefs about memory. We will suggest cognitive interventions designed to modify self-conceptions of memory and, thus, promote adaptive thought, affect and behavior to cope with memory problems. Finally, we will point to areas of needed research and suggest possible prevention programs.

Traditional Memory Training Programs

A great deal of effort has been devoted to developing training programs using strategies both to remediate and prevent memory loss in the elderly. Although training has been most successful for the remediation of minimal memory impairment (Hill, Sheikh, & Yesavage, 1986), there is some evidence that use of visual mnemonics or organizational strategies can help to compensate for impairment caused by neurological deficits (Poon, 1985).

Memory training programs typically focus on teaching organizational strategies and/or improving concentration and attention (Lapp, 1987; Yesavage, 1985). Research has indicated that the elderly are less likely than the young to generate spontaneously visual images or to organize the material when faced with a memory task (Poon, 1985). Programs designed to teach visualization strategies through verbal elaboration or visual imagery have been relatively successful. Two of the most popular mnemonic strategies are visual image associations for name-face recall and the method of loci for list learning (Lapp, 1987; Yesavage, 1985). The image association involves looking for a dominant feature in the person's face, transforming the person's name by finding meaning in it, and visualizing the feature and the name transformation together.

We will highlight the method of loci because we are currently using it in our research. Method of loci involves making an association between a list of items or concepts to be remembered and a predetermined list of locations. First, subjects are asked to learn to visualize a series of locations in a familiar sequence (e.g., the route one takes when one enters one's home). Next subjects visualize the items from the word lists in the various locations (e.g., banana on the doormat). When asked to recall the items from the list, the subject visualizes each of the locations. This facilitates recall of the items which should be associated with each of the locations.

It has been found that combining method of loci with pretraining in making visual or verbal associations increases the effects. For example, when method of loci is combined with verbal elaboration or emotional impressions, the effects on memory performance are greater. Verbal judgments serve to augment the depth of processing of visual material through verbal elaboration (Yesavage, 1985) and lead to broader transfer effects than method of loci training alone (Hill et al., 1986). These judgments can take the form of image associations or emotional impressions (Lapp, 1987). For example, if a banana is visualized on the doormat, one could make the image association, "Don't step on the banana or it will be a mashed banana" and the emotional impression, "It would be a shame if someone slipped on the peel!"

Another common pretraining technique is relaxation training designed to reduce anxiety (Yesavage, 1985). Strategy training has been found more effective when combined with relaxation training. Although the effects of training on memory are enhanced, the transfer still is limited. It is possible that relaxation training, while reducing anxiety and arousal which are detrimental to memory, is not more effective because it does not modify the cognitions about memory aging and performance which underlie the anxiety.

In summary, training programs focused on memory and on other cognitive abilities (e.g., fluid intelligence) have been relatively successful in improving some aspects of memory and intellectual performance (Baltes & Willis, 1982; Poon, 1984; Willis, in press; Yesavage, 1985). Nevertheless, the effects of memory training have been limited. The major weaknesses cited are that the effects apply only to tests that are highly similar to the training materials, the strategies are not used outside of the laboratory, and the effects are short-lived (Greenberg, 1986; Poon, 1984, 1985). Attempts to improve memory training have typically combined multiple methods of training, included a pretraining program, or modified the training in accordance with individual differences in variables such as IQ or anxiety (Yesavage, 1985). These modifications do indeed result in improvements but only in that the effects for the trained tasks are stronger or there is transfer to a wider range of laboratory tasks. Existing training programs have thus failed to produce generalized, sustained improvements in memory.

Given the apparent ability of the elderly to benefit from memory training programs, what factors might account for poor generalization of training effects? Non-ability-related cognitive factors, such as beliefs and inferences about memory performance, may play an important role in influencing these patterns. Negative cognitions about memory capabilities can cause anxiety and interfere with task-related attention, resulting in performance and motivational deficits. It has been suggested that subjects in memory training studies have failed to apply newly-learned strategies in everyday settings because they are not motivated to do so (Hill, Sheikh, Yesavage, & Ponich, 1986; Poon, 1985). One possible source of poor motivation is the elderly's belief that they cannot do anything to improve their memory.

Self-Conceptions of Memory Aging

A growing body of evidence indicates that successful functioning requires not only skills, but also self-conceptions that foster effective use of these skills (Bandura, 1987; Rodin, Cashman, & Desiderato, 1987). Self-conceptions of memory include a set of beliefs concerning one's memory capabilities; the degree to which one can exercise control over one's memory; and whether aging results in irreversible memory loss. Based on research in other areas of cognitive functioning, there is every reason to believe that such self-conceptions should have significant impact on how well the elderly use their memory capabilities. Indeed, in their review of intervention programs for enrichment and prevention in the elderly, Rodin and her colleagues (1987, p. 162) concluded, " the data support the assertion that cognitive interventions which affect subjects' feelings of control may lead to more generalized effects than other types of cognitive intervention."

Does traditional memory training alone influence self-conceptions about memory? Most training studies have failed to assess self-conceptions. Overall, there is little evidence that current forms of memory training have an impact on the trainees' sense of control or efficacy regarding their memory (Hill, Sheikh, Yesavage & Ponich, 1986). There is, however, some evidence to suggest that if training includes some cognitive restructuring, memory self-confidence may be increased (Lachman & Dick, 1987).

To the extent that one can instill and strengthen in the elderly the belief that memory can be changed and controlled, it should enhance their motivation to apply strategies to solve memory problems, promote adaptive attributions, and facilitate their performance on memory tasks. We will present a framework for elucidating how self-conceptions mediate attributions and, in turn, cognitive performance. First, however, we will review studies demonstrating that the elderly are especially prone to problematic attributions and control beliefs and that modifying these attributions and control beliefs has positive consequences.

Age differences in attributions and control beliefs. A great deal of research has found that attributing failures to internal stable factors and successes to external factors is maladaptive and is associated with depression, low self-esteem, and poor subsequent performance (Abramson, Seligman, & Teasdale, 1978).

There is evidence that the elderly make less adaptive attributions for cognitive performance than do the young (Blank, 1982; Banziger & Drevenstedt, 1982; Lachman & McArthur, 1986). When faced with failure, the elderly are prone to blame it on internal, stable, and global factors, such as low ability. When they experience success they are less likely to take credit for it and are prone to attribute it to external, unstable factors. This attributional pattern is associated with decreased motivation, low effort expenditure, and poor performance following failure on cognitive tasks. Not surprisingly, the elderly also believe they have less control over their cognitive functioning (Lachman, 1986) and their memory (Hultsch, Hertzog, & Dixon, 1987). Moreover, attributions and control beliefs are related to cognitive performance in the elderly (Lachman, Steinberg, and Trotter, 1987).

Interventions to modify attributions and control beliefs. There have been a number of studies in which the actual controllability of the environment has been modified, with positive effects on psychological and physical functioning (e.g., Langer & Rodin, 1976; Schulz & Hanusa, 1978). However, only a few studies have modified the elderly's beliefs about control or attributions (Rodin & Langer, 1980; Rodin, 1983). Change in personal belief systems is important if the effects are to generalize across situations (Rodin et al., 1987). Rodin (1983) modified beliefs about efficacy and control in elderly nursing home residents, using a cognitive-behavioral technique designed to instill confidence and perceived control. Gaining confidence in one's competence and controllability over outcomes resulted in dramatic improvements in recall and activity level, and reductions in stress level and cortisol levels.

After documenting that the elderly are more likely to make self (internal) attributions than environmental (external) attributions for negative outcomes, Rodin and Langer (1980) designed an intervention to modify attributions. For example, they told elderly nursing home residents that the reason they were tired was because they were forced to rise early rather than that they were getting old, and that the reason they had trouble walking was because the tile floors were slippery rather than that they were suffering from aging-related motor problems. After the reattribution training, the elderly adults became more active, more sociable, and healthier.

Lachman and Dick (1987) demonstrated that combining memory training with an attributional persuasion retraining technique led to increased confidence in memory ability in elderly adults, whereas memory training alone did not. Method of loci has been found to be a relatively successful mnemonic strategy for the elderly. In this pilot study, they investigated whether method of loci training affects beliefs about memory in the elderly. The study was also designed to examine whether a brief attributional retraining technique would enhance the effects of memory training. As expected, the method of loci training itself was effective in improving memory performance and increasing performance predictions on the task trained. However, due to a ceiling-effect the effects were attenuated. The attribution training in conjunction with memory training was effective in improving memory performance and in improving confidence about memory. The group who received attribution training also developed more adaptive attributions for the transfer task, although not for the trained task (possibly due to a ceiling effect problem). There was, however, no transfer of training effects to a far transfer task, text recognition. These results suggest that the use of attributional retraining in conjunction with method of loci training may enhance not only memory performance but also attitudes and beliefs about memory, the ingredients deemed necessary for generalizability outside the laboratory.

Although the Lachman and Dick study provides preliminary evidence that beliefs about memory can be changed, the results also suggest that modifying attributions alone does not produce the broad effects desired. We propose that a broader program of cognitive restructuring specifically aimed at modifying self-conceptions of memory and more core motivational components is needed. Changing these self-conceptions and more basic underlying mechanisms is expected to have a more enduring and widespread effect on both attributions and memory performance.

A Framework for Linking Self-Conceptions and Performance

Goals predict patterns of performance. The Lachman and Dick study (1987) as well as other studies indicate that attributional retraining results in increased persistence and improved performance on the trained intellectual task (Andrews & Debos, 1978; Chapin & Dyck, 1976; Dweck, 1975; Rhodes, 1977), but these changes are not necessarily maintained or generalized to other tasks (Forsterling, 1985; Rodin, 1983).

We propose that to help the elderly deal effectively with memory problems, one must orient them toward a constellation of adaptive thought, affect, and behavior, and not simply adaptive attributions.

Research on achievement motivation and performance has clearly documented adaptive and maladaptive approaches to intellectual tasks. The adaptive ("mastery-oriented") pattern is characterized by meeting intellectual tasks head on, effective persistence in the face of difficulty, and continued positive affect in the pursuit of mastery. In contrast, the maladaptive ("helpless") pattern is characterized by avoidance and giving up in the face of difficulty.   Individuals displaying this pattern tend to evidence negative affect (such as anxiety),   negative   self-referent   cognitions,   and   dysfunctional attributions when they encounter obstacles (e.g., Ames, 1984; C. Diener & Dweck, 1978, 1980; Dweck & Repucci, 1973; Nicholls, 1975). Although individuals displaying these different patterns often do not differ in intellectual ability, these patterns have strong effects on cognitive performance (Dweck, 1986).

The bases of these patterns lie in the goals that are adopted for achievement tasks (Dweck & Elliott, 1983).   Elliott and Dweck (1988) demonstrated that when children are oriented toward performance goals, in which they seek to demonstrate to themselves and/or others that they are competent, *and* they believe themselves to lack ability, they display the maladaptive pattern on intellectual tasks.   When children are oriented toward a learning goal, in which they seek to develop ability, they display an adaptive approach, regardless of level of perceived ability.

These divergent effects were accompanied by substantial differences in performance.

Several conclusions can be drawn from these studies:

1)   Dysfunctional attributional and performance patterns arise when people are oriented toward a performance goal (i.e., *documenting* their abilities to themselves and/or others) *and* doubt their competence.   Adaptive patterns emerge when they are oriented toward a learning goal (i.e., developing their abilities).

2)   Dysfunctional attributions for failure are part of a stream of self-referent thought that detracts from focusing on task demands.   Those showing adaptive patterns rarely make attributions during task performance; they are focused on overcoming failure rather than accounting for it.

3)   Structuring environments to promote learning goals is likely to foster skill acquisition and facilitate performance.

This research has implications for the conceptualization and treatment of many chronic achievement difficulties, motivational problems, test and performance anxieties, avoidance reactions in evaluative settings, and stress reactions.   These psychological problems can be viewed as manifestations of performance goals combined with low perceived ability in the domain in question.   Presumably, helping individuals shift to a learning goal would ameliorate these problems, both relieving subjective distress and enhancing performance.   This strategy should prove more effective than attributional retraining, because attributions are a product of achievement goal/perceived ability interactions.   In fact, attributional retraining may conceivably represent a band-aid approach to modifying problematic inference patterns. It may help people ward off the conclusion that they lack ability when they encounter obstacles and thus bolster their confidence that they can do it. It is not likely, however, to alter the performance goal that predisposes them to focus on evaluating their ability in the first place. By helping people become learning-oriented, it should be possible to predispose them to evaluate the adequacy of their problem-solving strategies rather than the adequacy of themselves, and thus to keep them task-focused.

Evidence that people tend to make negative ability attributions for failure on memory tasks as they age suggests that they become increasingly performance-oriented with respect to memory functioning. That is, they appear to become oriented towards evaluating their memory capacity, rather than towards developing or maintaining it. This orientation, combined with the implicit belief that memory capacity decreases with age, may underlie the vulnerability to patterns of negative self-referent thought, poor problem-solving, and deficient performance when confronted with memory problems. A cognitive intervention designed to help the elderly become learning-oriented in coping with memory difficulties should be an effective way to enhance the acquisition and generalized use of memory strategies.

Self-conceptions of ability orient individuals to goals. How do individuals become oriented toward different goals? M. Bandura & Dweck (1988) showed that children's conceptions of ability orient them toward different goals: children who believe ability is a fixed trait or "entity" tend to seek favorable judgment of that trait (performance goals), whereas children who believe ability is a malleable quality strive to develop it (learning goal). These goals, in turn, foster different approaches to intellectual tasks.

They found that a key difference between children oriented toward performance and learning goals was the rules they used to draw inferences about their abilities. The performance-oriented, who seek judgments of competence, judged themselves capable when they easily outperformed others on normatively difficult tasks. The learning-oriented, who seek to develop competence, judged themselves most capable when they improved their skill through their efforts on personally challenging tasks.

Effort and high ability inferences appear to be inversely related within a performance goal perspective (i.e., "The harder you try, the less ability you possess."), and positively related within a learning goal perspective (i.e., "The harder you try, the smarter you get."). These different ways of assessing ability were related to different patterns of standard setting, task choice, interpretations of mistakes and effort expenditure, and affective reactions in achievement situations. Table 1 summarizes these diverse effects of goal orientations. These findings shed light on the cognitive schemas

Table 1

Model of Relationships Among Conceptions of Intelligence, Achievement Goals, and Patterns of Achievement-Related Thought, Affect and Behavior

Conceptions of Intelligence

Entity View	Incremental View
Intelligence is a fixed, unchangeable quantity.	Intelligence is a set of skills and body of knowledge that can be increased through effort expenditure.

Achievement Goal

Performance Goal	Learning Goal
To maintain positive judgments of competence	To increase competence

Cognitive, Affective, & Behavioral Patterns

	Performance Goal	Learning Goal
Definition of success:	High outcome/low effort relative to others	Increased competence relative to past performance
Errors:	Signify lack of competence	Information for improvement
Performance Standards:	Stringent, rigid	Flexible, attainable
Effort Expenditure:	Threatening	Positively valued
Affective Reactions:	Pride or relief, anxiety	Excitement, enthusiasm, boredom, disappointment
Task Choice:	Maximizes display of competence	Maximizes learning opportunities

underlying the different reactions accompanying learning- and perfor-
mance-orientations found by Elliott and Dweck (1988).

Table 1 also includes a factor found to be associated with
achievement goals -- children's beliefs about intelligence. Children
viewing intelligence as a fixed, stable attribute, the quantity of
which is revealed through performance (entity conception), tended to
favor performance goals. They sought to validate that their ability
was high and to avoid evaluation that it was low. In contrast,
children viewing intelligence as a changeable attribute -- as a set of
skills and knowledge that can be increased through effort (incremental
conception) -- favored a learning goal. They sought to develop their
intellectual skills. Beliefs about the stability and controllability
of intelligence appear to predispose children toward different goals.

Recent research by Wood and A. Bandura (1987) showed that adults
who performed a challenging decision-making task under an induced
entity conception of ability suffered a loss in perceived self-
efficacy, lowered their goals, and became less efficient in their
analytic strategies. In contrast, those who performed the task under
an acquirable skill conception of ability sustained their perceived
efficacy, continued to set challenging goals, and used effective
analytic strategies.

Extending the framework to memory performance of elderly adults.
This framework can be fruitfully extended to the elderly and memory
functioning. There is evidence that older adults view memory capacity
and function from an "entity perspective." That is, memory capacity
is seen as an uncontrollable attribute that "shrinks" with age
(Hultsch et al., 1987; Lachman, Baltes, Nesselroade, & Willis, 1982).
Hence, as people age they believe their memory abilities decrease, and
that losses are irreversible and uncontrollable. They may also believe
that poor performance on one memory task indicates deterioration in
all aspects of memory. These beliefs would predispose them to become
less confident and more performance-oriented with respect to memory
function. This performance goal - low perceived ability combination
is especially likely to impede learning and problem-solving. A
cognitive intervention that instills a learning orientation towards
memory functioning would promote an "incremental" conception of
memory. Within this conception memory capacity is controllable and
memory can be improved through effort. Table 2 illustrates the
predicted relationship among beliefs about memory, goals, and
responses to memory problems.

In sum, as people age they will be increasingly prone to evaluate
their memory capacities negatively rather than to attempt to improve
them. That is, they become especially vulnerable to the belief that
their memory ability has begun to deteriorate irreversibly. As a
consequence their goal is to monitor and evaluate the extent of the
deterioration. Within this view, any memory problem is seen as a sign
of inevitable and uncontrollable decline and is met with low persist-

Table 2

Predicted Relationships Among Beliefs About Memory,

Goals, and Response to Memory Problems

Beliefs about Memory	Goal	Responses to Memory Problems
Memory capacity is an entity that automatically and irreversibly deteriorates with age. (Shrinking Entity)	Performance Goal: Evaluate one's ---> memory capacity. --->	Attributed to loss of memory and aging, Low use of compensatory strategies, Low persistence, Avoidance of difficult tasks, Dysphoric mood
Memory is multi-faceted. Although some facets of memory may decline, with effort and compensatory strategies, memory can be improved.	Learning Goal: Develop strategies ---> for improving --->atus memory.	Attributions to insufficient effort or ineffective strategies, Development and use of compensatory strategies, High persistence, Involvement in challenging tasks

ence in the search for compensatory strategies. We hypothesize that by helping the elderly critically evaluate the belief that memory is a "shrinking entity", and by promoting a view of memory as controllable, we can foster a learning orientation towards memory problems. That is, by promoting a view that memory is multifaceted and that use of effort and compensatory strategies improves it, elderly persons will become oriented toward the goal of finding ways to develop their capacities. Thus memory problems will trigger increased effort in a search for effective strategies. In short, this will foster an orientation that is associated with thought patterns and affective reactions that will enhance memory performance.

We are using this framework to develop interventions to be described later. First, however, we describe preliminary work testing and validating the framework.

Testing and Validating Theoretical Underpinnings with Elderly Adults

Ideally, prior to developing interventions, some correlational and experimental work would be done to test the framework we have presented. We, along with Mary Bandura, are conducting such empirical work.

Although there is evidence that older persons believe that memory decline is irreversible and uncontrollable, we are currently examining the relationship between self-conceptions of ability and goals and reported and actual memory performance. We are refining a scale which taps a view of memory as an uncontrollable entity that shrinks over time (e.g. "Once your memory starts to go, there isn't much you can do about it") versus a view of memory as controllable and that can be improved (e.g. "If you work at it you can improve your memory"). A memory goal scale is also being developed that is designed to assess learning and performance goals with respect to memory, e.g., "When I think about doing memory problems I hope: that they are a challenge for me so I can learn new ways of remembering things" (learning goal); or "that they are easy for me" (performance goal). It is predicted that having a view of memory as a shrinking entity is associated with performance goals, and lower reported and actual memory performance.

We also have designed an experiment to test the effectiveness of cognitive restructuring programs. The proposed project involves two forms of training. The first is memory training designed to teach mnemonic strategies. Specifically, the method of loci and verbal elaboration by making judgments about the word stimuli will be trained (Lapp, 1987; Yesavage & Rose, 1984). As described above, method of loci has been found to be one of the most successful mnemonic strategies for the young and the elderly. However, the effects of training are limited to list learning. Combining method of loci with pretraining in making verbal judgments has been found to be even more effective, but still shows limited generalizability across tasks (Yesavage & Rose, 1984). The second type of training involves cognitive restructuring of self-conceptions of memory. Self-conceptions of memory include a set of beliefs concerning one's memory capabilities; the degree to which one can exercise control over one's memory; and whether aging results in irreversible memory loss. The research will examine the effects that memory training and cognitive restructuring have, both singly and in combination, on self-conceptions of memory and memory performance. Of special interest is the extent to which changes are generalized across memory tasks and maintained over time.

Young (ages 18 to 30) and elderly (ages 63 to 75) subjects will be randomly assigned to one of five treatment groups: memory training, cognitive restructuring, cognitive restructuring with memory training, a practice control group, and a no-contact control group. It is expected that both young and elderly adults will benefit from memory training and that the elderly adults will achieve greater benefits from cognitive restructuring than the young, largely because the young already have more adaptive control beliefs and attributional patterns regarding their memory performance. The young are expected to outperform the elderly on all memory tasks. Although memory training with cognitive restructuring will not eliminate the age differences, it is expected to minimize the differences.

Memory training should improve memory performance more on tasks that are closely related to those trained (near transfer tasks) than on far transfer tasks, but these circumscribed benefits will dissipate with time. Those who receive cognitive restructuring with memory training, however, are expected to show greater amounts of transfer across near and far tasks, and more long-term effects of training. Training effects will be assessed immediately following training and one month and six months following training. These memory gains are expected because the cognitive restructuring program focuses on instilling a learning orientation toward memory ability, which should in turn lead to greater perceived control and more functional attributional patterns. Although the method of loci technique is not easily applied to the far transfer tasks, transfer is expected because of the newly acquired adaptive self-conceptions and the experience of success in improving performance. The cognitive restructuring program alone should have much greater impact on beliefs than on memory performance, because success experience and performance feedback on memory tasks is additionally needed to achieve improvements in memory. The practice control group is expected to show some small improvement on memory tasks due to practice effects. However, the effects should be limited to the tasks that were practiced and no transfer to other tasks or to self-conceptions is expected. This group is included to compare the effects of practice and contact with those of training because in other cognitive training studies (Baltes & Willis, 1982; Rodin et al., 1987), practice has produced significant improvement in performance. The no-contact control group is expected to show very little improvement, although there may be a minimal amount due to the experience of taking the memory tasks at the pretest and three posttests. Neither the control groups nor the memory training alone should produce significant changes in self-conceptions of memory.

Assessment of Memory Complaints in the Elderly Prior to Treatment

Memory complaints and depression. As indicated previously, physical and psychological factors may be involved in the etiology of the older adult's memory problems (Eisdorfer & Stotsky, 1977). Before any treatment is begun for memory problems, a careful evaluation of the elderly client is needed. An assessment should be made to determine if the memory deficits are associated with depression, drug reactions, or physical problems. The elderly adults' complaints about memory problems are more often associated with depression than with impaired function (Kahn, Zarit, and Hilbert, 1975). The Geriatric Depression Scale (Yesavage,1987) and the Beck Depression Inventory (Beck, Rush, Shaw, & Emery, 1979) have been found to be valid measures of depression for the elderly.

Memory complaints and organic brain syndrome. Clients, of course, should also be asked to bring in all their medications and should have had a recent physical exam. The *Mental Status Questionnaire* and the *Face-Hand Test* are two instruments that may be used for screening intellectual deficits that are associated with organic brain syndrome in the elderly (Zarit, Miller, & Kahn, 1978). These instruments are not definitive. Unfortunately, diagnosis of Alzheimer's remains complex (see Crook & Miller, 1985; Khachaturian, 1985). Definitive diagnosis can only come with brain tissue autopsy. It is often very difficult to know whether an individual is in the early stages of Alzheimer's or is experiencing a mild and relatively stable form of memory impairment (Crook & Miller, 1985).

Cognitive Restructuring Interventions

Using cognitive restructuring in conjunction with other interventions. Although these factors should be assessed, the presence of depression or organic brain syndrome does not rule out the use of cognitive-restructuring treatments for memory problems. If depression is detected it should be treated first, e.g., with cognitive therapy techniques (Beck et al., 1979) adapted for elderly adult populations (see Emery, 1981; Thompson, Davies, Gallagher & Krantz, 1986), prior to introducing cognitive restructuring interventions for self-conceptions of memory. If an organic brain syndrome is suspected, given their variable progression, and given that misdiagnosis as an irreversible condition is quite common, i.e. 10%-30% (Khachaturian, 1985), cognitive restructuring plus memory strategies and possibly pharmacological treatments could be used to ameliorate the deterioration in the early stages.

Rationale for using cognitive restructuring for memory and aging.
We hold that even the discovery of a pharmacologic treatment for
memory loss may not obviate the need for cognitive intervention. This
suggestion is derived from research findings in depression demonstrating that even with endogenous depression (e.g., depressions that
respond to biological interventions), a combination of medication and
cognitive therapy may be more efficacious than either one alone
(Blackburn, 1985).

Work currently being done in evaluating different treatment
approaches to depression may further inform our thinking. Parallels
may be drawn between matching treatments for depression (Beck et al.,
1979) and matching treatments for memory problems in the elderly. It
seems that in regard to response to treatment, depressions are
heterogeneous (Beck et al., 1979; Simons, Lustman, Wetzel, & Murphy,
1985; Zimmerman & Coryell, 1986). Pharmacological agents can be very
valuable in the acute treatment of some depressions. Other depressions appear to respond to cognitive therapy alone (Rush, Hollon,
Beck, & Kovacs, 1978). For others a combination of cognitive therapy
and anti-depressants may work best (Blackburn, 1985). Beck et al.
(1979) suggest that even when a careful assessment is made in order to
select a particular treatment, gaps in our understanding of the
etiology of depression limit the clinicians ability to specify the
optimal treatment. Although strides are currently being made in
matching treatment with type of depression (e.g., Simons et al., 1985;
Zimmerman & Coryell, 1986; Zimmerman, Coryell, & Pfohl, 1986), an
empirical trial-and-error approach is often needed. A thorough
initial evaluation may suggest a particular approach (e.g., anti-
depressants), but careful re-evaluations of that approach are needed
to determine if the patient is responding. If the response is not
satisfactory, modification of the treatment may be necessary (e.g.,
change medication, add cognitive therapy, or try cognitive therapy
alone) until improvement is achieved.

It appears that specifying treatment for memory complaints shares
many problems in common with specifying treatment for depression. The
cause of memory problems is multifactorial and much work in psychological and biological assessment needs to be done before clients can be
matched to optimal treatments. Here too, initially, an empirical
approach may be needed.

Compared to drug treatments for depression, a pharmacologic
intervention for the prevention of memory loss associated with senile
dementia is still in its infancy. The cholinergic system is believed
to be a possible locus of memory impairment related to Alzheimer's
disease. Studies have shown a deficiency of the enzyme choline
acetyltranferase associated with Alzheimer's (Bowen, White, &
Spillane, 1979; Davies & Maloney, 1976; Mash, Flynn & Potter, 1985;
Perry, Perry, & Blessed, 1977; Perry, Perry, & Blessed, 1978; Perry,
Tomlinson, & Blessed, 1978). The cholinergic system has been

implicated in memory processes (Reisberg, Ferris, & Gershon, 1981). For example, it is known that anticholinergic substances like scopolamine produce amnesia. Agents that enhance cholinergic functioning, e.g., physostigmine are being investigated. Currently there is no known drug treatment capable of modifying memory loss from Alzheimer's disease (Crook, 1986; Harbaugh, 1987; Reisberg, Borenstein, Franssen, Shulman, Steinberg, & Ferris, 1986). None of the cognitive acting drugs have been demonstrated to have a significant long-term impact in reversing or retarding intellectual impairment (Reisberg, Ferris, DeLeon, 1985; Reisberg, Ferris, & Gershon, 1981).

Some who have reviewed the pharmacologic research have begun to attend to the relatively neglected clinical changes accompanying Alzheimer's disease. Eisdorfer and Stotsky (1977) suggest that treatment of disorders associated with organic brain syndrome, e.g. depression, remains the most significant clinical strategy. Reisberg et al. (1986) suggest that clinical symptoms appear to result from two primary interacting processes -- neurochemical changes and the psychological impact of cognitive losses. They suggest that paranoid and delusional ideation associated with Alzheimer's, e.g. that people are stealing things, may stem from memory problems such as not recalling the location of household objects. These researchers suggest that these symptoms may be amenable, to some extent, to psychotherapeutic interventions.

It appears that the elderly experiencing memory loss problems are generating patterns of beliefs and attributions that are even being noted by those who are searching for pharmacologic treatments. We suggest that future research look at the efficacy of combining psychotherapeutic interventions such as the one we described with pharmacologic agents in the amelioration of Alzheimer's disease.

Clearly, not every elderly client with memory complaints will benefit from a cognitive restructuring program. Because the restructuring techniques we are about to describe are rooted in cognitive therapy techniques, Rosenbaum's *Self Control Schedule* (1980) may be useful in assessing the appropriateness of using cognitive restructuring for particular clients. Researchers (Simons et al., 1985) have found that depressed patients who score high on this scale which measures learned resourcefulness seem to benefit most from cognitive therapy techniques. Future research needs to determine if this scale or others may be used to predict the elderly client's response to cognitive restructuring procedures.

The cognitive interventions that follow are rooted in our previously described conceptual framework and cognitive therapy techniques. We are currently in the process of testing these interventions. As yet, we have no data to support their efficacy, but there is a wealth of evidence supporting the use of cognitive therapy techniques in the modification of dysfunctional beliefs associated with depression (see Blackburn, 1985, for a review). Given that we hypothesize that dysfunctional beliefs about memory are central to many memory problems, there is good reason to support the use of this type of intervention in the modification of these beliefs. Clearly, however, research must validate their effectiveness and tease apart the pieces of the interventions that are related to change in memory performance.

What might a cognitive restructuring program for memory and aging look like? Let us first describe one we have begun to develop with Mary Bandura for our research. In this program we are using a group format to restructure self-conceptions of memory and goals.

Group cognitive restructuring program. The purpose of the cognitive restructuring component of the study is to help the elderly adopt a learning goal when confronted with memory tasks. A group format will be used because it has been effective for the elderly (Yost, Buetler, Corbishley & Allenden, 1986). Emphasis will be placed on modifying their beliefs about memory functioning, because beliefs are likely to play a critical role in influencing goal orientation. This cognitive restructuring program will therefore focus on: (1) educating the elderly about two different views of memory (i.e., as a shrinking entity versus a controllable attribute, that can be improved with effort), and how these conceptions influence people's orientation toward memory tasks; (2) promoting the view of memory as controllable through effort; (3) training in self-instructional strategies that support a learning orientation toward memory tasks; and (4) structuring opportunities to generate novel strategies useful in solving memory problems. This latter step is designed to provide experience in generating solutions to memory difficulties, so as to increase the likelihood that the participants will apply strategies to everyday problem situations. The cognitive restructuring will be conducted in 4 one-hour sessions.

The educational session will consist of didactic instruction, group discussion, and video presentation. The trainer will discuss different views of memory ability. A sample of such a protocol might be "People seem to have different beliefs about memory and what happens to it as they get older. Some people think that as they grow old they begin to lose their ability to remember things and there just isn't much they can do about it. Others believe that although there are some changes in memory as they grow older, these are not so terrible, and that they can prevent memory problems by extra effort and developing some new ways to remember things." These characterizations will serve as the impetus for group discussion concerning subject's conceptions of memory; how people with equal ability but different conceptions of memory might approach difficult memory tasks; and the effects of these orientations on memory functioning.

Participants will be shown a videotape with two models. The elderly subjects will see elderly women models. A voice-over will explain that the two women depicted have scored equally well on IQ and ability tests.   An interview with each woman will reveal that one believes memory declines with aging, whereas the other believes that she can exercise some control over her memory.   Each will then be shown working on a difficult memory task and encountering failure. They will portray the associated patterns of affect, thought, and behavior during performance and during a final interview. This video will also provide a basis for discussion of conceptions of memory and their effects.

In a subsequent session participants will generate performance- and learning-oriented responses to memory tasks and problems.   This will provide them with the opportunity to identify thoughts and reactions that are associated with these different orientations. Self-instructional materials will be devised reflecting learning- oriented coping responses.   This will serve as a vehicle for promoting a problem-solving focus and persistence in overcoming memory difficul- ties.   Learning-oriented self statements will be written on prompt cards, so that they will be readily accessible for practice.   An example of a learning-oriented self statement might be: "When a problem seems like it is more than I can handle, it's important to try to figure out one small thing I can do to begin to solve it."

In order to provide participants with an opportunity to practice using the adaptive conceptions and cognitions, they will be asked to generate common memory problems, and strategies to cope with them. During these exercises the relationship between a view of memory as controllable, adaptive self-statements, and problem-solving behavior will be emphasized.

Individual cognitive restructuring program.   Individual training programs to restructure self-concepts and goals might also be developed when time and resources are ample.   Individual cognitive therapy (Beck, Rush, Shaw, & Emery, 1979) developed to modify depressogenic belief systems might serve as a model.   Cognitive therapy techniques would be especially useful when depression is concomitant with memory problems, as is often the case (Kahn, Zarit, & Hilbert, 1975).   During cognitive therapy the client is taught to write down his/her dysfunctional thoughts and then counter them by writing out more adaptive ones.   Thus, a depressed individual would be asked to write out his/her thoughts in situations that are upsetting to them.   For example, if a friend does not return a call s/he may think "no one cares about me, I'm destined to live a lonely life." This individual would be trained by the therapist to generate a more realistic and adaptive thought to talk back to the negative ones, e.g., "There is no evidence for this.   Maybe my friend got tied up with something else.   I'll give him another call if I don't hear from him soon.   Besides, I just received a call from Susan yesterday.   I have other friends."

This technique could be adapted for elderly clients who have episodes of forgetting and then feel helpless and depressed.   The client could be trained to write out thoughts when this occurs, identify them as performance or learning oriented, and then replace performance with learning-oriented thoughts, if needed. The trainer could help the client make the shift by providing an index card with learning-oriented prompt questions, e.g., "What step could I take the next time to help me remember this?" Using the index card questions as a guide, the client could generate adaptive responses in the actual situation.

For clients who are unable or resistant to writing out thoughts during a memory loss incident, an oral point-counterpoint technique could be used in the training session. First the trainer elicits a list of typical thoughts that the client may have had during such an episode. The client is then asked to read one of these performance-oriented thoughts and the trainer counters with a learning-oriented thought. Once the client finishes the list, the roles are reversed with the trainer countering the client's performance-oriented thoughts and the client actively engaged in generating learning-oriented thoughts. A sample of such a dialogue might look like the following:

Client: "I'm always forgetting things."

Trainer: "That's not true. I do forget some things but there are a number of things I remember."

Client: "I'm getting old, I'm losing my memory and I'm going downhill."

Trainer: "It's true I'm getting older, but not everything is going downhill. I do remember some things and I can learn some new ways of coping with my aging."

Client: "An old dog cannot learn new tricks."

Trainer: "That's not true. I've just learned this technique of talking back to my self-defeating thoughts. I can learn other things."

Client: "I won't remember how to talk back when I'm alone."

Trainer: "What could I do to help me remember? What steps could I take? Maybe I could get the trainer to help me write out on a card some helpful things to say to myself when I get discouraged."

These types of cognitive techniques have been shown effective in the modification of depressive belief systems. In fact numerous studies have shown them to be as effective or more effective than the use of antidepressant medication for some forms of depression (Blackburn, 1985). The efficacy of cognitive restructuring in the treatment of depressions which may have a biological basis lends some credence to our hypothesis that cognitive restructuring may impact on memory loss problems regardless of the etiology. This technique may be most effective when used in conjunction with other treatments.

Trainers. One note of importance that must be included under cognitive intervention concerns the beliefs of those training the elderly. Those who intervene must examine their own beliefs about the elderly and memory problems. Trainers must first deal with their own dysfunctional beliefs about aging--e.g. "Old people are too old to learn new things and need to be cared for." As Emery (1981) points out, change agents working with the elderly must challenge their own maladaptive beliefs about the elderly in order to effectively impart useful techniques. Perhaps elderly persons who hold positive beliefs would make the best trainers.

Secondly, the trainer must establish a helpful therapeutic relationship. Prior to imparting useful techniques, the trainer needs to deal with the elderly's misconceptions about training. There is a stigma which is often associated with coming in for treatment. This is especially true if the individual is pressured to be there by significant others. For example, the individual might fear that s/he is about to be institutionalized or that s/he is losing her/his mind. The trainer can elicit these concerns and dispel them, e.g. by suggesting that the client will be learning more systematic ways of dealing with memory problems.

Prevention

We have presented cognitive restructuring interventions for those elderly individuals afflicted with memory problems. We now would like to turn to issues of prevention. One may first ask, how do elderly adults come to a view that memory loss is an inevitable and irreversible part of aging? Of particular relevance is research conducted by Chanowitz and Langer (1981) on premature cognitive commitment. They proposed that the context of initial exposure to information impacts on its subsequent use. When individuals are exposed to information that appears irrelevant to them, that information is not critically evaluated. For example, a woman may learn that a victim of rape provokes it, or a wealthy individual may learn that the poor are worthless. This information, because it does not seem applicable to them, is not processed mindfully. This is an efficient way of processing in that time and energy are not wasted on irrelevant material. When, however, circumstances change, e.g., the woman is raped, or the wealthy individual loses her fortune, the information is retrieved as an unconditional truth. It does not occur to them to search for alternative explanations. Chanowitz and Langer demonstrated the impact of premature cognitive commitments on intellectual performance. Subjects were given information about a "perceptual deficit" that the experimenters called field dependence. To manipulate the relevance of this information half the subjects were told that there was a high incidence of this condition in the population, and half were told that there was a low incidence in the population. In addition, half were told to think about ways to cope with such a deficit and half were not given these instructions. All subjects were then informed that they had the deficit. Their actual performance was then measured on an embedded figures task. In support of their hypothesis, those who processed the information under irrelevant conditions (low incidence/no think instructions) performed more poorly on the perceptual task. As the researchers point out, these results have implications for how the young process information about aging. More specifically, with reference to memory loss we can hypothesize that in our culture, old age is not associated as much with an increase in wisdom but of deterioration. The belief that memory loss in old age signals the beginning of an inevitable deterioration seems widespread. Individuals are exposed to this shrinking entity view of memory when they are young, and accept it mindlessly because it is irrelevant. This self-concept of memory is dormant until they are older and have forgotten something. Just like those with the imaginary deficit, that belief may impact on their cognitive performance regardless of actual impairment.

This work on premature cognitive commitment has implications for education and prevention. Clearly, much needs to be done in the way of education about memory problems. Efforts are already underway to educate the public about Alzheimer's disease (Gatz & Pearson, 1988). Although the intent behind these messages is admirable, the research on premature cognitive commitment suggests caution is called for in designing these educational messages. Many times information about Alzheimer's is essentially presented by a medical authority in the form of a list of symptoms. Given that for non-elderly, non-afflicted individuals, this information will usually be irrelevant, research on premature cognitive commitment (Chanowitz and Langer, 1981) suggests it will be mindlessly processed. Furthermore, a subsequent memory loss in middle adulthood or in old age may trigger the unconditional belief that they have the symptom, and, therefore, have Alzheimer's disease. This belief may result in some actual deterioration in performance, even when there is no organic cause. Moreover, even if there is an organic etiology, more deterioration may occur than is merited by the disease. In terms of prevention, we suggest that researchers investigate the impact of various ways of disseminating information about Alzheimer's. Public messages could be developed that might make people more mindfully process the symptom information. For example, it may be important to underline clearly that memory loss does not always signal Alzheimer's, or perhaps the media could show case examples where memory loss is a symptom of Alzheimer's and instances where it is not, e.g. depression.

Additionally, the media could be of help in presenting elderly role models with memory problems who are actively implementing strategies for coping with impairment. It may also be useful to educate the public about the many facets of memory in order to minimize the impact of the belief about a global "shrinking" entity; that is, to inform them that although there are aspects of memory that may decline, other aspects may remain intact.

As Gatz and Pearson (1988) point out, the media tends to present an overly pessimistic (e.g., frail, forgetful) and more recently an overly optimistic (e.g., healthy, wise, well-off) stereotype of the elderly. Clearly a more balanced view is needed; that is, a depiction of the elderly as experiencing the inevitable difficulties and challenges of aging but that recognizes that a mastery-orientation in the face of these difficulties can optimize functioning in later life.

Conclusions

The search for solutions to memory problems in the elderly has been dominated by psychopharmacological treatment and training in memory strategies. Relatively little work has been done examining the role of attributions and control beliefs regarding memory. We believe that the intervention proposed in this chapter has the potential to produce more widespread and sustained memory improvement. The intervention is unique in that it is rooted in a framework that elucidates a constellation of cognition, affect, and behavior that impacts on memory performance. Attribution and control beliefs are viewed as a part of that constellation. Within this framework, self-conception of memory ability is the key to this constellation. A self-conception of memory as a shrinking entity opens the door to a constellation that impairs memory performance. It orients one toward evaluating the extent of decline and unlocks the door to maladaptive thought (attributions of helplessness and expectations of little control), affect (anxiety, depression), and behavior (low persistence, low use of compensatory strategies). A self-conception of memory ability as multifaceted and subject to increases through effort orients one to improving memory capacity and opens the door to adaptive thought (attributions to insufficient effort, expectations of control), affect (feelings of mastery, challenge), and behavior (high persistence, use of effective strategies). Targeting these self-conceptions for change using cognitive restructuring techniques should be an efficient way to produce generalized improvement in memory performance. Further, it is expected that cognitive restructuring will be most effective when used in combination with memory strategy training (e.g., method of loci). This should provide performance feedback and direct experience with memory improvement which are important for the process of modifying self-conceptions of memory. Work is currently underway to test the validity of this approach.

References

Abramson, L. Y., Seligman, M. E. P., & Teasdale, J. D. (1978).

Learned helplessness in humans: Critique and reformulation. *Journal of Abnormal Psychology, 87,* 49-74.

Ames, C. (1984).   Achievement attributions and self-instructions under competitive and individualistic goal structures.   *Journal of Educational Psychology, 76,* 478-487.

Andrews, G. R., & Debos, R. L. (1978).   Persistence and the causal perceptions of failure: Modifying cognitive attributions.   *Journal of Educational Psychology, 70,* 154-166.

Baltes, P. B., & Willis, S. L. (1982).   Enhancement of intellectual functioning in old age: Penn State's Adult Development and Enrichment Project (ADEPT).   In F. I. M. Craik & S. E. Trehub (Eds.), *Aging and cognitive processes* (pp. 353-384).   New York: Plenum Press.

Bandura, A. (1987, in press).   Self-regulation of motivation and action through goal systems.   In V. Hamilton, G. H. Bower, & N. H. Fryda (Eds.), *Cognition, motivation and affect: A cognitive science view.*   Dordrecht: Martinus Nijhoff.

Bandura, M. M., & Dweck, C. S. (1988, submitted for publication).   The relationship of conceptions of intelligence and achievement goals to patterns of cognition, affect, and behavior.

Banziger, G., & Drevenstedt, J. (1982).   Achievement attributions by young and old judges as a function of perceived age of stimulus person.   *Journal of Gerontology, 37,* 468-474.

Beck, A. T., Rush, A. J., Shaw, B. F., & Emery, G. (1979).   *Cognitive therapy of depression.*   New York: Guilford Press.

Blackburn, I. M. (1985).   Depression.   In B. P. Bradley & C. Thompson (Eds.), *Psychological applications in psychiatry* (pp. 61-93).   New York: Wiley & Sons.

Blank, T. O. (1982).   *A social psychology of developing adults.*   New York: Wiley & Sons.

Bowen, D. M., White, P., & Spillane, J. A. (1979).   Accelerated aging or selective neuronal loss as an important cause of dementia? *Lancet, 1,* 11-14.

Chanowitz, B., & Langer, E. J. (1981).   Premature cognitive commitment.   *Journal of Personality and Social Psychology, 41,* 1051-1063.

Chapin, M., & Dyck, D. G. (1976).   Persistence in children's reading behavior as a function of *n* length and attribution retraining. *Journal of Abnormal Psychology, 85,* 511-515.

Crook, T. H. (1986). Drug effects in Alzheimer's disease. *Clinical Gerontologist, 5,* 489-502.

Crook, T. H., & Miller, N. E. (1985). The challenge of Alzheimer's disease. *American Psychologist, 40,* 1245-1250.

Davies, P., & Maloney, A. J. F. C. F (1976). Selective loss of cholinergic neurones in Alzheimer's disease. *Lancet, 2,* 1403-1407.

Diener, C. I., & Dweck, C. S. (1978). An analysis of learned helplessness: Continuous changes in performance, strategy, and achievement cognitions following failure. *Journal of Personality and Social Psychology, 36,* 451-462.

Diener, C. I., & Dweck, C. S. (1980). An analysis of learned helplessness: II. The processing of success. *Journal of Personality and Social Psychology, 39,* 940-952.

Dweck, C. S. (1975). The role of expectations and attributions in the alleviation of learned helplessness. *Journal of Personality and Social Psychology, 21,* 674-685.

Dweck, C. S. (1986). Motivational processes affecting learning. *American Psychologist, 41,* 1040-1048.

Dweck, C. S., & Elliott, E. S. (1983). Achievement and motivation. In E. M. Hetherington (Ed.), *Socialization, personality, and social development* (pp. 643-691). New York: Wiley & Sons.

Dweck, C. S., & Reppucci, N. D. (1973). Learned helplessness and reinforcement responsibility in children. *Journal of Personality and Social Psychology, 25,* 109-116.

Eisdorfer, C., & Stotsky, B. A. (1977). Intervention, treatment, and rehabilitation of psychiatric disorders. In J. E. Birren & K. W. Schaie (Eds.), *Handbook of the psychology of aging* (pp. 724-748). New York: Van Nostrand Reinhold.

Elliott, E. S., & Dweck, C. S. (1988). Goals: An approach to motivation and achievement. *Journal of Personality and Social Psychology, 1,* 5-12.

Emery, G. (1981). Cognitive therapy with the elderly. In G. Emery, S. D. Holland, & R. C. Bedrosian (Eds.), *New directions in cognitive therapy* (pp. 84-98). New York: Guilford Press.

Forsterling, F. (1985). Attributional retraining: A review. *Psychology Bulletin, 98,* 495-512.

Gatz, M., & Pearson, C. G. (1988). Ageism revised and the provision of psychological services. *American Psychologist, 43,* 184-188.

Greenberg, C. (1986, August). *Methodological problems of research on memory interventions for the elderly*. Paper presented at the meeting of the American Psychological Association, Washington, DC.

Harbaugh, R. E. (1987). Intracerebroventricular cholinergic drug administration in Alzheimer's disease: Preliminary results of a double-blind study. In R. J. Wurtman, S. H. Corkin, & J. H. Growden (Eds.), *Alzheimer's disease: Advances in basic research and therapies. Proceedings of the fourth meeting of the International Study Group on the Pharmacology of Memory Disorders Associated with Aging* (pp. 315-323). Zürich, Switzerland, January 16-18, 1987.

Hill, R. D., Sheikh, J. I., & Yesavage, J. A. (1986). *Three pretraining methods enhance mnemonic training in the elderly*. Unpublished manuscript, Stanford University, Stanford, CA.

Hill, R. D., Sheikh, J. I., Yesavage, J. A., & Ponich, P. (1986). *The effect of mnemonic training on perceived recall confidence.* Stanford University, unpublished manuscript.

Hultsch, D. F., Hertzog, C., & Dixon, R. A. (1987). *Age differences in metamemory: Resolving the inconsistencies* (CRGCA Technical Report No. 1). Atlanta, GA: Georgia Institute of Technology, Collaborative Research Group on Cognitive Aging.

Kahn, R. L., Zarit, S. H., & Hilbert, N. M. (1975). Memory complaint and impairment in the aged: The effect of depression and altered brain function. *Archives of General Psychiatry, 32*, 1569.

Khachaturian, Z. S. (1985). Progress of research on Alzheimer's disease. *American Psychologist, 40*, 1251-1255.

Lachman, M. E. (1986). Locus of control in aging research: A case for multidimensional and domain-specific assessment. *Psychology and Aging, 1*, 34-40.

Lachman, M. E., Baltes, P. B., Nesselroade, J. R., & Willis, S. L. (1982). Examination of personality-ability relationships in the elderly: The role of the contextual (interface) assessment mode. *Journal of Research in Personality, 16*, 485-501.

Lachman, M. E., & Dick, L. (1987). *Does memory training influence self-conceptions of memory aging?* Paper presented at the Gerontological Society of America, Washington, DC.

Lachman, M. E., & McArthur, L. (1986). Adulthood age differences in causal attributions for cognitive, social, and physical performance. *Psychology and Aging, 1*, 127-132.

Lachman, M. E., Steinberg, E. S., & Trotter, S. D. (1987). The effects of control beliefs and attributions on memory self-assessments and performance. *Psychology and Aging, 2,* 266-271.

Langer, E. J., & Rodin, J. (1976). The effects of choice and enhanced personal responsibility for the aged: A field experiment in an institutional setting. *Journal of Personality and Social Psychology, 34,* 191-198.

Lapp, D. (1987). *Don't forget.* New York: McGraw Hill.

Mash, D. C., Flynn, D. D., & Potter, L. T. (1985). Loss of M2 muscarine receptors in the cerebral cortex in Alzheimer's disease and experimental cholinergic deservation. *Science, 228,* 1115-1117.

Nicholls, J. G. (1975). Causal attributions and other achievement related cognitions: Effects of task outcome, attainment value, and sex. *Journal of Personality and Social Psychology, 31,* 379-389.

Perry, E. K., Perry, R. H., Blessed, G. (1977). Necropsy evidence of central cholinergic deficits. *Lancet, 1,* 189-192.

Perry, E. K., Perry, R. H., & Blessed, G. (1978). Changes in brain cholinesterases in senile dementia of the Alzheimer type. *Neuropathology and Applied Neurobiology, 4,* 273-277.

Perry, E. K., Tomlinson, B. E., & Blessed, G. (1978). Correlation of cholinergic abnormalities with senile plaques and mental test scores in senile dementia. *British Medical Journal, 2,* 1457-1459.

Poon, L. W. (1985). Difference in human memory with aging: Nature, causes, and clinical implications. In J. Birren & K. Schaie (Eds.), *Handbook of the psychology of aging* (second ed., pp. 427-462). New York: Van Nostrand Reinhold.

Poon, L. W. (1984). Memory training for older adults. In J. P. Abrams & V. J. Crooks (Eds.), *Geriatric mental health* (pp. 136-150). New York: Grunet Stratton.

Reisberg, B., Borenstein, J., Franssen, E., Shulman, E., Steinberg, G., & Ferris, S. (1986). Remediable behavioral symptomology in Alzheimer's disease. *Hospital and Community Psychiatry, 37,* 1199-1201.

Reisberg, B., Ferris, S. H., & DeLeon, M. J. (1985). Age-associated cognitive decline and Alzheimer's disease: Implications for assessment and treatment. In M. Berganer, M. Ermini & H. B. Stahelin (Eds.), *Thresholds in aging* (pp. 112-121). London: Academic Press.

Reisberg, B., Ferris, S. H., & Gershon, S. (1981). An overview of the pharmacologic treatment of cognitive decline in the aged. *American Journal of Psychiatry, 138,* 593-600.

Rhodes, W. A. (1977). *Generalization of attribution retraining.* Unpublished doctoral dissertation, University of Illinois, Champaign, IL.

Rodin, J. (1983). Behavioral medicine: Beneficial effects of self-control training in aging. *International Review of Applied Psychology, 32,* 153-181.

Rodin, J., Cashman, C., & Desiderato, L. (1987). Psychosocial interventions in aging focusing on enrichment and prevention. In M. Riley, A. Baum, & J. Matarazzo (Eds.), *Perspectives on behavioral medicine IV: Biomedical and psychosocial perspectives of aging* (pp. 149-172). New York: Wiley & Sons.

Rodin, J., & Langer, E. (1980). Aging labels: The decline of control and the fall of self-esteem. *Journal of Social Issues, 36,* 12-29.

Rosenbaum, M. (1980). A schedule for assessing self-control behaviors: Preliminary findings. *Behavior Therapy, 11,* 109-121.

Rush, A. J., Hollon, S. D., Beck, A. T., & Kovacs, M. (1978). Depression: Must pharmacotherapy fail for cognitive therapy to succeed? *Cognitive Therapy and Research, 2,* 199-206.

Schulz, R., & Hanusa, B. H. (1978). Long-term effects of control and predictability-enhancing interventions: Findings and ethical issues. *Journal of Personality and Social Psychology, 36,* 1194-1201.

Simons, A. D., Lustman, P. J., Wetzel, R. D., & Murphy, G. L. (1985). Predicting response to cognitive therapy of depression: The role of learned resourcefulness. *Cognitive Therapy and Research, 9,* 79-89.

Thompson, L. W., Davies, R., Gallagher, D., & Krantz, S. (1986). Cognitive therapy with older adults. In T. Brink (Ed.), *Clinical gerontology* (pp. 101-114). New York: Haworth Press.

Willis, S. L. (in press). Cognitive training and everyday competence. In K. W. Schaie (Ed.), *Annual review of gerontology and geriatrics: Vol. 7.* New York: Springer.

Wood, R., & Bandura, A. (1987). *Impact of conceptions of ability on complex decision-making.* Unpublished manuscript, Stanford University, Stanford, CA.

Yesavage, J. A. (1985). Nonpharmacologic treatments for memory losses with normal aging. *American Journal of Psychiatry, 142,* 600-605.

Yesavage, J. A. (1987). The use of self-rating depression scales in the elderly in assessment research. In L. Poon et al., (Eds.), *Handbook of clinical memory assessment of older adults* (pp. 213-217). Washington, DC: APA.

Yesavage, J. A., & Rose, T. L. (1984). Semantic elaboration and the method of loci: A new trip for older learners. *Experimental Aging Research, 10,* 155-159.

Yost, E. B., Buetler, L. E., Corbishley, M. A., & Allenden, J. R. (1986). *Group cognitive therapy: A treatment approach for depressed older adults.* Elmsford, NY: Pergamon Press.

Zarit, S. H., Miller, N. E., & Kahn, R. L. (1978). Brain function, intellectual impairment, and education in the aged. *Journal of the American Geriatrics Society, 26,* 2.

Zimmerman, M., & Coryell, W. (1986). Dysfunctional attitudes in endogenous and non-endogenous depressed inpatients. *Cognitive Therapy and Research, 10,* 339-346.

Zimmerman, M., Coryell, W., & Pfohl, B. (1986). The validity of dexamethasone suppression test as a marker for endogenous depression. *Archives of General Psychiatry, 43,* 347-355.

Psychological Perspectives of Helplessness
and Control in the Elderly, P.S. Fry (ed.)
© *Elsevier Science Publishers B.V. (North-Holland), 1989*

Chapter Thirteen

CREATING PSYCHOLOGICAL AND SOCIETAL DEPENDENCY IN OLD AGE

Jon HENDRICKS

Oregon State University

Cynthia A. LEEDHAM

University of Kentucky

Abstract

In this chapter, the authors focus on shared cultural values
and social policies which create dependency in old people,
rather than on the internal dynamics of psychological
control and dependency, using Achenbaum's postulate that
certain value conflicts such as self-reliance/dependency,
expectation/entitlement, work/leisure, individual/family,
private/public, and equity/adequacy feed into the stereotype
of older persons as being dependent. The authors argue that
negative connotations of ageism may be incorporated into
older people's self-image, thus leading to behaviors which
reinforce the stereotype. Conceptual frames for considering
ways in which social policy and its implications create
dependencies in aged individuals, and ways in which
individuals may be empowered are discussed. The authors
propose an interactional model to examine ways in which
values, social policies, and resultant social structures
reinforce dependency or empowerment in older persons.
Empowerment is defined as political activism and social
goods and a process of achieving balance and interdependence
between one's own needs and the needs of other generations.
The ways in which income and health policy tend to foster
dependency, particularly in the marginal elderly, are
examined. Implications of existing social policies are
discussed with reference to dependency in old age. In
conclusion, the authors advocate that rather than framing
the debate in terms of intergenerational inequity in current
distribution of resources, it may make more sense to ask
what is a decent minimum of resources, sufficient to
forestall dependency at different times in our lives. A
cradle-to-grave approach which seeks to provide access to a
decent minimum of health care and income within the limits
of resource constraints is proposed as means of empowering

*people of all ages. Policies directed specifically to the
elderly should seek to maximize functioning by providing
adequate services and opportunities for participatory
control in decisions, while avoiding over-protectiveness.*

Introduction

Societal Factors Promoting Dependency in Older People

All too frequently being old is equated with dependency and helplessness.   Among some social scientists it is maintained causal attribution of dependency must be set in the broader situational context
where it occurs, and analyzed as growing out of a dynamic interplay of
values, social policies, economic and environmental factors, rather
than from psychological processes of the elderly alone.   Such a view
is clearly congruent with dialectical models of life-span developmental psychology (Norris, 1987; Riegel, 1975).   The tremendous variety
among older people and the contexts in which they grow old must also
be recognized.   Consideration should be given both to preventing the
creation of dependency in elderly persons capable of high levels of
functioning and participation, and to maximizing remaining functional
capacity for those with impairments.   Accordingly, while models of
learned helplessness and the literature on life events have a real
part to play in understanding conceptions of dependency, we contend
they must be set within the rubric of value conflicts, negotiated
social policies through which these are expressed, and their impact on
everyday lives.

The animal model of learned helplessness--in which exposure to a
situation where no course of action seems to effect outcomes, thereby
leading   to   ineffectual   response   patterns   (Overmier & Seligman,
1967)--has received widespread application.   Seemingly the uncontrollability of an occurrence results in an apathetic attitude of "Why do
anything?"   The outcome is passivity in the face of events that might
otherwise be averted.   Broad ranging generalizations of the model have
been applied in analyses of school failure (Dweck & Reppucci, 1973),
lower class resignation (Bresnahan & Blum, 1971), studies of victimization (Peterson & Seligman, 1983) and a host of other situations.   The literature on morale and life satisfaction has also drawn
on theories of learned helplessness.   Among the more fruitful applications are a variety of increasingly sophisticated models for explaining depression (Abramson, Seligman & Teasdale, 1978; Peterson &
Seligman, 1984, 1985; Seligman, 1972, 1975).   These models have
obvious appeal for explaining the mechanisms of the creation of
psychological dependency in the elderly.   Our focus, however, is on
societal factors liable to lead to learned helplessness, rather than
on the details of learned helplessness *per se*.

The stereotype of the elderly as dependent is prevalent in
western societies.   If behavior seemingly corresponds to expectations

lodged in the stereotype, we attribute negative characteristics to the actor. Consequently, we may look only at the individual, thus overestimating his/her role in dispositional causes of action (Ross, Amabile & Steinmetz, 1977). When examined in light of societal forces, presumed dependency may turn out to be partially a result of cultural patterning which promotes a complex of values and attitudes that casts older persons in unfavorable lights, thus fostering dependency. As we shall note below, social gerontologists themselves have not always been cognizant of the influence social factors have had in their own research. Early gerontological theories served to reaffirm societal values without questioning their impact. Looking at those attitudes and values thought to characterize the perception of the elderly in western cultures, and the United States in particular, it is possible to identify a range of themes conducive to creating dependency. According to Achenbaum (1983) and others (Tropman & McClure, 1980), acknowledging the role of values in shaping not only policies but the very warp and woof of the lifeworld of the elderly, will help highlight the normative dimensions of their lives. Like conceptual spectacles of any type, values color the way the world is perceived. Reflecting states of societal and cultural development, value choices pervade our very being. If we are to make sense of what happens to older people we must have some idea of the values that help shape their lives.

As Achenbaum (1983) notes, "Because value choices pervade all aspects of life, their impact in the realm of policymaking can hardly be exaggerated" (p. 18). The same is true to a large extent for attitudes toward the elderly. While we should not underestimate the plurality of values in modern industrialized societies, we may usefully draw on Achenbaum's (1983) typology, developed with specific reference to the United States. Looking at the United States over the 20th century, Achenbaum (cf. Tropman & McClure, 1980) identifies seven sets of paired global value dilemmas affecting the elderly. *(1) Self-reliance/dependency*: underlines the strain between self-sufficiency and relying on others. Throughout history and most of the life-course we stress the former, and social policy in the United States tends to emphasize people's responsibility for providing for their old age so that they will not be dependent. While Social Security provides a minimum upon which to build for one's old age, it is only extended to those who have proven their self-reliance by working the requisite period (Achenbaum, 1983; Tropman & McClure, 1980). Considerable stigma is attached to the development of dependency in old age. "To be deemed dependent was to be perceived as different....isolated conceptually and socio-economically from the mainstream of society" (Achenbaum, 1983, p. 20). *(2) Expectation/Entitlement*: Expectation refers to striving toward goals, whatever they may be, whereas entitlement means being guaranteed certain components of those goals by virtue of categorical membership. *(3) Work/Leisure*: refers to the conflict between productive activities and those not deemed productive. People in many western societies tend to emphasize the work ethic, so that lesser status is accorded those not engaged in

the world of work. *(4) Individual/Family*: highlights the balancing
of personal goals or aspirations with those of the larger family unit.
With the emphasis on individuality, the tendency has been to separate
individual needs from those of families and other social groups.
Whether to provide benefits on the basis of individual need, or within
the context of the family, is a crucial issue in the dependence or
independence of the elderly. The emphasis on individuality is no place
more apparent than in the treatment of aging as something that happens
to individuals simply because of their biology (Levin & Levin, 1980).
(5) Private/Public: underscores the distinction between private and
public responsibility. Historically, in the United States, there has
been a tendency towards privatism, with the issue of support for the
elderly seen primarily in those terms. This trend was mitigated, but
not reversed, during the New Deal. Absence of broad-based government
entitlement programs tends to lead to dependency and impoverishment,
particularly for the marginal elderly. *(6) Equity/adequacy*: Should
equal treatment be accorded to all or should resources be reserved
only for the most needy? Seemingly, the former has taken precedence
over the latter, at least in the United States. The emphasis has been
on equity of opportunity rather than on results in terms of facilitating adequate living conditions for all. Again, this stance may lead
to dependency among the most disadvantaged. *(7) Novelty/tradition*:
Should individuals or groups seek new approaches or rely on tried and
true alternatives in dealing with issues? The American quest for
novelty, argues Achenbaum, leads to a devaluation of the experience
and potential of the elderly. Within a whole range of value conflicts, Achenbaum contends the values that predominate tend to be
antithetical to empowerment of the elderly.

The Reality of Old Age

The early gerontological literature amply demonstrates discussions of
declines thought to characterize aging--a trend which is currently
being rectified (Labouvie-Vief, 1985; Rowe & Kahn, 1987). Physiological, psychological and cosmetic changes were described largely in
terms of decline. Add to these social changes couched in the values
already discussed, and the thrust toward conceiving aging in terms of
dependency and learned helplessness becomes apparent. Among gerontologists, ascription of negative attributes to a person merely
because of age or the manifestation of age-related changes is referred
to as *ageism*. Ageism not only colors the perception of others, but of
the self as well. In both cases it entails a pernicious and pejora-
tive view.

The formulation of self-concept, or in the case of older persons,
age-identity, incorporates more than simple chronological age. A
fluid concept, to be sure, self-image includes personal assessments of
myriad role involvements, recognition of age-norms, and age-appro-
priate behavior, underpinned by the types of values discussed above,
social and anticipated timetables, health and physical limitations,

and interaction patterns in both formal and informal relationships (Hendricks, 1987).

Kuypers & Bengtson's (1973) *social breakdown* theory provides a valuable perspective on the interdependency between older people and their social world, and how dependency may be fostered. Borrowing from Zusman's (1966) social breakdown syndrome of psychiatric patients, they assert negative feedback when facing the portent of failure exacerbates that risk, and initiates what becomes a self-fulfilling prophecy. What is the fate of older persons dealing with role losses, unfamiliar situations, physical impairments or other drastic changes against a backdrop of societal prejudices? As they reach out for cues as to how they should act, they are treated as the personification of failing capacities in need of benign intervention, or worse. As they seek interaction, older persons may insidiously adopt as their own the negative characteristics attributed to them, and slip further into dependencies as the cycle repeats. In discussing how the model may help explain behavior, Kuypers and Bengtson maintain that continuing adherence to middle-age values, such as visible productivity, assures the attribution of negative characteristics.

Neither the original authors nor those who have applied the breakdown model (Breytspraak, 1984) contend it is inevitable. In nearly all cases it is suggested that intervention predicated on restructuring the social environment, and development of problem-solving capacities may enable older people to break the spiral. Improving environmental supports and lessening social isolation while facilitating the expression of personal strengths, if in no other way than allowing older people to make independent decisions, will go a long way toward lessening dependency (Hendricks & Hendricks, 1986; Lawton, 1983; Looft, 1972). Let us turn now to an examination of theories in social gerontology which have, or have not, been conducive to an understanding of how dependencies are created and maintained.

Gerontological Theory and the Psychology of Helplessness

By their segmentation of social structure and the lifeworld of individuals, early theories in social gerontology reinforce the ageist implications of societal value themes. Structural imperatives are either given primacy, with the individual seen as passively adapting to them; or ignored in favor of a tight focus on individuals. Either way, aging persons are implicitly treated as passive consumers of policies, goods and services, rather than as active moral agents, with rights to participation in the social construction of public policy (Ladd, 1973). More recent gerontological theories provide a way to transcend the structure-meaning dichotomy (Dreyfus & Rabinow, 1983), facilitating an examination of the dynamic between political and economic factors, culture, meaning and intentionality. This paves the way for considering how policy constrains the life world of individ-

uals fostering dependency; and how people can, in turn, shape their
world, and have an impact on social policy and its implementation.

    While such a schematization obviously does not do justice to the
complexities and contributions of individual theories, it is useful to
conceptualize the generational emergence of gerontological theory in
dialectical terms of thesis, antithesis, and synthesis (Hendricks &
Hendricks, 1986; Hendricks & Leedham, 1987).   First phase theories
focused on aging at the level of the individual, taking structural
factors as given.   Disengagement theory (Cummings & Henry, 1961),
grounded in functionalism, held mutual withdrawal or disengagement
from society was desirable in the interests of optimum levels of
personal gratification and of ensuring an uninterrupted continuation
of the social system--which would thus be spared disruptions caused by
deaths of elderly people in key positions.   Activity theory (Havighurst & Albrecht, 1953; Maddox, 1970), in contrast, held continuance
of a moderately active lifestyle has a marked preservative effect on
well-being.   Early versions of activity theory were, however,
criticized for tending to define activity in terms of pastimes geared
to what were thought to be older people's interests and abilities,
rather than in terms of meaningful participation (Gubrium, 1973;
Phillips, 1957).   Second generation theories such as modernization or
age-stratification theory--the antithesis--focused on social organization to the neglect of cultural factors and individual intentionality,
by positing universally found structural factors with their own
dynamic.   This exclusive concentration on the structural level still
cast the older people in a passive role, and did not make for a
critical examination of the relationship between social policy and the
aged as intentional persons. Nancy Foner's (1982) allusions to the
ways in which age systems structure opportunity, however, presents a
preliminary move towards attending to the interplay between structure
and individual lifeworlds.   In reaction to the emphasis on social
structure, some psychologically oriented gerontologists moved toward a
predominantly subjective approach, developing personality theory and
continuity theory focusing on individual personality differences
(Bultena, 1969; Covey, 1981; Fox, 1981; Neugarten, 1977; Neugarten,
Crotty, & Tobin, 1964; Neugarten, Havighurst, & Tobin, 1968).   Again,
however, they concentrate on individual-level factors, to the
exclusion of the import of social organization.

    More recent theories--the synthesis--provide a theoretical
framework for examining the relationship between psychological
dependency--or empowerment--and structural factors. Theories grounded
in political economy (Estes, Swan, & Gerard, 1982) concentrate on
ways in which social institutions are shaped by individual and
corporate actors, and in turn circumscribe their lifeworld of
individuals.   Certain social-psychological perspectives (Marshall,
1981; 1986) examine constraints imposed by structure from the
individual level, focusing on their meaning for particular individuals, and options available within them.   Kuypers and Bengtson's
(1973) model discussed above, and Breytspraak's (1984) development of

it are cases in point. Both perspectives provide a means of linking structural and individual levels, though with slightly different emphases. Taken together they allow for a multidimensional analysis of the interplay between societal constraints, cultural meanings, individual meaning-giving and social power which constitutes the continually renegotiated fabric of social structure. They provide us with a framework for considering ways in which social policy and its implications create dependencies in aging individuals--and ways in which those individuals may be empowered.

The Power of Social Policy

How Social Policy Establishes the Arena Within Which Old Age Is Lived

In explaining behavior, observers are always at risk of making attribution errors if they do not acknowledge all factors which may affect it. In keeping with our emphasis on broader social currents, and as a means of integrating perspectives grounded in political economy and social psychology in examining the mutual influence of social and individual factors, we propose a modification of a framework formulated by Billings and Moos (1985). The original model was designed to facilitate examination of ways in which social background factors such as socioeconomic status and gender influenced depression through their impact on personal and environmental resources, environmental stressors, appraisal and coping mechanisms. Rather than taking social background factors as given, we expand the model to include consideration of how they are socially constructed by the interplay between social policy, economic and material conditions, and societal values. We also emphasize the bidirectional nature of the process. Not only may policies and social values shape lives of individuals: Individuals may help fashion policies, and ultimately values.

Values, public policies, and material conditions influence individuals' personal resources--both psychological and economic-- through their impact on the structure of labor markets. In turn, labor markets, provide differential opportunities for saving and accruing pension rights clearly tied with adjustment during the retirement years. Education, too, has been shown to be relevant as it influences both problem-solving and interpersonal skills. Together both labor market and education underpin factors affecting health, such as access to health care, nutrition, and living conditions. Environmental resources--the organizational contexts of people's lives, and physical and architectural features of the community (Moos & Mitchell, 1982), as well as informational, material and emotional support provided by intimates--may be more, or less supportive of autonomy in the elderly, depending on the social policies and values in which they are grounded. Environmental stressors--both stressful events, or major negative life changes, such as forced retirement or

Figure 1:   An Integrative Framework for Analysis of the Influence of Social Policy on
            Adaptive Processes and Dependency *

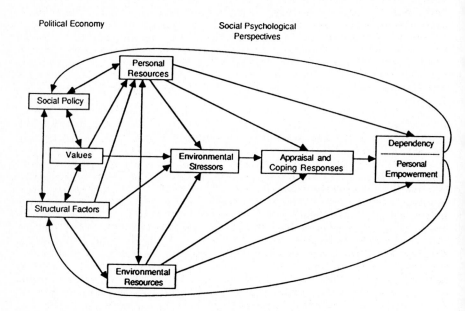

*Adapted from Billings & Moos, 1982

From: Psychosocial Theory and Research on Depression:
An Integrative Framework and Review. *Clinical Psychology
Review, 2*, 213-237, by A. G. Billings and R. H. Moos.
Copyright 1982 by Pergamon Journals Ltd. Reprinted by
permission.

residential relocation; and life strains, such as stresses that come
with limited finances resulting in an inability to maintain acceptable
lifestyles--can be said to be largely shaped by social policy. On the
individual level, coping strategies, reflecting the dynamic interplay
between appraisal--the perception and interpretation of environmental
stimuli--and coping responses--those behavioral strategies used to
deal with stimuli (Billings & Moos, 1985; Lazarus, 1981)--are each
shaped by structural determinants. To illustrate: The degree to which
individuals are likely to adopt a proactive rather than a passive
stance toward an issue will be influenced by types of services available, knowledge of and ability to obtain information about options,

and ability to pay or obtain third party payment, as well as the degree to which others regard them as competent.

Socially reinforced negative self-concepts, or a lack of resources, may lead to passive responses to problems in living and thereby into situations which reinforce dependency (cf. Kuypers & Bengtson, 1973). Yet, as Kuypers and Bengtson (1973) suggest, development of an individual's problem-solving and coping skills, and provision of adequate resources may lead to reduced dependence through a process of social reconstruction. Linking the insights of the political economy of aging and social psychological approaches concentrating on intentional individuals and how they are influenced by social policy, the revised Billings and Moos model shown in Figure 1 may be useful both in analyzing ways in which societal processes disenfranchise aging individuals, and how they can be enfranchised as co-shapers of social policy.

In addressing the nature of empowerment, Clark's (1987) four-fold scheme is relevant to our discussion here. The first of Clark's four dimensions is social goods and political activism. It "...does little good to speak of personal empowerment without at least initial consideration of the need to provide sufficient social resources to enable individuals to exercise choice in their lives" (Clark 1987). Acknowledging both the role of social policy in patterning life choices, and the need to involve older people in the policy process is a first step. Secondly, empowerment is effective deliberation: the ability to think consciously about complex actions. Yet to do so requires a certain amount of education, and sufficient information to make decisions. The implication is that the elderly must be treated as autonomous adults, given access to adequate information about key decisions and policies surrounding them, and, where necessary, education in decision-making. Thirdly, Clark reminds us that empowerment is a long-term process. The conditions of dependency and its grounding in social policy stretch across the lifecourse rather than beginning fresh in old age. The interplay between social policy, environmental and personal resources, environmental stressors, coping styles, and dependency has its roots in an individual's whole biography and in the history of society: It has implications for future options. Finally, Clark sees empowerment as balance and interdependence, an ability to come to terms with the realities of one's personal history, present situation, and needs for support and assistance while maintaining a measure of freedom and independence. It calls for a balancing of needs and visions of one's own generation and those of others, within existing resource constraints.

In the next two sections, we focus on the relationship between income, health policy and dependency. Generally speaking, personal resources can be said to fall along three dimensions, social-familial, personal-physiological and a fiduciary axis (Hendricks & Hendricks, 1986). Our discussion here will be limited to the latter two, since health and economic well-being, augmented by an array of social

supports, undergird both personal mastery and perceived efficacy.   In
the United States, there are approximately 100 diverse federal
programs which have a direct impact on the everyday life of old
people.   We will discuss two in an effort to underscore the way
policies relate to dependencies.   Then we turn to the issue of
intergenerational equity, examining it from a lifecourse perspective.
To set it in broad perspective, we discuss the interdependence of
generations, diversity occurring within generations, alternative
definitions of equity and their implications for dependency.   Finally,
in considering future directions, we propose a model of empowerment as
balance and interdependence: an alternative to the creation of dependency.

Income Policy: Adequacy or Dependency

Upon acceptance of retirement benefits, older people become members of
a legally defined category whether they like it or not.   We need only
reference the extent to which legal definitions of old age become
social definitions, to underscore their salience. In all bureaucratic
societies entitlement legislation is taken as normative, affecting the
social construction of the realities of old age.   Separated from the
work-a-day world and what had likely been a central component of their
self-concepts, older workers moving into retirement experience a
reduction in social status (Williamson, Shindul & Evans, 1985).
Without status it becomes increasingly difficult to negotiate from a
position of strength with others or events in the environment to
maintain a feeling of efficacy.   A key aspect of a sense of mastery
among the elderly is an ability to utilize personal resources in
dealing with various exigencies of life.

     Through various forms of entitlement legislation, society plays a
central role in shaping either adequacy or dependency in older
people's financial picture.   In societies where retirement has been
institutionalized, certain benefits are assured but at the expense of
renouncing participation in the world of work.   All industrialized
countries have some form of guaranteed benefit for the elderly either
based on previous earnings, or, if they were deficient for any reason,
a form of public welfare.   In either instance, the income picture for
older citizens is at least in part beyond their control.   By and
large, the wages of retirement reflect lifelong profiles of the wages
of work.   Deciding whether older people as a group face financial
dependency is not an easy question.   By some criteria they look fairly
well off; by others, headed for hard times.   Actual poverty rates in
the United States, based on income necessary for a subsistence diet
and multiplied by a factor of three to allow for other expenses,
include 14.1 percent of all persons over the age of 65.   If a level of
125 percent of the actual poverty level is used, to reflect additional
expenses for health care, the figure jumps to 22.4 percent of those
over 65 in dire economic circumstances.   Whatever these figures
currently represent, they do reflect an improvement over those of 25

or 30 years ago when they were roughly twice as high. Yet there is no room for complacency. Median income for householders over age 65 is less than half that of any other group in the United States, meaning older people are disproportionately represented among lower income groups. As is often the case, the risk is not spread equally. Older women, minorities, the chronically ill, those who have been widowed or otherwise live alone are generally at greater risk for economic dependence. Part of the reason they are more vulnerable is because of the web of social policies that shape their lifeworlds. What it means to be old is, to some extent, a policy decision.

In the United States, for example, the retired have a right to Social Security benefits, either based on their own earnings or as a dependent of a principal wage-earner, or to Supplemental Security Income--a form of welfare for those without Social Security or other income sufficient to assure an adequate standard of living. Tied to past earnings, Social Security also reflects a clear pattern of occupations. Beginning with those jobs deemed most central to the economy, it was only gradually expanded to cover more peripheral occupations. In fact, it was the early 1980s before more marginal pursuits were included. Domestics, seasonal workers, and those employed in small firms were among the last to be covered. These are exactly the workers whose lifetimes have been marked by low wages, and who would be least likely to be able to save for their old age. Many critics assert successive revisions to the Social Security Act were aimed at workers in monopoly industries where a stable workforce is important. In non-monopoly industries and in secondary labor markets, worker turn-over and seasonal employment are keys to profitability: Hence stable workforces are of no utility. As a rule of thumb, for those who draw Social Security only, replacement rates are a little over one-half of income in the years preceding retirement. Generally speaking, single people, women and minorities receive slightly less, while males, whites and couples receive slightly more than the average.

Earnings above a specified threshold in the years between retirement and age 68 result in an automatic reduction of benefits received. Above a maximum, benefits cease until the worker reaches age 70. This means, for lower and middle income elderly--those with annual wages between $8400 and $20,000--their federal Social Security benefits are discounted proportionately. The logic is simple enough, benefits are for the retired, not continuing workers. The consequence is, however, that those workers who might choose to remain active, and forestall potential dependence, are penalized most. The rich elderly, with income from sources other than wages, do not sacrifice any benefits.

The poor elderly, those retired without nonearned incomes or the possibility of working become dependent on the largess of the State for their economic needs. Should they incur expenses above those they can afford they have no choice but to declare their destitution, surrender any remaining resources, with exemptions for a homestead and certain other resources, and accept entitlement benefits for the medically or financially indigent. There are over 3.9 million of the latter whose sole income derives from Supplemental Security Income administered independently by individual states. Needless to say, there is a great deal of inequality in the way benefits are scheduled, yet without exception all recipients are at or below poverty levels.

Because of the way income policies are written, the benefit structure is such that pre-retirement social class alignments are not altered during retirement: the same relative inequities or advantages remain. To speak then of dependency prompted by insufficient resources in old age is to speak of a pattern that may well have been a lifetime in the making. In point of fact, over 80 percent of the social security recipients in the United States have no other source of income; only about 10 percent have earnings in excess of $8400 with the remainder earning less.

Obviously not all elderly are dependent on federal benefits. There are a huge number of private pension schemes available but only about one-half of the workers in the United States are eligible. For those who do receive a private annuity, replacement rates are between 60 and 75 percent of pre-retirement earnings. Earlier mismanagement, and abandonment of private programs in the face of stiff regulations brought on-line by the 1974 Employee Retirement Income Security Act (ERISA), have left a large proportion of the labor force without adequate pension protection.

With variations of this basic pattern common throughout many western industrialized economies, it is not surprising that Townsend (1986), writing in Britain, suggests retirement is itself a chief cause of dependency. Means-tested social assistance programs for older workers may create as many problems as their proponents maintain they solve. Even the pattern of retirement suggests, he maintains, a social class bias: those in the professions can forestall retirement while hourly and salaried employees have little sway in the face of bureaucratic requirements. Even with cost-of-living adjustments, spiralling inflation and the costs of health care practically ensure that for a large proportion of those elderly living too long into retirement the grim spectre of financial hardship awaits. And with it, a real and grinding dependency.

Health Policy and Dependency

Patterns of Coverage: Since their enactment in 1965, Medicare and Medicaid have considerably improved access to health care. Yet, they still embody serious problems in patterns of support for health and long-term care which make for a failure to maximize functioning, if not dependency. Ideally, effective health care would provide preventive services in the interests of maintaining high levels of functional independence in well elderly. For those with chronic impairments, it would furnish necessary supportive services in the least restrictive environment, to capitalize on people's strengths and prevent further deterioration. Involvement in choice between options for care, and rights to appeal adverse determinations are important. Current provisions fall short of these ideals due to problems in coverage, financial gaps in programs, a preoccupation with cost-cutting thereby eroding advances, and lack of information on coverage and appeal rights.

A fundamental problem with Medicare is that it is designed for acute illness rather than providing preventive services or supporting functioning in the face of chronic conditions. This is partially true of the recently passed catastrophic illness provisions. Medicare Part A is financed mainly by payroll deductions paid into a trust fund. It covers all those who are entitled to Social Security. Its main focus is on specified provisions for hospital care. Physician visits, and a limited number of other outpatient services, are covered by Part B--a voluntary program with a monthly premium, up to $24.80 by 1988: a sizable sum for those living close to poverty. Part B also includes deductibles and co-payments, thus placing further burdens on those with limited funds. Visual impairments and hearing deficits are among the most frequent and easily corrected functional problems of the elderly, making possible considerable improvement in quality of life. Yet eyeglasses and hearing aids are not covered under Medicare: The result is that many elderly go without. Many older people also lack access to adequate dental care which could prevent tooth loss, and resultant nutritional problems (U.S. Senate, Special Committee on Aging, 1987). Nursing home coverage under Medicare Part A is confined to a mere one hundred days of skilled care after acute hospitalization, but with co-payments after the twentieth day. The idea is that nursing home stays will provide rehabilitation and eventual return to the community. Those who require longer stays and lesser degrees of supportive care must pay out-of-pocket or spend down in order to be qualify for Medicaid. Home health care under Medicare is similarly restricted to rehabilitative benefits. Recipients must be housebound, and need the care of a skilled practitioner (such as a registered nurse) on a part-time or intermittent basis, in the interests of recovery. Medicare will not pay for home care to stable individuals. Hence, there is no possibility of obtaining payment for limited supportive care to remain relatively independent. Hospice benefits do, however, provide support for the terminally ill.

Medicaid is the major public payer for nursing home services. It is largely intended for those who qualify for Supplemental Security Income, and the medically indigent who need not be 65. Beginning in 1981, under a mandate by the Republican administration, expenditures were cut below those already approved. Throughout the mid-1980s, however, coverage was extended to additional categories by means of piecemeal legislation passed as amendments to other bills. Currently some 23.7 million people in the United States are on Medicaid, yet

fewer than half the nation's 32 million poor receive its medical
benefits. The estimated 1989 payout under Medicaid provisions will
total about $34.2 billion with half to over three quarters coming from
federal dollars, depending on relative affluence of states. Though
jointly financed by federal and state funds, it is administered by
states themselves: Consequently protection varies rather dramatically. In all instances, to qualify for Medicaid payments for nursing
home care, older persons must spend down their assets, leaving
themselves, and possibly a spouse destitute, thus creating financial
dependency in people who were relatively self-sufficient. The
personal needs allowance for Medicaid nursing home beneficiaries has
remained at a meager $25 a month since 1972, severely limiting
patients' ability to purchase basic necessities like toothpaste, eye
glasses, clothing, laundry, newspapers or phone calls (U.S. Senate
Special Committee on Aging, 1987). Under the 2176 waiver program,
some states do provide a limited amount of home care services through
Medicaid. The pressure in these programs is, however, to focus on
limiting costs by providing care in the community to those who would
otherwise be in skilled or intermediate care nursing facilities. This
precludes provision of services to prevent deterioration of functioning in those with lesser needs.

Some social services to preclude or reduce inappropriate institutionalization are provided under Title XX of the Social Security
Act, but these are constricted due to competing demands on Title XX
funds for services for non-elderly. Additionally there has been no
increase in Title XX funds since 1984. Title III of the Older
Americans Act provides some funding for supportive services, for
congregate nutrition services, and for home-bound nutrition services.
True to form, funds are limited, and agencies experience competing
demands for supportive care after discharge from hospital, and from
those needing long-term services to maintain independence. Approximately 19 percent of the community dwelling elderly living on
their own experience some limitations in activities of daily living
due to chronic conditions. Seventy percent of these rely on informal
care from family and friends. A large proportion of those who receive
paid care pay for it out-of-pocket, making payment for long-term care
a serious factor in impoverishment of the elderly (U.S. Senate,
Special Committee on Aging, 1987). The creation of viable protection
against long-term care expenses remains an important challenge and one
in which the United States lags behind the rest of the industrialized
world.

The Issue of Cost: Indeed, due to serious gaps in coverage,
health and long-term care expenditures together place a heavy burden
on older persons in the United States, particularly those whose
incomes have been limited throughout life. Those not eligible for
Social Security do not qualify for Medicare: Consequently in 1986,
the latest reporting year, there were approximately 389,000 persons
aged sixty-five and over without any form of insurance (U.S. Senate
Special Committee on Aging, 1987). Because of stringent eligibility

requirements for medical assistance under the Medicaid program, about two-thirds of the elderly poor are not covered. About one-third of the elderly near-poor are pushed into poverty by out-of-pocket medical expenditures, and premiums for private insurance (Commonwealth Fund Commission on Elderly People Living Alone, 1988). Part B premiums, deductibles and co-payments represent a sizable expenditure for those covered by Medicare, and have been increasing as part of the current budget-cutting efforts. In 1985, the first time, older people spent more for health care than they did when Medicare and Medicaid began: over 15 percent of their already limited incomes (U.S. Senate Special Committee on Aging, 1987).

Since the early 1980s, concern with the federal deficit, and resultant cost-cutting measures have threatened services providing support for the independence of the elderly. We noted above the stagnation in Title XX funds for social services to community elderly, and Title III funds for supportive services. There have also been pressures from both state and the federal government to keep Medicaid costs down, affecting payments for nursing care and 2167 waiver community care programs. At the same time, the Health Care Financing Administration has stepped up denials on home health services financed by Medicare. In 1983, Medicare Part A hospital reimbursement was switched to a prospective payment system whereby hospitals are paid regulated amounts for each of 471 disease related groups (DRGs), thus either losing or making money on hospitalizations according to their own cost controls. There is an obvious incentive for early discharge, and since inception of DRGs, a study performed for the Senate Special Committee on Aging, and numerous congressional hearings (U.S. Senate, Special Committee on Aging, 1985a, 1985b, 1985c; U.S. House of Representatives, Committee on Education and Labor, Subcommittee on Human Resources, 1986; U.S. House of Representatives, Select Committee on Aging, 1985; U.S. House of Representatives, Select Committee on Aging and Task Force on the Rural Elderly, 1985) have indicated the elderly are being discharged into the community "quicker and sicker."   The U.S. Senate Special Committee on Aging (1987) also notes a dramatic increase in Medicare admissions to nursing homes in the same period. This at least raises questions of whether early discharge under adverse conditions creates dependency and impedes return to former levels of functioning. Knowledge is another facet of quality care. The Senate Committee on Aging (1987) has inquired into the inadequacy of information about rights and mechanisms for elderly to appeal adverse decisions on hospitalization or eligibility for Medicare provisions. These findings are not encouraging, to say the least.

There are, then, serious gaps in health and long-term care services designed to support functioning of the elderly in the light of a focus on cost-containment threatening services even further. All would agree, cost is an important issue, and every effort should be made to ensure adequate services are rendered in a cost-effective manner. Yet cost cutting is itself costly: Especially if it promotes negative attitudes toward entire groups; or results in blaming those

who are the victims of ill-health for their plight. It also ignores
the fact that preventive services, and support designed to prolong
functioning of community elderly might actually save funds in the
long-run. Indeed, improvement of health care and preventive services
across the lifecourse may make for a healthier, less debilitating, and
less costly old age for those who will be old tomorrow or the day
after.

Dependency and Intergenerational Conflict: The Debate

Yet, in recent years, there has been a tendency to conceptualize
allocation of resources in terms of intergenerational inequity:
competition between generations for scarce resources. With a stagnant
economy, and rates of joblessness in the early 1980s approaching
levels not seen since the Great Depression, a new day dawned: The
elderly came to be seen as a burden on the economy, diverting
resources from younger generations (Davis & van den Oever, 1981;
Tigges, 1988). New edicts in the policy realm began countermanding
programs two generations in the making. Budgetary shortfalls and a
shifting political ideology came together. For the elderly, this
meant retrenchments on nearly every quarter and a great deal more
uncertainty than at any time since the Depression. 1983 saw the
beginning of a gradual increase in retirement age, a six month delay
in Social Security cost-of-living adjustments, and introduction of
prospective payment and other cost-cutting measures in Medicare.
Also affected were Medicaid, and social service programs under the
Older Americans Act. In attempting to alter the compact between
society and its older citizens, claims were made that younger
generations were suffering because of inequitable settling of
resources on the elderly (Longman, 1987). A viable claim, on the face
of it, but one which misrepresents not only the current situation, but
what lies ahead.

Focusing on intergenerational conflict diverts attention from
diversities and inequities within generations, and from interests
common to groups in all generations (Binstock, 1985). In 1984, income
inequality among the aged was higher in the United States than in any
other advanced industrial society. While some older people are indeed
wealthy, 30 percent of the elderly are economically insecure in that
their incomes are less than twice the poverty level, and the elderly
constitute 33 percent of the long-term poor. Across all age-groups,
the percent share of the total national income for the bottom three
fifths of U.S. families was lower in 1984 than at any time since
information was first collected in 1947 (Tigges, 1988). The challenge
to entitlement benefits thus forms part of what Piven and Cloward
(1982) term "the new class war" waged under the auspices of the Reagan
Administration. It is a war challenging rights of so-called "non-
productive" citizens to receive benefits, directed not only against
the elderly, but at social benefits throughout life. These have been
targeted as a cause of federal government deficits; yet a similar

logic is seldom used when referring to defense or other valued programs (Binstock, 1985; Kingson, Hirshorn & Cornman, 1986; Kingson, Hirshorn & Harootyan, 1986).

In portraying the elderly solely as recipients of economic transfers, the intergenerational equity perspective fails to acknowledge interdependence and reciprocity between generations and individuals across the lifecourse. While autonomy is important, it is also normal for individuals at all ages to have needs that may best be met by others or societal institutions. At the private level, the elderly make significant contributions to younger generations, both through income transfer, and through services in kind (Kingson, Hirshorn & Cornman, 1986; Kingson, Hirshorn & Harootyan, 1986; Morgan, 1983). Furthermore, the majority of older people have long paid in to Social Security and the Medicare trust fund. While the elderly, particularly the old-old, are more vulnerable to chronic conditions, there are functionally disabled persons in receipt of public benefits in younger generations, too; and older persons who continue to make real contributions, either through paid work or through voluntary community services.

Setting interdependence in a lifecourse perspective, serves to clarify the complex patterns of giving and receiving in which individuals participate over the time. During childhood and youth, people receive rather than give, although they may make significant contributions to family life. During young and middle adulthood, people give more than they receive, though they doubtless receive assistance, some from the elderly. During the later years, particularly advanced old age, individuals increasingly receive resources, without ceasing to be active contributors in the exchange (Morgan, 1983). Beginning early on, people benefit from cultural, scientific, and other social advances forged in earlier years by those who are now old. Persons in all generations may benefit indirectly from policies directed to the elderly, such as income support or home health programs. Furthermore, the face of aging for today's young will be shaped by the policies they construct for today's elderly (Kingson, Hirshorn & Cornman, 1986; Kingson, Hirshorn, & Harootyan, 1986). Without doubt, the seeds of dependency germinate across the lifespan. Today's marginal young are likely to be tomorrow's marginal elderly. A life of poor nutrition, lack of access to adequate health care, unemployment or low-paying peripheral jobs, portends poverty, chronic illness and perhaps even dependency in old age.

Rather than focusing on intergenerational inequity defined in terms of a narrow range of federal government transfers, it may make more sense to speak of equity of access to resources to forestall dependency at all ages. Leedham (1986) offers a basis for this approach in her use of concepts of equitable access outlined by the Office of Technical Assessment (U.S. Congress, Office of Technical Assessment, 1985) to develop an environmentally grounded approach to health care as process over time. The first definition of equitable

access: the right of citizens to fulfillment of all of their needs,
is unrealistic in view of limitations on resources, and the political
realities of a market economy.   The second, market-based approach,
asserts all citizens have the right to purchase fulfillment of their
needs at a price reflecting true costs to the supplier.   This perspective reinforces a competitive market ideology, failing to protect the
unemployed and those in marginal sectors of the economy.   The third
view holds that social policy should assure an adequate level or
decent minimum of access to resources for all citizens without
excessive hardships in attaining them.   This approach allows us to
adapt Clark's (1985) lifecourse perspective on the distribution of
goods, and to ask what we would consider to be a decent minimum of
resources, sufficient to prevent unnecessary dependency, at different
times in life.   It also permits a flexible approach to the diversity
of the elderly, and consideration of contextual factors which create
diverse needs, and differing hardships to be overcome.   To this should
be added the view of individuals as active participants in the
creation of resources and social policies.

Conclusions and Future Directions: Dependency or Empowerment

Part of the challenge in preventing stereotyping and the creation of
unnecessary dependence is to recognize the enormous diversity among
the elderly and the plasticity of aging (Labouvie-Vief, 1985; Rowe &
Kahn, 1987).   While there are significant numbers of old persons with
impairments requiring supportive services, there are more healthy
elderly who can and do contribute (Kingson, Hirshorn, & Harootyan,
1986).   Rowe and Kahn (1987) draw a distinction between two alternative modes of normal aging: "usual aging" and "successful aging."   In
usual aging, extrinsic environmental factors heighten potentially
negative effects of aging *per se*.   In successful aging, extrinsic
factors play either a neutral or positive role.   One of the negative
factors in usual aging is imposed loss of autonomy and control, due to
economic, health or other factors, which may lead to adverse effects
on emotional states, performance, subjective well-being and physiological indicators (Rodin, 1986; Rowe & Kahn, 1987; Shupe, 1985).
Considerable research has been amassed to buttress the notion that
heightening the elderly's sense of subjective control, even for those
who appear to be quite dependent, can result in significant gains in
cognitive, emotional and even physical well-being (Labouvie-Vief,
1985; Langer & Rodin, 1979; Schulz, 1976; Shupe, 1985; Wolk, 1976).

Labouvie-Vief (1985) further questions the validity of research
on supposed intelligence decline in aging on the grounds that it is
biased against cognitive maturity.   In so doing, she distinguishes two
approaches to problems.   Intrasystemic logical thought, the type most
frequently tapped in intelligence tests, isolates problems from their
context, and seeks to solve them in terms of universal principles.
Persons using this mode emphasize the search for the "correct"
solution; and are highly dependent upon those who define truth.   This

type of intelligence is undoubtedly highly adaptive vis-à-vis problems encountered in school, but less so in the real world. In intersystemic thought, characteristic of mature adults, the individual learns to order true and false assumptions from the perspectives of multiple systems, with allowance for uncertainty, which, in turn, opens the way for the development of new knowledge. Problems are considered in their social and environmental setting, giving salience to practical concerns. Birren (1969), for instance, found older adults tended to define problems in terms of maximizing benefits and minimizing risks for the system within which they operate, whereas younger adults tended to define them in more individualistic terms. These findings underline the importance of Ladd's (1973) claim regarding potential contributions of elderly as active co-creators of social policy.

Labouvie-Vief's (1987) intersystemic thought fits nicely with Clark's (1987) notion of empowerment as balance and interdependence: the balancing of needs and visions of one's own generation with those of others within the limits of social resources. It also ties in with House's (1980) conception of the public good as a negotiated rule structure to which people adhere even though it may run counter to their immediately desired satisfactions, if only to improve overall opportunities of obtaining satisfaction. For this to be true, however, empowerment must also be political activism and public goods (Clark, 1987): sufficient economic and health resources for the elderly to be active beneficiaries and participants in society. It implies access to information necessary to make informed choices; and stretches across the lifecourse.

The idea of empowerment as interdependence spans, and resolves to some degree, many of the value-dilemmas outlined by Achenbaum (1983). The ideal of rugged independence, and the resultant stereotyping of some as dependent, is replaced by a realization of interdependence between generations and persons. While individuals are seen as entitled to benefits by virtue of their membership in society, they strive to create conditions which make those benefits possible. Expectations are also tempered by a realistic appraisal of current economic conditions. Social justice is evaluated in terms of adequacy of results: what it takes to make possible a decent minimum standard of living for the individual, rather than quantitatively equal benefits for all. Innovative approaches to social problems are valued--but so are contributions of tradition which set them within broader historical and societal settings. Productive work as an option for some elderly, and leisure as a need of the middle-aged and young, are both recognized.

Implicit in the above discussion is a cradle-to-grave approach to health and income policies. This means ensuring a safety net for all within limitations of available resources. Such an approach would both improve current quality of life of marginal young and middle-aged persons, and, through its preventive impact, decrease the prospect of dependency as they age. Within this framework, policies for older people should be designed to maximize functioning. Income support, adequate housing, health care, and a range of community-based services should be there to enable those elderly who need them to cope creatively with limitations, but without infantilization through overly protective services. If failing capacities mandate an institutional environment, every effort should be made to foster a sense of control and a variety of options (Labouvie-Vief, 1985). A sense of control may also be reinforced by information and education alerting the elderly to plan ahead for possible declines, so they may exercise some choice if they have to confront long-term care (American Association of Retired Persons, 1986).

It is important, too, to recognize potential and actual contributions of the elderly. This implies making it possible for those who are willing and able to work to do so. We also need to be aware of private contributions of the elderly in terms of financial assistance and practical help to families and to each other. Finally, organizations should be structured to make it possible for the elderly to participate in formulating the policies and decisions which affect their lives. If we are to speak meaningfully of dependency at any age, we must be cognizant of how lives are lived, not in isolation, but in socially constructed contexts.

References

Abramson, L. Y., Seligman, M. E. P., & Teasdale, J. D. (1978) Learned helplessness in humans: Critique and reformulations. *Journal of Abnormal Psychology, 87,* 49-74.

Achenbaum, W. A. (1983). *Shades of gray: Old age, American values, and federal policies since 1920.* Boston: Little, Brown.

American Association of Retired Persons. (1986). *A matter of choice: Planning for difficult decisions.* Washington, DC: American Association of Retired Persons.

Billings, A. G., & Moos, R. H. (1985). Psychosocial stressors, coping and depression. In E. E. Beckham & W. R. Leber (Eds.), *Handbook of depression: Treatment, assessment and research* (pp. 939-974). Homewood: Dorsey Press.

Billings, A. G., & Moos, R. H. (1982). Psychosocial theory and research on depression: An integrative framework and review. *Clinical Psychology Review, 2,* 213-237.

Binstock, R. (1985). The oldest old: A fresh perspective on compassionate ageism revisited. *Milbank Memorial Fund Quarterly, 63,* 420-451.

Birren, J. E. (1969). Age and decision strategies. *Interdisciplinary topics in gerontology.* Basel: Karger.

Bresnahan, J. L., & Blum, W. L. (1971). Chaotic reinforcement: A socioeconomic leveler. *Developmental Psychology, 4,* 89-92.

Breytspraak, L. M. (1984). *The development of self in later life.* Boston: Little Brown.

Bultena, G. (1969). Life continuity and morale in old age. *The Gerontologist, 9,* 251-253.

Clark, P. G. (1985). The social allocation of health care resources: Ethical dilemmas in age-group competition. *The Gerontologist, 25,* 119-125.

Clark, P. G. (1987, November). *The philosophical foundations of empowerment: Implications for health care programs and practice.* Paper presented at a symposium on "Empowerment of the elderly in the health care system: Potential and pitfalls" at the 40th Annual Scientific Meeting of the Gerontological Society of America, Washington, DC.

Commonwealth Fund Commission on Elderly People Living Alone. (1987). *Medicare's poor: Filling the gaps in medical coverage for low-income elderly Americans.* Baltimore, MD: Johns Hopkins University.

Covey, H. C. (1981). A reconceptualization of continuity theory: Some preliminary thoughts. *The Gerontologist, 21,* 628-633.

Cummings, E., & Henry, W. E. (1961). *Growing old: The process of disengagement.* New York: Basic Books.

Davis, K., & van den Oever, P. (1981). Age relations and public policy in advanced industrial societies. *Population and Development Review, 7,* 1-18.

Dreyfus, H. L., & Rabinow, P. (1983). *Michel Foucault: Beyond structuralism and hermeneutics* (2nd ed.). Chicago: University of Chicago Press.

Dweck, C. S., & Reppucci, N. D. (1973). Learned helplessness and reinforcement responsibility in children. *Journal of Personality and Social Psychology, 25,* 109-116.

Estes, C. L., Swan, J., & Gerard, L. (1982). Dominant and emerging paradigms in gerontology: Toward a political economy of ageing. *Ageing and Society, 2,* 151-164.

Foner, N. (1982). Some consequences of age inequality in non-industrial societies. In M. W. Riley, R. P. Ables & M. S. Teitelbaum (Eds.), *Aging from birth to death: Vol. 2.   Sociotemporal perspectives* (pp. 71-86). Boulder: Westview Press.

Fox, J. H. (1981)   Perspectives on the continuity perspective. *International Journal of Aging and Human Development, 14,* 97-115.

Gubrium, J. F. (1973).   *The myth of the golden years: A socio-environmental theory of aging.* Springfield, IL: Charles C. Thomas.

Havighurst, R. J., & Albrecht, R. (1953). *Older people.* New York: Longmans, Green.

Hendricks, J. (1987).   Age identification.   In G. Maddox (Ed.), *Encyclopedia of aging* (p. 15). New York: Springer.

Hendricks, J., & Hendricks, C. D. (1986). *Aging in mass society: Myths and realities.* Boston: Little, Brown.

Hendricks, J., & Leedham, C. A. (1987).   Making sense of literary aging: Relevance of recent gerontological theory. *Journal of Aging Studies, 1,* 187-208.

House, E. R. (1980). *Evaluating with validity.* Beverly Hills: Sage.

Kingson, E. R., Hirshorn, B. A., & Cornman, J. M. (1986). *Ties that bind: The interdependence of generations.* Washington, DC: Seven Locks Press.

Kingson, E., Hirshorn, B., & Harootyan, L. K. (1986).   *The common stake: The interdependence of generations.*   Washington, DC: Gerontological Society of America.

Kuypers, J. A., & Bengtson, V. L. (1973).   Social breakdown and competence: A model of normal aging. *Human Development, 25,* 181-201.

Labouvie-Vief, G. (1985).   Intelligence and cognition.   In J. E. Birren & K. Warner Schaie (Eds.), *Handbook of the psychology of aging* (2nd ed.) (pp. 500-530). New York: Van Nostrand Reinhold.

Ladd, J. (1973). Policy studies and ethics. *Policy Studies Journal, 2,* 38-43.

Langer, E. J., & Rodin, J. (1979). The effects of choice and enhanced responsibility: A field experience in an institutional setting. *Journal of Personality and Social Psychology, 34,* 191-198.

Lawton, M. P. (1983).   Environment and other determinants of well-being in older people. *The Gerontologist, 23,* 349-357.

Lazarus, R. S. (1981). The stress and coping paradigm. In C. Eisdorfer, D. Cohen, A. Kleinman & P. Maxim (Eds.), *Models for clinical psychopathology* (pp. 177-214). New York: Spectrum.

Leedham, C. A. (1986, November). *Diagnosis-related groups: A theoretical critique.* Paper presented at the 39th Annual Scientific Meeting of the Gerontological Society of America, Chicago, IL.

Levin, J., & Levin, W. C. (1980). *Ageism: Prejudice and discrimination against the elderly.* Belmont, CA: Wadsworth.

Longman, P. (1987). *Born to pay: The new politics of aging in America.* Boston: Houghton Mifflin.

Looft, W. R. (1972). Egocentrism and social interaction across the life span. *Psychological Bulletin, 78,* 73-92.

Maddox, G. L. (1970). Themes and issues in sociological theories of human aging. *Human Development, 13,* 17-27.

Marshall, V. (1981). Societal toleration of aging: Sociological theory and social response to population. In *Adaptability and Aging. I.* (pp. 85-104). Paris: International Center of Social Gerontology.

Marshall, V. (1986). Dominant and emerging perspectives in the social psychology of aging. In V. Marshall (Ed.), *Later life: The social psychology of aging* (pp. 9-31). Beverly Hills: Sage.

Moos, R. H., & Mitchell, R. E. (1982). Conceptualizing and measuring social network resources. In T. A. Wills (Ed.), *Basic processes in helping relationships* (pp. 213-232). New York: Academic Press.

Morgan, J. N. (1983). The redistribution of income by families and institutions and emergency help patterns. In G. J. Duncan & J. N. Morgan (Eds.), *Five thousand American families: Patterns of economic progress: Vol. 10, Analyses of the first thirteen years of the panel study of income dynamics.* Ann Arbor: Institute for Social Research, University of Michigan.

Neugarten, B. (1977). Personality and aging. In J. E. Birren & K. Warner Schaie (Eds.), *Handbook of the psychology of aging* (pp. 626-649). New York: Van Nostrand.

Neugarten, B., Crotty, W., & Tobin, S. (1964). Personality types in an aged population. In B. Neugarten et al. (Eds.), *Personality in middle and late life* (pp. 158-187). New York: Atherton Press.

Neugarten, B., Havighurst, R. J., & Tobin, S. (1968). Personality and patterns of aging. In B. Neugarten (Ed.), *Middle age and aging* (pp. 173-177). Chicago: University of Chicago Press.

Norris, J. E. (1987). Psychological processes in the development of late-life social identity. In V. W. Marshall (Ed.), *Aging in Canada: Social perspectives* (pp. 60-81). Toronto: Fitzhenry & Whiteside.

Overmier, J. B., & Seligman, M. E. P. (1967). Effects of inescapable shock upon subsequent escape and avoidance learning. *Journal of Comparative and Physiological Psychology, 63*, 23-33.

Peterson, C., & Seligman, M. E. P. (1983). Learned helplessness and victimization. *Journal of Social Issues, 39*, 103-116.

Peterson, C., & Seligman, M. E. P. (1984). Causal explanation as a risk factor for depression: Theory and evidence. *Psychological Review, 91*, 347-374.

Peterson, C., & Seligman, M. E. P. (1985). The learned helplessness model of depression: Current status of theory and research. In E. E. Beckham & W. R. Leber (Eds.), *Handbook of depression* (pp. 914-939). Homewood, IL: Dorsey Press.

Phillips, B. S. (1957). A role theory approach to adjustment in old age. *American Sociological Review, 22*, 212-227.

Piven, F. F., & Cloward, R. A. (1982). *The new class war: Reagan's attack on the welfare state and its consequences.* New York: Pantheon Books.

Riegel, K. F. (1975). Toward a dialectical theory of development. *Human Development, 18*, 50-64.

Rodin, J. (1986). Aging and health: Effects of the sense of control. *Science, 233*, 1271-1276.

Ross, L., Amabile, T., & Steinmetz, J. (1977). Social roles, social control, and bias in social-perception processes. *Journal of Personality and Social Psychology, 35*, 485-494.

Rowe, J. W., & Kahn, R. L. (1987). Human aging: Usual and successful. *Science, 237*, 143-149.

Schulz, R. (1976). Effects of control and predictability on the physical and psychological well-being of the institutionalized aged. *Journal of Personality and Social Psychology, 33*, 563-573.

Seligman, M. E. P. (1972). Learned helplessness. *Annual Review of Medicine, 23*, 407-412.

Seligman, M. E. P. (1975). *Helplessness: On depression, development and death.* San Francisco: Freeman.

Shupe, D. R. (1985). Perceived control, helplessness and choice. In J. E. Birren & J. Livingston (Eds.), *Cognition, stress and aging* (pp. 174-197). Englewood Cliffs, NJ: Prentice-Hall.

Tigges, L. M., (1988). *The class basis of generational conflict in the 1980s.* Paper presented at the meeting of the Southern Sociological Society, Nashville, TN.

Townsend, P. (1986). Ageism and social policy. In C. Phillipson & A. Walker (Eds.), *Ageing and social policy: A critical assessment* (pp. 15-44). London: Gower.

Tropman, J. E., & McClure, J. K. (1980). Social values in the policy process. *Policy Studies Journal, 9,* 604-613.

U.S. Congress. Office of Technical Assessment. (1985). *Medicare's prospective payment system. Strategies for evaluating cost, quality, and medical technology.* Washington, DC: U.S. Government Printing Office.

U.S. House of Representatives. Committee on Education and Labor. Subcommittee on Human Resources. (1986). *Oversight hearing on Title III, Older Americans Act, and effects of medicare's DRG implementation.* Hearing. July 30, 1985. Washington, DC: U.S. Government Printing Office.

U.S. House of Representatives. Select Committee on Aging. (1985). *Health care cost containment: Are America's aged protected?* Hearing. July 9, 1985. Washington, DC: U.S. Government Printing Office.

U.S. House of Representatives. Select Committee on Aging and Task Force on the Rural Elderly. (1985). *Sustaining quality health care under cost containment.* Hearing. February 16, 1985. Washington, DC: U.S. Government Printing Office.

U.S. Senate. Special Committee on Aging. (1985a). *Medicare DRG's: Challenges for post-hospital care.* Hearing. October 24, 1985. Washington, DC: U.S. Government Printing Office.

U.S. Senate. Special Committee on Aging. (1985b). *Medicare DRG's: The Government's role in ensuring quality.* Hearing. November 12, 1985. Washington, DC: U.S. Government Printing Office.

U.S. Senate. Special Committee on Aging. (1985c). *News.* February 26, 1985. Washington, DC: U.S. Government Printing Office.

U.S. Senate. Special Committee on Aging. (1987). *Developments in aging: 1986: Vol. 1.* Washington, DC: U.S. Government Printing Office.

J. Hendricks and C. A. Leedham

Williamson, J. B., Shindul, J. A., & Evans, L. (1985). *Aging and public policy.* Springfield, IL: Charles C. Thomas.

Wolk, S. (1976). Situational constraint as a moderator of locus of control-adjustment relationship. *Journal of Consulting and Clinical Psychology, 44,* 420-427.

Zusman, J. (1966). Some explanations of the changing appearance of psychotic patients: Antecedents of the social breakdown syndrome concept. *The Milbank Memorial Fund Quarterly, 44,* 363-374.

Psychological Perspectives of Helplessness
and Control in the Elderly, P.S. Fry (ed.)
© Elsevier Science Publishers B.V. (North-Holland), 1989

Chapter Fourteen

CHOOSING TO IMPROVE PERFORMANCE

Lawrence C. PERLMUTER, *VA Outpatient Clinic, Boston, MA*

Steven H. GOLDFINGER, *VA Outpatient Clinic, Boston, MA*

Nancy R. SIZER, *VA Outpatient Clinic, Boston, MA*

Richard A. MONTY, *U.S. Army Engineering Laboratory
Aberdeen Proving Ground, MD*

Abstract

*Motivational levels are elevated when individuals believe
that they have control over tasks and over behavioral
outcomes. When individuals are permitted to make choices,
their perception of control increases. In addition, by
enhancing motivation, the exercise of choice facilitates
performance on a variety of cognitive tasks. However, with
advancing age or in the presence of a chronic disease such
as diabetes, the effectiveness of choice in improving
performance is attenuated. Despite these limitations on the
effectiveness of choice, cognitive performance can still be
improved significantly by the simple expedient of increasing
the perception of control. Increased motivation appears to
improve performance by suppressing interference from
background stimuli. That is, decreased concentration on
relevant target stimuli and increased interference from
less relevant background stimuli are characteristics of the
decline in cognitive function in the aged. This reflects a
decrease in differentiation, a putative cognitive process
that identifies target and background stimuli and appropriately proportions cognitive resources to them. When
differentiation is effective, interference from background
stimuli decreases. Because differentiation is an effort
demanding process, its effectiveness depends upon an
adequate level of motivation. Research indicates that the
degree to which an individual differentiates predicts
performance on a variety of cognitive tasks. Overall, these
findings are hopeful in demonstrating that choice can serve
as an effective motivational intervention for decreasing the
rate of cognitive decline and improving the quality of life
in vulnerable older individuals.*

Introduction

Opportunities for decision making and choice may decrease with advancing age as a result of physical and social restrictions, disease states and cognitive decline (Salthouse, 1982; Weisz, 1983). As the exercise of choice becomes less frequent, motivation levels decrease and cognitive performance declines (Perlmuter, Monty & Chan, 1986; Langer, 1983). Compromised cognition is likely to lower competence and self-esteem with the result that further efforts at control are diminished. Therefore, delineating the relationship among choice, motivation, and cognition is important both to the explanation and remediation of cognitive decline.

This chapter will examine the effectiveness of choice in enhancing motivation and cognitive function. Low levels of motivation are associated with diminished concentration on focal stimuli and increased susceptibility to interference from background cues, each of which contributes to poorer performance on cognitive tasks in the aged. We will attempt to show how motivation facilitates the appropriate allocation of cognitive resources to focal as well as to background stimuli.

Choice Increases Motivation, Improves Performance

Enhanced motivation improves cognitive performance in the young as well as in the aged (Perlmuter, Monty & Chan, 1986; Langer, Rodin, Beck, Weinman & Spitzer, 1979). In one study (Perlmuter & Smith, 1979), individuals were provided with the opportunity to make some choices within the task--a procedure that increases the perception of control (Perlmuter & Langer, 1983; Chan, Karbowski, Monty & Perlmuter, 1986). Men, aged 50-70 years, who had sought assistance for memory problems at the Veterans Administration Clinic in Boston, were presented with a paired associate task consisting of words that were low to moderate in meaningfulness (e.g., VICAR, PECAN) and thus relatively difficult to learn. Paired associate learning provides one of the most reliable indices of age-related changes in cognitive status (Erickson & Scott, 1977). Basically, the paired associate procedure involves learning of associations between a stimulus word and a response word. The test for learning involves the presentation of the stimulus word to determine whether the correct response word can be recalled.

After explaining and illustrating the procedure for learning paired associates to the participants, 10 stimulus words, each accompanied by two potential response words, were presented. In one condition (Choice), participants selected and circled one response word in each pair to be associated with the stimulus word. In the Force condition, one response word in each pair had been circled prior to presentation and participants drew another circle around it. Both groups studied the designated stimulus-response pairs and then received a cued recall test trial in which only stimuli were presented. Participants were to recall the response words and record these next to the respective stimuli. Study and test trials alternated until six tests were completed.

Table 1 presents the mean percentage of correct responses as well as the mean percentage of incorrect or misplaced responses (intrusions) on the first and last test trials. Individuals in the Choice group not only learned significantly better than those in the Force group, but the number of intrusions within the Choice group was relatively low in comparison to the number of correct responses. On the other hand, intrusions in the Force group were high relative to the number of correct responses (see Table 1).

Fleming and Lopez (1981) examined paired associate learning in a group of elderly community dwellers, the majority of whom were women. The Choice group performed significantly better than the Force group. Based on the overall results, it can be concluded that the beneficial effects of choice are not limited to men, nor to individuals complaining of memory problems.

Table 1

Mean Percent Correct Responses and Intrusions in a Paired Associate Task for Choice and Force Groups

	Trial 1		Trial 6	
	Choice Group	Force Group	Choice Group	Force Group
Mean % Correct	28	8	48	22
Mean % Intrusions	3	7	6	13

A Motivational Mechanism of Choice

One explanation for these findings is that when individuals are enabled to make meaningful choices they perceive an increased amount of control, and this in turn elevates motivation (Perlmuter, Scharff, Karsh & Monty, 1980). Indeed, there is a substantial body of evidence showing that performance improves as motivation increases, at least up to a point (Kleinsmith & Kaplan, 1963). On the other hand, these studies do not disallow the possibility that in the Choice condition, participants selected response words which had idiosyncratic mnemonic properties that facilitated their association with stimulus words. Such an advantage is less likely in the Force group. Despite its intuitive appeal, the idiosyncratic explanation does not fully account for the benefits of choice, since it has been shown that the opportunity to exercise a meaningful choice (Monty, Geller, Savage & Perlmuter, 1979; Savage, Perlmuter & Monty, 1979) has more influence on performance than the particular items that have been selected.

Choice improves performance on portions of the task over which no choice had been permitted and even generalizes to tasks that are unrelated to the one on which the choices had been made. In a paired associate study (Monty, Rosenberger & Perlmuter, 1973), college-age participants were presented with 12 stimulus words each accompanied by five potential response words. One response word in each set was to be associated with the respective stimulus word, either selected by the participant (Choice group) or the experimenter (Force group). The novel feature of the experiment was that while one group chose 100% of their response words, two other groups chose only 25% of the responses, with the remainder assigned by the experimenter. Participants in the Early Choice group selected their responses to the first three stimuli, while those in the Late Choice group selected responses to the final three stimuli in the sequence; the remaining nine responses were assigned by the experimenter. A fourth group (Force) had all the response words assigned by the experimenter.

Results showed that the 100% Choice group learned significantly better than the Force group, replicating previous findings with aged subjects. More importantly, the Early Choice group learned as well as the 100% Choice group, while the Late Choice group performed similarly to the group offered no choice at all. The identical amount of choice at the conclusion of the task failed to benefit performance relative to the Force group. Apparently, the opportunity for choice at the commencement of the procedure enhanced motivation which in turn may have strengthened the development of stimulus response associations.

Using a similar early versus late choice procedure, White (reported in Perlmuter & Monty, 1977) showed that performance on a reading comprehension task was improved significantly by allowing choice at the start of the task. These results were found with grade school children, supporting the notion that the opportunity for control may have measurable effects on motivation, even in young children (deCharms, 1979; Renshon, 1979).

To examine how choice on one task affects performance on an unrelated task not involving choice, college-age participants either chose or were assigned response words to be learned on a paired associate task (Perlmuter et al., 1980). With the start of the paired associate learning trials came an unanticipated simple reaction time task in which participants were required to release a key as quickly as possible in response to presentations of a tone. Results showed that not only was paired associate learning facilitated by choice, but reaction times were also significantly faster in the Choice group. The opportunity to choose response words in advance of the paired associate task produced motivational effects that improved performance on the reaction time task.

Despite improved performance on both the paired associate and reaction time tasks pursuant to choice, it remains possible that the facilitation of reaction times was only indirectly affected by choice-induced motivation. Feedback from performance on the paired associate task would have been more positive in the Choice group, and thus motivated faster reaction times. To eliminate differential feedback from performance in the two groups, another experiment was run in which the reaction time task was introduced following the Choice/Force procedure but *before* the paired associate learning trials. As predicted, reaction times were significantly faster for Choice than for Force participants. These data provide the most direct evidence for the notion that the effects of choice are mediated by an increase in motivation--a theoretical mechanism especially suited to explaining the energization and facilitation of speeded behaviors (Brown, 1961).

Age-related Changes in the Effectiveness of Choice

While the effects of choice and control have been observed in young and in old (Monty & Perlmuter, 1987), little is known about the *relative* effectiveness of choice in young and old. To examine this relationship, young (18-35 years) and older participants (55-74 years) were presented with a paired associate task consisting of stimulus words each accompanied by two response words (McGlinchey, Perlmuter, Sizer & Nathan, 1985). Participants selected one response word to be learned to the respective stimulus words. Each of the stimulus-response pairings were available for study for about five seconds.

Following the study trial, the stimulus words were displayed and subjects were instructed to recall and record the response words. Performance was poor for both groups with young participants correctly recalling 21% of the response words and older participants recalling only 7%--a highly significant difference. More importantly, participants rated on a 1-7 scale (1 = none, 7 = a lot) how much choice they had in making their selections. However, because the self-reports of freedom to choose were assessed following the cued-recall test, performance levels may have influenced the reported perception of control. Nevertheless, older subjects (mean = 3.6) reported feeling significantly less free than younger subjects (mean = 5.4).

The Effectiveness of Choice in Aged Diabetics

Although paired associate performance declines with advancing age (Erickson & Scott, 1977), the opportunity to make choices within the task has beneficial effects for young as well as old. The magnitude of the improvement may decrease with advancing age. Is the effectiveness of choice further attenuated by the presence of a chronic disease such as non-insulin dependent diabetes? This question is especially relevant because diabetes affects upwards of 10% of the population over 65 years of age (Lipson, 1986), and because diabetics, like those with other chronic diseases, tend to have elevated depression scores (Berkman, Berkman, Kasl, Freeman, Leo, Ostfeld, Huntley & Brody, 1986). Depressed individuals, because of psychological factors such as sense of helplessness and detachment, and physiological factors including altered metabolic functioning, may be less susceptible to the benefits of choice (Freedman, Bucci & Elkowitz, 1982). Since diabetics must continuously monitor their disease and modify their behavior accordingly, an effective motivational procedure may be useful in enhancing compliance with regimen. Increased motivation may improve cognitive functioning and alleviate the more frequent everyday memory problems experienced by these individuals (Tun, 1987).

To assess the effectiveness of choice in improving performance and the extent to which background stimuli interfere with target learning, a group of 55-74 year old diabetics were compared with age-matched non-diabetics on a recognition memory task. Specifically, the 20 target words to be learned were displayed on lines containing either one or three additional background words, all of which were minimally related to each other. On half of the lines, individuals chose their target word, while on the remaining lines, target words were assigned. Choice and Force lines were randomly interspersed.

Instructions required the learning of target words; no explicit mention was made regarding background words. To determine how choice affected the intentional learning of targets and the incidental learning of background words, each 'old' word was presented individually. To provide a measure of false alarms, an equal number of new words was also presented. Participants indicated whether each word was "old" or "new"--i.e., had or had not appeared previously.

The recognition test showed that for all individuals self-chosen target words (mean % correct = 80±21) were learned significantly better than those which were assigned (mean % correct = 60±26). Moreover, background words from Choice lines (mean % correct = 50±25) were recognized significantly better than comparable words from Force lines (mean % correct = 36±22). Thus, choice facilitated the learning of both target *and* background words; the improved learning of targets on Choice lines did not occur at the expense of learning background words. Similar results have been found with college-age subjects (Monty, Perlmuter, Libon & Bennet 1982). The increment in motivation appears to enable the individual not only to learn better, but also to learn more.

An evaluation of the diabetes variable revealed that target recognition was significantly poorer for diabetics. More importantly, a comparison of performance on Choice and Force lines revealed that the improvement attributable to choice was less in diabetics than in non-diabetics. Apparently, one of the sequelae of a chronic disease may be to inhibit the effectiveness of a motivational intervention. These results, however, do not eliminate the possibility that a more intensive motivational intervention may allow disease-impaired individuals to reach the performance levels of age-matched controls.

Overall, these results are consistent with respect to the effectiveness of choice: normal aging attenuates the effectiveness of a motivational intervention, as does the presence of a chronic disease such as diabetes. Thus, impairments associated with some diseases in the aged may maintain the perception of control at a low level. In turn, chronically depressed levels of control render motivational interventions less effective than they are for younger and healthier individuals.

The Nature of Compromised Cognition in the Aged

Results from the recognition test described above may be useful in further explicating the frequent finding that old learners have increased difficulty in suppressing irrelevant information (Layton, 1975). This difficulty may be responsible for degraded cognitive performance in the aged. For example, elderly adults attend more strongly to irrelevant stimuli in a multiple-item recognition task than do young adults (Kausler & Kleim, 1978). Farkas & Hoyer (1980) found poorer performance in the aged in a perceptual grouping task, which they attributed to distraction from background stimuli. In a paired associate task involving release from proactive interference (PI), young people were less vulnerable to PI than were older people who lived at home, who in turn were less vulnerable than institutionalized older people (Winocur & Moscovitch, 1983). Erber (1986) found greater interference on coding and copying tasks for older as compared to younger subjects.

Additional evidence for the relationship between contextual interference and performance derives from the Stroop procedure. When presented with the unusual requirement of attending to conventional background cues (ink color), while suppressing attention to conventional target cues (color name), interference was found to be greatest in the aged (Comalli, Wapner & Werner, 1962). On the other hand, when materials were presented tachistoscopically, irrelevant background cues showed no evidence of differential interference for young or old (Wright & Elias, 1979).

There are some inconsistent findings in this literature. For older people but not for college students, memory for the spatial location of target drawings was enhanced when irrelevant drawings were present during learning (Park, Puglisi & Lutz, 1982). A later study (Park, Puglisi & Sovacool, 1984), however, reported conflicting results; while young adults benefitted from the presence of background cues (i.e., context) in a test of memory for cartoon characters, the performance of elderly adults was slightly better when such background cues were absent.

There are two seemingly paradoxical findings in the literature relating to the increased susceptibility of the aged to background cues. The first of these derives from a memory experiment in which individuals were to learn, in serial order, a list of letters. One letter in the list was made distinctive by being oversized. |While the memory performance of the young benefitted from this manipulation (Von Restorff Effect), that of the old did not (Cimbalo & Brink, 1982). Thus, while the old are less able to suppress interference from background stimuli, they appear less able to utilize background stimuli to enhance performance. Second, in young and old, suscep- tibility to interference from the context does not disrupt performance when motivation levels are increased. To illustrate this point we will return to the recognition study with diabetics and non-diabetics. In that task, background stimuli would be expected to interfere with target recognition, especially in the Choice condition where increased commerce with background stimuli is necessitated by the process of choosing targets. Contrary to expectation, choice enhanced the recognition of both target *and* background words in young and old. Thus, despite the increased potential for interference from background stimuli, such stimuli are better learned and less disruptive to target learning pursuant to choice. We will further examine this finding.

Choice and Differentiation

The process that helps to insulate against interference from back- ground stimuli and facilitates the appropriate allocation of process- ing resources to the primary stimuli we refer to as *differentiation*. Conceptually, a task may be considered to contain a finite number of target stimuli, defined by the learner or by instructions; amorphous background cues exist in vast amounts. Hence, the indiscriminate learning of background cues 'parri passu' with targets would be expected to dissipate cognitive resources required for target learning (Schulman, 1975).

Differentiation is presumed to be a graded and effort-demanding process that involves the implicit identification of both the target and background stimuli as such. Further, differentiation facilitates the learning of target as well as background stimuli, albeit to different levels. The equivalent or even greater attention to

background stimuli relative to targets reflects failed differentiation.   Differentiation is indexed by the difference in target and
background learning scores (target minus background).   The larger the
difference between target and background learning, the stronger is
differentiation.

Differentiation is illustrated in a number of experimental
paradigms, such as the incidental learning of "place-on-a-page"
(background) that occurs simultaneously with target learning.   As
background learning increases, target learning also increases.
However, high levels of background learning are associated with a
decrement in target learning.   While these relationships have been
observed in college-age subjects (Schulman, 1975), in the aged, as
background learning levels increase, target learning decreases
(Kausler & Kleim, 1978).   Thus, an explication of the relationship
between target and background learning may help to account for
age-related declines in cognitive performance.

Evidence Supporting the Differentiation Hypothesis

The relationship between choice and differentiation was examined
initially in a recognition task which was included in a test battery
that evaluated changes in cognitive function associated with aging and
non-insulin-dependent diabetes mellitus (Perlmuter, Hakami, Hodgson-
Harrington, Ginsberg, Katz, Singer & Nathan, 1984).   The hypothesis
examined was that choice improves recognition memory by facilitating
differentiation between target and background items, i.e., by
increasing the difference between target and background recognition
scores (target minus background).   In addition, it was proposed that
the degree of differentiation is a relatively stable individual
difference variable, such that high differentiators are expected to
perform better than low differentiators on other cognitive tasks.   The
test of the differentiation notion derived from a re-analysis of the
data from the recognition task described previously.   Specifically,
the difference in recognition scores (target minus background) was
calculated separately for Choice lines and for Force lines.   As
predicted, differentiation scores were significantly greater in the
Choice condition (mean % difference = 30 ± 23) than in the Force
condition ($25\pm22\%$), $t(247) = 2.98$, $p < .005$.   Thus, choice not only
facilitates both target and background recognition, but more importantly, increases the absolute difference between the two.

Predictive Utility of Differentiation Scores

If higher differentiation is associated with more effective cognitive
functioning, differentiation scores should decrease with advancing age
and should also be lower for members of a population with demonstrated
cognitive deficits (Tun, Perlmuter, Russo & Nathan, 1987).   Contrary
to expectations, no significant associations were found between age

and differentiation scores--an outcome that might have been conditioned by the relatively restricted age range, namely 55-74 years. In support of the hypothesis, differentiation scores were lower among diabetics (mean = 26±19%) than among non-diabetic age-matched controls (mean = 33±11%), $t(246)$ = 2.23, $p < .05$. This finding is consistent with the generally poorer learning and greater number of everyday memory problems encountered by diabetics (Tun et al., 1987).

Differentiation scores, if they index reliable individual differences, should predict performance on various cognitive tasks. The recognition task provided differentiation scores from Force as well as Choice lines. Baseline levels of differentiation are provided by performance on Force lines; scores from Choice lines are significantly elevated by the opportunity to make choices and thus do not reflect habitual levels of differentiation. Therefore, differentiation scores from Force lines should be more useful as predictors.

To examine the predictive utility of differentiation, participants were divided at the median differentiation score on Force lines into low and high differentiation groups. Performance of these groups was compared on a variety of cognitive tasks. A parallel set of analyses was performed with medians derived from Choice lines. Because of the observed differences in performance between diabetics and controls, and because of the limited number of non-diabetics, these analyses were limited to diabetics only.

Since the speed of behavior is one of the markers for cognitive decline, we predicted that increased slowing would be associated with low differentiation--an effortful and presumably time dependent process. Simple reaction time measures were derived from a task in which individuals released a key in response to a tone on each of 30 trials. Mean lift (key release) time was analyzed separately from mean movement time--the time required to reach a key located 13 cm to the right of the first key. As predicted, low differentiators on Force lines showed slower lift times (Table 2).

A speed component as well as a measure of distractibility is found in the Digit Symbol Substitution Task (DSST) (Wechlser, 1944), in which rows of digits must be replaced with paired symbols as rapidly as possible. Results on the DSST paralleled those on the reaction time task, with high differentiators on Force lines correctly transcribing significantly more symbols (Table 2). Performance on the Backward Digit Span (Wechlser, 1944), which requires individuals to hold digits in memory long enough to reverse their order prior to report, was significantly better for high differentiators than for low differentiators (Table 2). This finding extends the predictive utility of differentiation scores to untimed tasks. On the other hand, two measures that are relatively unaffected by practice or learning--Forward Digit Span (Perlmuter et al., 1984), a measure of working memory capacity; and movement time (described above)--were not related to differentiation scores (Table 2).

To the extent that differentiation is a basic cognitive process, it should be related to those variables which reflect cognitive functioning outside as well as inside the laboratory.   It was hypothesized that subjects with more years of formal education and with higher vocabulary levels (Wechsler, 1944) would have higher differentiation scores.   Although the direction of causality is unclear, it was found that those with high differentiation scores on Force lines had more years of formal education (low, mean = 11.6±3.6; high, mean = 12.7±2.8; t(207) = 2.40, p < .05), as well as sig-nificantly higher vocabulary scores (low, mean = 39.2±14.9; high, mean = 48.5±14.7; t(198) = 4.43, p < .001) than subjects with low differentiation scores.

Table 2

Performance of Low and High Differentiators on Force and Choice Lines (Diabetics Only)

	Force		Choice	
	Low	High	Low	High
Simple Reaction	476±100	437±88	468±101	446±90
Time (msec)	t(167) = 2.69*		t(167) = 1.51	
Digit Symbol	37.5±11.8	42.6±10.8	39.3±11.2	41.0±11.9
Substitution	t(200) = 3.20**		t(200) = 1.08	
Digit Span	4.22±1.45	4.87±1.39	4.60±1.54	4.50±1.36
Backward	t(204) = 3.28**		t(204) = 0.49	
Digit Span	6.71±1.36	6.62±1.46	6.72±1.51	6.61±1.32
Forward	t(204) = 0.44		t(204) = 0.57	
Movement Time	477±177	432±158	481±191	431±144
(msec)	t(167) = 1.75		t(167) = 1.97	

* p < .05   ** p < .01

The analyses described in Table 2 examined the relationship of choice and differentiation in individuals with chronic disease and measurable cognitive impairment.   To evaluate the effectiveness of choice in improving differentiation in relatively healthy individuals across a broader age-span, a young (17-29 years) and an old (58-88 years) group were compared.   Half of the young and half of the old were placed in a Force group; the remainder were placed in a Choice group.   A discrimination task similar to the recognition task described earlier was used.   Twenty lines were presented, each with two or four words.   One word on each line served as the target and the remainder were considered as background words. Half of the young and half of the old participants chose their own target words to be learned, while for the remaining participants targets were assigned. Subjects were instructed to learn the target words; no mention was made of the background words.   A week after the learning phase, a discrimination test was used in which an old word (target or background) and a new word were presented in pairs.   Individuals indicated which word in each pair was old.

Young individuals, because of higher baseline levels of motivation, should be more effective than older individuals in differentiating between target and background stimuli.   Based on this hypothesis, it was predicted that in the Force group, more young than old people would be good differentiators, i.e., target discrimination scores greater than background scores.   In the Choice group, where motivation is enhanced, the ratio of good to poor differentiators (background discrimination scores greater than or equal to target scores) should be more nearly equal for young and old.

Table 3

Number of Good and Poor Differentiators
by Age and Force/Choice Groups

	Force Group		Choice Group	
	Young	Old	Young	Old
Good Differentiators				
	9	2	14	8
(Targets > Background)				
Poor Differentiators				
	6	14	2	6
(Targets $\leq$ Background)				

$$\chi^2 = 5.70, \ p < .05 \qquad \chi^2 = 2.14, \quad p > .05$$

Results indicated that in the Force group, a significantly greater proportion of young than old subjects were good differentiators; in the Choice group, the ratio of good to poor differentiators was not different for young and old, with both age groups showing a majority of good differentiators (Table 3). In fact, among the old, the proportion of good differentiators in the Choice group resembles the proportion of young individuals who are good differentiators in the Force group. Overall, these findings extend those seen with diabetics and implicate choice and motivation in differentiation.

Summary and Conclusions

Advancing age and chronic disease are associated with the decline in the perception of control. Diminished levels of control reduce motivation and, in turn, degrade cognitive performance. Decreased cognitive function lowers the individual's sense of competence and self-esteem, a set of consequences that--in a downward spiral--further decrease the perception of control.

When individuals are provided with the opportunity to make some choices, the perception of control is strengthened and performance improves. However, advancing age and chronic disease (diabetes) progressively attenuate the effectiveness of an intervention to enhance the perception of control. Nevertheless, even for the aged with chronic disease, the opportunity to make some choices significantly improves performance.

Decreased concentration on relevant (target) information and increased interference from less relevant (background) information are characteristic of the age-related decline in cognitive performance. Differentiation facilitates concentration on targets and suppresses attention to background stimuli, and is indexed by the difference in the level to which target and background stimuli are learned. Since differentiation is thought to be an effort-demanding process, the level of motivation must be sufficiently high for differentiation to be effective. Thus, young individuals, whose baseline levels of motivation are generally higher than those of old individuals, differentiate more effectively. With advancing age, problems such as chronic disease and depression may attenuate motivation levels and adversely affect differentiation.

Research and clinical experience show that choice can be a potent facilitator of cognitive performance. The findings discussed here elucidate the mechanism of choice and have significant implications for educational and training programs. The discovery that cognitive decline can to some extent be reversed in the aged provides a hopeful note for improving the quality of life in vulnerable older individuals.

Acknowledgments

The preparation of this chapter was assisted by support from VA Medical Research Services.   Special thanks to Anne Shore for assistance with the preparation of this chapter.

References

Berkman, L. F., Berkman, C. S., Kasl, S., Freeman, D. H., Leo, L., Ostfeld, A. M., Huntley, J. C., & Brody, J. A. (1986). Depressive symptoms in relation to physical health and functioning in the elderly. *American Journal of Epidemiology, 124,* 372-388.

Brown, J. S. (1961). *The motivation of behavior.* New York: McGraw-Hill.

Chan, F., Karbowski, J., Monty, R. A., & Perlmuter, L. C. (1986). Performance as a source of perceived control. *Motivation and Emotion, 10,* 59-70.

Cimbalo, R. S., & Brink, L. (1982).   Aging and the von Restorff isolation effect in short/term memory. *The Journal of General Psychology, 106,* 69-76.

Comalli, P. E., Wapner, S., & Werner, H. (1962).   Interference effects of Stroop color-word test in childhood, adulthood, and aging. *Journal of Genetic Psychology, 100,* 47-53.

deCharms, R. (1979).   Personal causation and perceived control.   In L. C. Perlmuter & R. A. Monty (Eds.), *Choice and perceived control* (pp. 29-40). Hillsdale, NJ: Lawrence Erlbaum Associates.

Erber, J. T. (1986).   Age-related effects of spatial contiguity and interference on coding performance. *Journal of Gerontology, 41,* 641-644.

Erickson, R. C., & Scott, M. L. (1977). Clinical memory testing: A review. *Psychological Bulletin, 84,* 1130-1149.

Farkas, M. S., & Hoyer, W. J. (1980).   Processing consequences of perceptual grouping in selective attention. *Journal of Gerontology, 35,* 207-216.

Fleming, C. C., & Lopez, M. A. (1981).   The effects of perceived control on the paired associate learning of elderly persons. *Experimental Aging Research, 7,* 71-77.

Freedman, N., Bucci, W., Elkowitz, E. (1982). Depression in a family practice elderly population. *Journal of the American Geriatrics Society, 30,* 372-377.

Kausler, D. H. (1982). *Experimental psychology and human aging.* New York: Wiley & Sons.

Kausler, D. H., & Kleim, D. M. (1978). Age differences in processing relevant versus irrelevant stimuli in multiple-item recognition learning. *Journal of Gerontology, 33,* 87-93.

Kleinsmith, L. J., & Kaplan, S. (1963). Paired-associate learning as a function of arousal and interpolated interval. *Journal of Experimental Psychology, 65,* 190-193.

Langer, E. J. (1983). *The psychology of control.* Beverly Hills, CA: Sage Publications.

Langer, E. J., Rodin, J., Beck, P., Weinman, C., & Spitzer, L. (1979). Environmental determinants of memory improvement in late adulthood. *Journal of Personality and Social Psychology, 37,* 2003-2013.

Layton, B. (1975). Perceptual noise and aging. *Psychological Bulletin, 82,* 875-883.

Lipson, L. G. (1986). *The older diabetic.* Lexington, MA: Lexington Books.

McGlinchey, R. E., Perlmuter, L. C., Sizer, N., & Nathan, D. (1985). *Effects of aging in type II diabetes on decision making and perceived control.* Presented at the Eastern Psychological Association Meeting.

Monty, R. A., Geller, E. S., Savage, R. E., & Perlmuter, L. C. (1979). The freedom to choose is not always so choice. *Journal of Experimental Psychology: Human Learning and Memory, 5,* 170-179.

Monty, R. A., & Perlmuter, L. C. (1987). Choice, control and motivation in the young and aged. In M. L. Maehr & D. A. Klieber (Eds.), *Advances in motivation and achievement, Vol. 5* (pp. 99-122). Greenwich, CT: JAI Press.

Monty, R. A., Perlmuter, L. C., Libon, D., & Bennet, T. (1982). More on contextual effects on learning and memory. *Bulletin of the Psychonomic Society, 20,* 293-296.

Monty, R. A., Rosenberger, M. A., & Perlmuter, L. C. (1973). Amount and locus of choice as sources of motivation in paired associate learning. *Journal of Experimental Psychology, 97,* 16-21.

Park, D. C., Puglisi, J. T., & Lutz, R. (1982).   Spatial memory in older adults: Effects of intentionality. *Journal of Gerontology, 37,* 330-335.

Park, D. C., Puglisi, J. T., & Sovacool, M. (1984).   Picture memory in older adults: Effects of contextual detail at encoding and retrieval. *Journal of Gerontology, 39,* 213-215.

Perlmuter, L. C., Hakami, M. K., Hodgson-Harrington, C., Ginsberg, J., Katz, J., Singer, D. E., & Nathan, D. M. (1984).   Decreased cognitive function in aging non-insulin-dependent diabetic patients. *The American Journal of Medicine, 77,* 1043-1048.

Perlmuter, L. C., & Langer, E. J. (1983).   The effects of behavioral monitoring on the perception of control. *Clinical Gerontologist, 2,* 37-43.

Perlmuter, L. C., & Monty, R. A. (1977).   The importance of perceived control: Fact or fantasy? *American Scientist, 65,* 759-765.

Perlmuter, L. C., Monty, R. A., & Chan, F. (1986).   Learning, choice, and control.   In M. M. Baltes & P. B. Baltes (Eds.), *The psychology of control and aging* (pp. 91-118).   Hillsdale, NJ: Lawrence Erlbaum Associates.

Perlmuter, L. C., Scharff, K., Karsh, R., & Monty, R. A. (1980).   Perceived control: A generalized state of motivation. *Motivation and Emotion, 4,* 35-45.

Perlmuter, L. C., & Smith, P. (1979).   *The effects of choice and control on paired-associate learning in the aged.*   Presented at the New England Psychological Association Meeting.

Renshon, S. A. (1979).   The need for personal control in political life: Origins, dynamics, and implications.   In L. C. Perlmuter & R. A. Monty (Eds.), *Choice and perceived control* (41-63).   Hillsdale, NJ: Lawrence Erlbaum Associates.

Salthouse, T. A. (1982).   *Adult cognition: An experimental psychology of human aging.*   New York: Springer-Verlag.

Savage, R. E., Perlmuter, L. C., & Monty, R. A. (1979).   Reductions in the amount of choice and perception of control.   In L. C. Perlmuter & R. A. Monty (Eds.), *Choice and perceived control* (pp. 91-106).   Hillsdale, NJ: Lawrence Erlbaum Associates.

Schulman, A. I. (1973).   Recognition memory and the recall of spatial location. *Memory and Cognition, 1,* 256-260.

Tun, P. A., Perlmuter, L. C., Russo, P., & Nathan, D. M. (1987). Memory self-assessment and performance in aged diabetics and non-diabetics. *Experimental Aging Research, 13,* 151-157.

Wechsler, D. (1944). *The measurement of adult intelligence* (3rd ed.) Baltimore: Williams & Wilkins.

Weisz, J. R. (1983). Can I control it? The pursuit of veridical answers across the lifespan. In P. B. Baltes & O. G. Brim, Jr. (Eds.), *Life span development and behavior, Vol. 5.* New York: Academic Press.

Winocur, G., & Moscovitch, M. (1983). Paired-associate learning in institutionalized and non-institutionalized old people: An analysis of interference and context effects. *Journal of Gerontology, 38,* 455-464.

Wright, L. L., & Elias, J. W. (1979). Age differences in the effects of perceptual noise. *Journal of Gerontology, 34,* 704-708.

Psychological Perspectives of Helplessness
and Control in the Elderly, P.S. Fry (ed.)
© *Elsevier Science Publishers B.V. (North-Holland), 1989*

Chapter Fifteen

PSYCHOLOGICAL PERSPECTIVES OF HELPLESSNESS
AND CONTROL IN THE ELDERLY: OVERVIEW AND APPRAISAL

Prem S. FRY
The University of Calgary

Abstract

*This chapter presents an overview and appraisal of the areas
of helplessness and control as related to aging, and
attempts to elucidate the degree of integration achieved
between the psychology of aging and psychology of control.
Major areas of deficits in control and aging are reviewed,
and conceptual advances made in the field of psychology of
control and aging are discussed with special reference to
their implications for educational, clinical and training
programs for older adults.*

Introduction

Considering how difficult it is to summarize and critically appraise
the major constructs of control within the separate fields of aging
and psychology of control, it is perhaps almost futile to attempt a
review of the two areas within a single chapter. Nevertheless the
final chapter is dedicated to this mission. One rider should be
noted, however. My remarks with regard to each issue are highly
selective and even idiosyncratic, and concentrate on the ways in which
the various contributors to this volume link their thinking with one
another.

This volume illustrates rather nicely the steady growth and
emergence of a new field concerned with studying the interface of a
psychology of control and a psychology of aging. The field cuts
across many of the traditional areas of the psychology of control
(e.g., locus of control, choice, control attributions, learned
helplessness, autonomy and power) having particular relevance to the
mental health and social, emotional and psychological well-being of
older adults. Knowledge of control and the related developmental

processes have clear implications also for morale, life-satisfactions and self-efficacy in older adults.

Although the contributors to this volume represent many different vantage points, a few critical issues and concerns have surfaced a number of times. The volume has highlighted the issues that I believe to be both substantive and pervasive in the field as it stands today. Controversies surrounding issues of dependence versus independence, personal autonomy versus interdependence, personal control versus environmental control, and personal adaptation versus environmental adaptation, have been addressed.

Toward this end, each individual chapter has attempted to integrate and address theoretical issues, research issues and issues of intervention. While earlier studies of adult control have attempted to study control or personal causation in contrived settings, most interestingly, gerontologically-oriented researchers and practitioners concerned with studying the experience of control (causation) and the visual experience of control (perceived control) have attempted to go straight to the real-life macroenvironments in which individual behavior and experience are embedded. Throughout this volume, I have been impressed by the range of real-life phenomena of aging to which theorizing about choice, responsibility, internality, helplessness and control etc. has been applied. It is clear that research in the psychology of control and aging has already proved useful in determining various strategies for helping elderly persons in the context of daily functioning and within nursing homes, institutions and long-term care facilities. The fields of aging and control have also been of aid in illuminating fresh and new possibilities for the training of geriatric professionals and their staffs, and caregivers of the elderly.

There is at least one other important area of application in which work has started and that should be highlighted. This has to do with the developmental course of controllability and how individuals may assume personal responsibility and initiative toward the control of their own development and growth. There are already some potential avenues of inquiry that may be fruitful to pursue. It is possible that certain programs of reattributional training and cognitive restructuring strategies applied hitherto to youth, but not sufficiently to older adults, will illuminate the source of motivational style in older persons and show how control can be achieved over memory decline and other cognitive functions such as recognition, recall and information processing. Some of these programs, as discussed in this volume, are based on the hypothesis that loss of control in old age is less genetic and more learned, and that decline in cognitive controls and information processing is perhaps less intellectual and more motivational. Some programs of intervention developed for older persons within a social cognitive framework have already been pioneered and have become very important to the cognitive functioning and learning of older persons.

The results of several control-enhancing intervention programs designed for older persons substantiate our belief that the psychology of control, as related to the psychology of aging, is inextricably linked with the well-being of older persons and is developing rapidly as a justified academic field of inquiry. It is justified not only by its theoretical and conceptual endeavors but ultimately by its applications to the welfare of older individuals. Older adults have come stereotypically to be viewed as helpless, weak and lacking in capabilities for being productive and competent. However, the more recent investigations of subjective control orientations of elders provide confirmation of the notion that the elderly are in fact not as helpless or dependent as we might think. Furthermore, the desire for autonomy and personal control does not appear to decline with old age. Indeed, having a sense of personal control and having access to some choices and options is very important to the mental well-being of older persons. Fear of declining controls is most devastating in old age especially since it carries with it broad implications against the individual's self-worth. Issues such as these figure prominently throughout the volume and future work should help to refine and disentangle existing confusions between perceived controls and actual controls in old age.

Summary and Conclusions

Let me now summarize my comments by providing a brief overview of the state of the field of aging and control as it presently exists and the scope of the undertakings.

First and foremost, we must acknowledge and applaud the fact that we now have a psychology of control with situation-specific and control-specific dimensions having wide applicability to the functioning of older adults in a more controlled and autonomous manner.

While space constraints made it impossible to produce, in this one volume, a concrete case for the wide range of intervention work being done towards enhancing cognitive and social controls in older persons, a few chapters in this volume illuminate the control processes that come in to play in improving motivation, memory and learning. Studies discussing control-enhancing interventions that are significantly related to reducing vulnerability states, depression and excess disability in the elderly are also discussed.

The inception of control, autonomy and power as an area of study in the psychology of aging can be likened to the inception of dialectic discourse as a field of analysis. Just as a variety of interests in linguistics, logic, philosophy, cognitive psychology and metapsychology are represented in the development of discourse analysis, similarly there are increasing numbers of geneticists, physicians, biologists, psychologists, economists and political scientists concerned with providing the older adults with increased opportunities for enhancing autonomy, participatory control, responsibility and choices.

However, the field of the psychology of control as related to aging has a very limited history, and there are still quite a few glaring deficits that must be encountered.

The *first* major deficit is the lack of conceptual clarity as to the kinds of control constructs that are particularly applicable to older adults as distinguished from younger adults. For example, a brief overview of control constructs as used in the research studies with older adults makes it quite clear that learned helplessness and affective uncontrollability and dependence are control constructs that are more frequently associated with aging and old age. The prevailing view in the literature on aging and control is that perceived control declines in later life because of the numerous assaults and constraints associated with biological aging. A greater potential for frustration exists in old age when individuals are encouraged to believe that they *are* and *should be* increasingly responsible for their functioning while simultaneously they are being deprived of the instruments of control in their environments.

The operations of control that are deemed to be more desirable in the later years stress functions of participatory control, proxy control, instrumental and secondary control as differentiated from primary control. What is still missing, however, is a rational taxonomy of control operations that apply more critically to the later stages of human development as distinguished from the earlier stages. This constitutes a *second* major deficit in the field of control and aging.

A *third* major deficit is the absence of a coherent theory of the biological, genetic, social and environmental factors involved in stress production. There is still no confirmed view on how much of the stress, anxiety and difficulty in coping experienced in late life is a function of biological age *per se* and how much stress is psychologically induced (i.e., is a direct outcome of perceived levels of control, attributional styles, motivations and lack of free choice). Although there is a well-articulated view of why choice and control are important to youth, there is no similar coherent explanation for why control and choice are so inextricably linked to the well-being of older adults, and why even frail and chronically ill elderly persons experience a decrease in stress when they have opportunities for choice and control. In studies examining changes in control patterns through the life cycle it is now more evident that individuals' sense of power and control changes with corresponding changes in actual control and competency judgments. As is true of earlier stages of development, the sense of control in the later years continues to be a combination of both the changing capacity of the individual to emit effective responses (competence) and the responses of the environment (contingency). Unfortunately, as compared to natural environments of younger adults, the environments of older adults tend to be much more deterministic, restraining and at times coercive. In old age, especially, individuals are inclined to underestimate outcome contingency and personal competency, and one may therefore speculate that although there may be little or no change in actual control, older adults show greater vulnerability to learned helplessness. Only those adults who work to increase their competence and at the same time are able to maintain illusions of contingency and competence have been found to be well-adjusted and free of depression. The basic proposition stressed in the control literature on aging is that it is important to preserve some sense of personal control even if in reality there is a substantial decrease in actual controls, contingencies and competency. In view of the great range of individual differences in the general decline in status, activity and biological health of older adults, it is difficult to ascertain the optimal level of desired control for the elderly. Depending on environmental contingencies, cultural differences and personality factors of older persons, it is to be expected that optimal control may sometimes be above the real or actual level of contingencies and competence, but also considerably lower than the maximum. The salutary effects of enhanced control have been demonstrated especially with the institutionalized aged, by introducing very simple activities over which the elderly could exert some measure of personal control. On the other hand, there are frequent occurrences or situations in which expectancies for control exceed the limits of human control that can be expected of frail and dependent elderly, and where some measure of dependency would not only be appropriate but should also be supported. What is missing therefore is a rational explanation of what are optimal levels of control that *can* and *should* be expected of older adults as distinguished from younger adults. This constitutes the *fourth* major deficit in the field of aging and control.

When dealing with control constructs as applied to the sick and frail elderly, the literature suggests an interplay between two aspects of control: control and responsibility for the cause of problems, and control over the solution to the problems. Accordingly, investigations using control-relevant interventions with elderly persons have suggested that interventions stressing expectations of responsibility and control over *both* the *cause* of problems and their *solutions* may be more detrimental than conducive to a positive sense of control. Expectancies for control over both the cause of the problem and the solution to the problem may be particularly detrimental for frail elderly because individuals are made to feel in control, and failing to achieve control may more likely precipitate negative reactance and greater helplessness following failure to control. Therefore judgments of *perceived* and *actual control* raise unexplored ethical issues which deserve investigation. Although it is not a major contention of the aging and control literature, the argument has been presented by some writers in this volume that helping and caregiving activities are best appreciated as two-edged swords in the

lives of many elderly. Caregiving has the potential to both aid and
harm the elderly recipient. Depending upon the physical health of the
older person and the setting in which he/she lives, the same helping
activities may either enhance perceptions of control or create excess
disability.

Although most of the authors of this volume share the philosophy
that a high level of control enhances well-being, some authors have
also pointed out that if high levels of personal and primary control
over causes and outcomes are expected of aging individuals, negative
consequences may result as well. Given the best of circumstances, it
must be remembered that the elderly are an *at risk* population and may
not have the necessary biological and psychological resources required
to function at expected levels of control and self-regulation.

Compared to other areas of the functioning of older persons,
considerably greater study has been done on correlates of personal
control in institutional settings. While some researchers suggest
that enhancement of control in institutional settings may lead to
positive psychosocial outcomes for elderly residents, others have
warned that efforts to increase autonomy and independence in individuals living in institutional settings may have a "boomerang"
effect, particularly if such control-enhancing interventions are not
supported on a long-term basis.

To address these questions further research will have to be done
to decide what defines optimal autonomy for older persons living in
health care settings and what are realistic expectancies for role
competency, responsibility and efficacy for frail elderly persons.
The absence of research to determine which models of helping, responsibility or control are optimally effective for what groups of
elderly, and under what circumstances, constitutes the *fifth* major
deficit in the field of aging and control.

Overall, the limitations and strengths of some types of control-
enhancing interventions in institutional settings are reflected in
various chapters of this volume. One of the major criticisms noted
about such interventions is that they relate to very circumscribed
aspects of institutional living and have few practical implications or
applications for reducing feelings of helplessness in the general
population of older persons. In summary, it has been postulated that
interventions which waive the expectancy for primary control and
stress aspects of secondary control are much more safe and realistic.
Various kinds of secondary control procedures (e.g., predictive
control, participatory control and interpretive control) as differentiated from primary control have been associated with many positive
outcomes among elderly individuals, especially frail elderly living in
total care institutions, or dependent elderly persons living in
constrained and unalterable circumstances.

It should be noted that most of the work in control and aging, although not all of it, has been done among older adults living in democratic Western societies in which beliefs about internal control, choice, potential choice and personal autonomy are based on values inferred from democratic principles. There are still no coherent and well-differentiated data coming from cross-cultural studies of aged persons from diverse subcultures or ethnic groups. The field of aging *per se* abounds in cross-cultural speculations but the decisive data for confirming the cross-cultural reliability and validity of significant control constructs having relevance to aging are missing. Before it is possible to confirm whether individuals' sense of power and perceptions of control change with changes in their actual control throughout the life cycle, we need to supplement our knowledge with developmental data on control from cultures other than the Western democratic culture. Thus the *sixth* major deficit revolves around the lack of cross-cultural data on developmental changes in control and motivations for control.

A final and *seventh* deficit is related to our ignorance about the permanence of the effects of choice and control in elderly individuals. We still do not know whether older adults' need for personal control is transient and fluctuates from day to day or from situation to situation, or whether it is foundational as opposed to superficial. It is recognized that opportunities for decision making and responsible choice may decrease with advancing age as a result of physical and social restrictions, disease states and decline in cognitive skills. As such, it is to be expected that motivation levels decrease with age because of diminishing opportunities for exercising choice and control. As the exercise of choice becomes less frequent, decreasing motivation levels are reflected in lowered self-esteem, with the result that further efforts at control are diminished. Also, with increasing age individuals must gradually become ready for institutional life where restrictions and demands for conformity are prevalent. If individual expectancies for high levels of control and autonomy in late life are not gradually modified, they may produce greater disappointments and may eventually result in long term adverse sequelae. Further research will have to be done in order to address the question of what constitutes optimal levels of motivation and choice for older persons. The lack of research in this area constitutes a major deficit in our understanding of control processes in aging.

From the perspective of this volume, the problems and issues mentioned represent the most salient deficits in the field of aging and control.

On the other hand, the field of control in aging has made considerable advances and can justifiably be proud of its contributions to interventions promoting the well-being of older adults. Let us touch on a few of the advances that have been accomplished.

First, it is now known that control and choice, however they are operationalized, almost invariably have positive effects on the cognitions, stress perceptions, emotions and performance efforts of older adults. Moreover, this has been shown to be the case for a wide variety of situations and manipulations (e.g., coping with stress, improving memory and learning, enhancing activity levels and participatory tasks, and last but not least reinforcing self-esteem and self-confidence). The psychology of control field has uncovered these benefits, and this is a substantial contribution to the developmental and clinical psychology of aging.

Second, there presently exist three or more conceptual frameworks (e.g., social learning framework, cognitive framework, developmental framework, and clinical framework) within which to consider the effects of autonomy, choice and control. From the perspective of a clinical psychology of aging there is evidence to suggest that interventions aimed at increasing choice and control produce reductions in depression, stress, passivity and negative ideations. By optimizing opportunities for control experiences, older adults can be expected to overcome excess disability and generalized helplessness and depression. However, unless elderly persons are helped to make cognitive and affective accommodations successfully, they may succumb to ineffective, helpless and escapist strategies leading to still further enhanced perceptions of stress and anxiety.

Third, from the perspective of a developmental psychology of aging there is evidence that individuals are producers of their own future development and goals, and capable of a relatively self-determined way of life for an increased period of time. This discovery provides a hopeful note for individuals being able to improve the quality of their own functioning.

From the perspective of a social psychology of aging, experiences of control and power have implications for the interpersonal relationships of older adults with their friends, caregivers, physicians and legal advisors.

Fourth, a major conceptual advance in the psychology of control is reflected in the person-environment fit conceptualization (P-E fit) of control and autonomy as it pertains to the environments of older adults. Recent conceptualizations of control have focused not merely on constructs of individual control, competence and autonomy of the individual but also on aspects of restrictive, constraining and coercive environments which diminish the individual's sense of influence and self-efficacy. The P-E fit concept permits a more flexible alternative to intervention which would target change in expectancies for control in both individuals and environments in order to increase congruence between persons and their environments. High-energy individuals may use instrumental strategies to control their environment and increase its congruence with their needs. Conversely, low-energy individuals may use a variety of intrapsychic strategies to accommodate their needs and perceptions of control to fit the existing situation. Within a P-E fit framework the individual may work actively to maximize his/her freedom in the physical environment. At the same time, the environment may be modified to increase the individual's perceived freedom by allowing more choice, privacy and territoriality. These trends have several important implications for practitioners and social policy planners who must consider not only the elderly persons' efforts at choice and control, but also attend to designing environments which favor internality, privacy, choice, and the experience of participatory control for the individual.

Fifth, in contradistinction to the idea that the need to control is permanent and unchanging in old age, it has been suggested that the conscious desire for control is not a penultimate articulation of most older persons' personality. As noted by some authors in this volume, declining physical and mental energies in old age may, realistically speaking, prompt a change in high-energy action-oriented coping strategies that were effective in the past. To some extent, older persons may wish to put more distance between themselves and the events that are potentially intrusive. Some elderly may develop a sense of "philosophical detachment". It is postulated that by maintaining a certain level of control in old age and by desiring to exercise a reasonable level of choice, older individuals, not unlike younger individuals, are testing their coping abilities to deal effectively with a changed and changing environment. Upon attaining a certain level of influence and control in important situations and over some significant others, most older persons are quite happy to discontinue further testing and evaluation of their influence and to adapt to a more routinized schedule in which reasonable accommodations of social dependence and interdependence serve as a source of gratification and vicarious fulfillment. Although still capable of a considerable degree of actual control, many older persons may consciously wish to replace active control and mastery strategies with gradual and dignified acceptance of some aspects of later life realities. These notions represent a significant conceptual advance. As several authors in this volume have contended, people experience choice if they seem in one way or another to decide when they want dependency and when they want autonomy, and especially if they can identify situations and alternatives that seem best for them at their stage of development. Such a concept of choice and control is not easily subject to empirical proof. Nevertheless, it represents a conceptual advance in the field of aging and control. It is, however, one of the unresolved themes in the area of perceived control that needs to be pursued further.

Obviously there are a number of different strands and psychological frameworks represented in this volume. At this point it is important to recognize that these differing viewpoints are complementary and axiomatic to the need for understanding control processes in older persons. It is important, therefore, for the psychology of control and the psychology of aging to attempt to unify these approaches.

As a closing comment, I believe that this volume contains in it the seeds of a unique integration of cognitive, motivational and sociological approaches to the application of control constructs to the daily lives of older persons. Action-theoretical perspectives of life-span development suggest that humans actively seek to control their environments that in turn alters their motivational levels as well as their perceptions of control. The authors of this volume have discussed two possible windows on the role of the individual and the role of the environment, namely, (1) the study of older individuals' needs, motivations and goals for control and individual action; and (2) the environmental influences that enhance or deflate perceptions of control or actual control in older adults.

Implied throughout the volume is the assumption that the construction and modification of control expectancies continue throughout the life-span and change with age. With the rapid growth in the number of elderly and the increasing incidence of depression, helplessness and excess disability in this age group, an important social policy consideration for the 1980s and 1990s is how to train the elderly to function more autonomously and effectively in matters of physical and mental health care. The environmental factors influencing control, autonomy or choice in old age may vary from person to person depending on individual differences in reserve capacity and level of maximum functioning. On a more cautious note it must be concluded that if frail and vulnerable elderly persons are pushed beyond their reserve capacities and limits of functioning to attain control, the push for autonomy can have deleterious consequences. What is ideally needed is for older persons to achieve a fine balance between the putative need for autonomy and personal influence on the one hand, and the need for dependence and interdependence on the other hand.

AUTHOR INDEX

SUBJECT INDEX

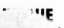